Fundamentals of Anaesthesia and Acute Medicine

# Intensive Care Medicine

Fundamentals of Anaesthesia and Acute Medicine

# Intensive Care Medicine

*Edited by*

Julian Bion
*Reader in Intensive Care Medicine, University Department of Anaesthetics and Intensive Care, Queen Elizabeth Hospital, Birmingham*

*Series editors*

Ronald M Jones
*Professor of Anaesthetics, St Mary's Hospital Medical School, London*

Alan R Aitkenhead
*Professor of Anaesthesia, University of Nottingham*

and

Pierre Foëx
*Nuffield Professor of Anaesthetics, University of Oxford*

First published in 1999
by BMJ Books, BMA House, Tavistock Square,
London WC1H 9JR

**British Library Cataloguing in Publication Data**

A catalogue record for this book is available from the British Library

ISBN 0-7279-1076-0

Typeset by Apek Typesetters, Nailsea, Bristol
Printed and bound by Redwood Books, Bath

# Contents

# Acknowledgments

I would like to acknowledge the patience and efficiency of Mary Banks and Alex Stibbe at BMJ Books, and in particular the forbearance and support of my wife and family, during a prolonged editorial gestation.

# Contributors

**P J D Andrews**
Consultant in Neuroanaesthesia and Intensive Care
Western General Hospital
Edinburgh, UK

**J F Bion**
Reader in Intensive Care Medicine
University Department of Anaesthesia and Intensive Care
Queen Elizabeth Hospital
Birmingham, UK

**G Bishop**
Director of Intensive Care
Liverpool Health Service
Liverpool, Australia

**M A Branthwaite**
Barrister-at-law
London, UK

**S J Brett**
Consultant in Intensive Care Medicine and Anaesthesia
Department of Anaesthesia and Intensive Care
Hammersmith Hospital
London, UK

**P Bristow**
Staff Intensivist
Liverpool Health Service
Liverpool, Australia

**T Clutton-Brock**
Senior Lecturer in Anaesthesia and Intensive Care
Queen Elizabeth Hospital
Birmingham, UK

**J H Coakley**
Consultant Physician in Intensive Care
St Bartholomew's Hospital
London, UK

**J O Defraigne**
Department of Cardiovascular Surgery
University of Liège
Belgium

**T W Evans**
Professor of Intensive Care Medicine
Imperial College School of Medicine
Consultant in Thoracic and Intensive Care Medicine
Department of Respiratory Medicine
Royal Brompton Hospital
London, UK

**S J Fairclough**
Department of Pharmacy
Royal Liverpool Children's NHS Trust
Liverpool, UK

**R E Ferner**
Consultant Physician
City Hospital
Birmingham, UK

**C S Garrard**
Intensive Therapy Unit
John Radcliffe Hospital
Oxford, UK

**J W M Greve**
Academisch Ziekenhuis
Maastricht, The Netherlands

**L Harper**
Registrar in Nephrology
Queen Elizabeth Hospital
Birmingham, UK

**M T E Heafield**
Consultant Neurologist
Queen Elizabeth Hospital
Birmingham, UK

**P E Hersch**
John Farman Intensive Care Unit
Addenbrooke's Hospital
Cambridge, UK

**J Hill**
Consultant Surgeon, Department of General and Colorectal Surgery
Manchester Royal Infirmary
UK

**K Hillman**
Professor and Chairman, Department of Anaesthetics and Intensive Care
Liverpool Health Service
Liverpool, Australia

**M Itaglietta**
Professor, Department of Applied Mechanics and Engineering Science
University of California
USA

**B E Keogh**
Consultant in Cardiothoracic Surgery
Queen Elizabeth Hospital
Birmingham, UK

**K-L Kong**
Consultant Anaesthetist
City Hospital
Birmingham, UK

**I Mackie**
Senior Lecturer in Haematology
University College London
London, UK

**T Mcleod**
Consultant Anaesthetist
Birmingham Heartlands Hospital
Birmingham, UK

**G McMahon**
Lecturer/Senior Registrar in Emergency Medicine
Hope Hospital
Salford, UK

**M Manji**
Consultant, Anaesthesia and Intensive Care Medicine
Queen Elizabeth Hospital
Birmingham, UK

**K Messmer**
Professor, Klinikum Grosshadern
Munchen, Germany

**G R Park**
Director of Intensive Care
John Farman Intensive Care Unit
Addenbrooke's Hospital
Cambridge, UK

**G A Pearson**
Consultant in Paediatric Intensive Care
Birmingham Children's Hospital
Birmingham, UK

**A J Petros**
Department of Anaesthesia and Intensive Care
Great Ormond Street Hospital for Children NHS Trust
London, UK

**J Pincemail**
Department of Cardiovascular Surgery
University of Liege
Belgium

**M Poeze**
Academisch Ziekenhuis
Maastricht, The Netherlands

**M V Prescott**
Consultant in Accident and Emergency Medicine
North Staffordshire Hospital
Stoke-on-Trent, UK

**G Ramsay**
Associate Professor, Academisch Ziekenhuis
Maastricht, The Netherlands

**A D Redmond**
Professor of Emergency Medicine
North Staffordshire Hospital
Stoke-on-Trent, UK

**N T Richards**
Consultant Nephrologist
Queen Elizabeth Hospital
Birmingham, UK

**J H Rommes**
Department of Intensive Care
Ziekenhuiscentrum Apeldoorn
The Netherlands

**K Rowan**
Director of Audit and Research
ICNARC
London, UK

**M P Shelly**
Consultant in Anaesthesia and Intensive Care
NHS Trust South Manchester University Hospital
Manchester, UK

**P F X Statham**
Consultant Neurosurgeon
Western General Hospital
Edinburgh, UK

**A P H Steele**
Registrar in Anaesthesia
Kingston Hospital
London, UK

**M A Stokes**
Senior Lecturer in Paediatric Anaesthesia and Intensive Care
Birmingham Children's Hospital
Birmingham, UK

**J Takala**
Professor of Anaesthesiology/Director
Department of Anaesthesiology and Intensive Care
Kuopio University Hospital
Kuopio, Finland

**S J H van Deventer**
Department of Experimental Internal Medicine
Academic Medical Centre
Amsterdam, The Netherlands

**H K F van Saene**
Consultant/Reader in Medical Microbiology
Department of Clinical Microbiology
Royal Liverpool Children's NHS Trust
Liverpool, UK

**A P Tometzki**
Department of Paediatric Cardiology
Royal Hospital for Sick Children
Edinburgh, UK

**J-L Vincent**
Department of Intensive Care
Erasme University Hospital
Brussels, Belgium

**P G M Wallace**
Consultant Anaesthetist
Intensive Therapy Unit
Western Infirmary
Glasgow, UK

**B N J Walters**
Consultant Physician, Obstetric and General Medicine
Department of Internal Medicine
Royal Perth Hospital/King Edward Memorial Hospital for Women
Perth, Western Australia

**A Webb**
Consultant Physician and Clinical Director
Department of Intensive Care
UCL Hospitals
London, UK

**J Wendon**
Senior Lecturer, Institute of Liver Studies
King's College Hospital
London, UK

**D W Yates**
Professor, Department of Emergency Medicine
Hope Hospital
Salford, UK

# Foreword

## The Fundamentals of Anaesthesia and Acute Medicine Series

The pace of change within the biological sciences continues to increase and nowhere is this more apparent than in the specialties of anaesthesia, acute medicine, and intensive care. Although many practitioners continue to rely on comprehensive but bulky texts for reference, the accelerating rate of biomedical advances makes this source of information increasingly likely to be dated, even if the latest edition is used. The series *Fundamentals of Anaesthesia and Acute Medicine* aims to bring to the reader up to date and authoritative reviews of the principal clinical topics which make up the specialties. Each volume will cover the fundamentals of the topic in a comprehensive manner but will also emphasise recent developments of controversial issues.

International differences in the practice of anaesthesia and intensive care are now much less than in the past, and the editors of each volume have commissioned chapters from acknowledged authorities throughout the world to assemble contributions of the highest possible calibre. Three volumes will appear annually and, as the pace and extent of clinically significant advances varies among the individual topics, new editions will be commissioned to ensure that practitioners will be in a position to keep abreast of the important developments within the specialties.

Not only does the pace of advance in biomedical science serve to justify the appearance of an international series of this nature, but the current awareness of the need for more formal continuing education also underlines the timeliness of its appearance. The editors would welcome feedback from readers about the series, which is aimed at both established practitioners and trainees preparing for degrees and diplomas in anaesthesia and intensive care.

RONALD M JONES
ALAN R AITKENHEAD
PIERRE FOËX

# Preface

The process of trying to care for a critically ill patient without adequate prior training usually generates considerable anxiety amongst medical and nursing staff, as well as being dangerous for the patient, a source of distress to relatives, and expensive for the hospital when errors result in litigation. One of the main benefits of intensive care is the clinical training which it offers in resuscitation, preventative care, applied pharmacology and physiology, diagnosis, and ethics. Trainees (both medical and nursing) who have gained experience in the intensive care unit generally find that they have become much more confident in recognising critical illness in its early stages, and find it easier to interpret clinical signs, take appropriate initial action, and call for help before the patient is moribund. In this book we have tried where appropriate to focus on early signs of organ system dysfunction, and preventative management. The text has been written for trainees from a variety of backgrounds but with a common interest in acute medical care. It is not intended as a recipe book, and given its size cannot be comprehensive; but it should provide an introduction to the subject and offer the reader a succinct companion to clinical practice.

Julian Bion

# PART ONE

# INTRODUCTION AND BACKGROUND

# 1: Intensive care: history, challenges, and definitions

J F BION

## How intensive care started

Intensive care usually dates its origins from the polio epidemics of the 1950s, when hospitals had to cope with large numbers of patients presenting with ventilatory failure. The epidemic that afflicted Copenhagen was described by the epidemiologist Professor Lassen[1] in an article still worth reading, not least because of its lack of jargon and complex statistics. Those polio victims who developed respiratory failure were initially managed using "iron lung" ventilators in different areas of the hospital. Within a few weeks, about 100 patients had been received. The mortality rate of 90%, combined with the lack of adequate numbers of these ventilators, suggested the need for a new approach, and so advice was sought from the anaesthetist Professor Björn Ibsen. He showed, using the relatively new technique of arterial blood gas analysis, that the patients were dying from hypoxaemic ventilatory failure. He performed a tracheostomy on a 12-year-old girl, using a cuffed tracheal tube: the girl survived.

After this three important changes were introduced: patient care was centralised within the hospital; airway control was provided via surgically formed tracheostomies; and the patients' lungs were ventilated with oxygen-enriched air using manual positive pressure provided by teams of medical students. This resulted in a reduction in the mortality rate to 40%. Lassen noted the psychological benefits of having a dedicated attendant permanently by the bedside, but also pointed out that this was more expensive. He also showed that, although the new system of management produced many more survivors, it delayed death among patients destined not to survive. The old (cuirass) method allowed more patients to die faster, and therefore at lower cost.

## Costs and outcomes

The polio story focuses our attention on some of the challenges for intensive care. Resource constraints and implicit rationing were common then; today we have "cost containment" of much larger budgets, but the increase in expectations makes rationing feel even more acute. There is wide disparity in the funding of intensive care, even among Western countries:

the USA allocates around 20–30% of acute hospital costs, or 1% of the gross domestic product, GDP[2]), whilst the UK spends only 6·2% of her GDP on health care generally, and a mere 1–2% of the (much smaller) hospital budget on intensive care.[3] Rationing intensive care is common,[4] with the result that only the most severely ill patients are admitted, usually at an advanced stage in their illness when the chances of producing a rapid improvement in their condition are much reduced. Scarce resources are thus concentrated on patients who may not be able to benefit from them.

Achieving better outcomes depends on understanding the pathophysiology of disease and providing appropriate and timely treatment: multidisciplinary collaboration between basic science and clinical medicine is fundamental to this process. Arterial blood gas measurement was not a routine technique in the 1950s, but its application in poliomyelitis ventilatory failure produced a simple change in clinical management which saved many lives. Since then, the technology associated with intensive care has transformed clinical practice, but this has not necessarily been accompanied by better outcomes for all patients. Indeed, organ-system support can actually make things worse by deferring but not preventing death, with the result that it can cost twice as much to produce a non-survivor as a survivor from critical illness.[5] In part, this is because the patient population has changed. Intensive care now deals with older, sicker patients with more advanced and complex disease, in whom the acute physiological derangement can be reversed, but not the underlying chronic ill health. As the main function of organ-system support is to buy time for specific therapy to reverse the disease process, if this is delivered too late, or if the disease cannot be cured, organ support will either be prolonged or ineffective. Similarly, new treatments based on inadequate understanding of the basic disease process will also be ineffective, as the anti-cytokine trials have demonstrated.

## Determinants of outcome

These interrelationships of physiological reserve, acute disease, and organ support and therapy are shown in Figure 1.1, which illustrates the concept that perceived severity of illness (the factor that influences our clinical judgment most strongly) is actually the product of two variables that we cannot measure accurately: the magnitude and nature of the acute disease and the patient's physiological reserve. For any given "insult" – trauma, surgery, infection – patients with more reserve are likely to cope better than those with impaired health, who may also be more susceptible to severe illness. We tend to respond to evolving critical illness by providing delayed reactive treatment, whereas we should be offering earlier proactive intervention in patients at risk of critical illness. For example, there is evidence[6] that many patients requiring emergency admission to intensive care receive substandard management on the ordinary wards beforehand, and it is a common experience that patients who have a cardiorespiratory arrest had documented changes in vital signs many hours previously. To improve this situation, we need to develop methods of identifying patients with limited reserve or evolving critical illness, and to intervene promptly. How can we do this?

## Early identification of the sick patient

The first and most important practical message is that patients with unstable or deteriorating physiology, particularly those with hypoxaemia, hypotension, tachypnoea or a metabolic acidosis, should be assumed to be critically ill and to need experienced management. The second point is that critical illness is often preceded by a systemic oxygen debt which, in high-risk surgical patients at least, can be reversed by intravascular volume expansion[7] and supplementary oxygen. Many patients also have impaired myocardial function,[8] and benefit from adjunctive inotropic agents.[9] The detection and prevention of incipient organ system dysfunction is thus

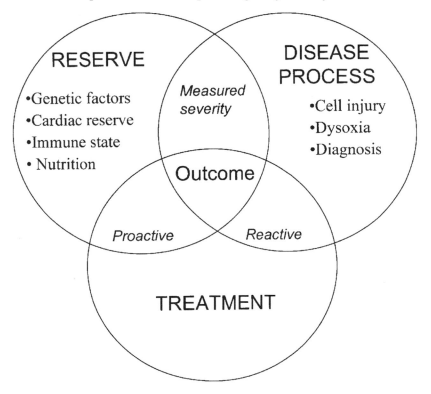

Fig 1.1   Factors influencing outcome from critical illness

relatively simple, and certainly within the ability of most medical and nursing staff. More complex, and the subject of growing research interest, is the interplay between genetic and acquired (including lifestyle) factors which limit physiological reserve and determine susceptibility to infection and cardiovascular dysfunction. Until methods are developed for quantifying risk in these terms, we are obliged to use surrogate measures such as family history, physical appearance to assess biological as opposed to chronological age, the degree of physical independence for activities of daily living, and social factors.

## When should patients be referred to intensive care?

Patients identified as being at risk of critical illness require prompt referral, not necessarily for admission to the intensive care unit (ICU), but for accurate diagnosis and treatment of the disease process, and to establish appropriate treatment goals. This might involve deciding that a patient should not be admitted to the ICU, for example, based on medical assessment of likely benefit and documentation of the patient's wishes. All too often these complex decisions are not discussed beforehand, with the result that patients are often subjected to inappropriate resuscitation and life-sustaining treatment.[10-12]

Criteria for admission to intensive and high-dependency care have been developed in the UK using the requirement for organ-system support (Box 1.1).[13] Patients who need advanced respiratory support (intubation and mechanical ventilation), or those with acute failure of two or more organ systems, should be admitted to intensive care, whereas single acute non-respiratory organ-system failures can be managed in a high-dependency

---

**Box 1.1** *Criteria for admission to intensive care or high-dependency care[13]*

Intensive care is appropriate for patients who:
- need or are likely to need advanced respiratory support alone
- need support of two or more organ systems
- have chronic impairment of one or more organ systems sufficient to restrict daily activities and who also require support for an acute reversible failure of another organ system

High-dependency care is appropriate for patients who need:
- support of a single failing organ system, excluding advanced respiratory support
- step-down care after discharge from intensive care
- more detailed observation or monitoring than can safely be provided on a general ward, including postoperative monitoring for longer than a few hours

---

environment (for example, renal failure in a dialysis unit, myocardial infarction in a coronary care unit, and so on). These criteria and the associated definitions of organ-system failure and support may be useful for categorising severity: a patient who is tachypnoeic, hypoxaemic, and hypotensive should be categorised as having two acute organ-system failures until disproven, and evidently meets the criteria for intensive care referral.

## Learning from experience

Managing critical illness without adequate training can be frightening for medical and nursing staff, dangerous for the patient, and expensive for the hospital when errors result in litigation. One of the main benefits of intensive care is the clinical training which it offers in resuscitation, applied pharmacology and physiology, diagnosis, and ethics. This experience is of considerable value when dealing with an acutely ill patient outside the ICU. An increasing number of countries are introducing multidisciplinary intensive care training and specialty status,[14] and this should be reflected by improved standards of practice both in the ICU and throughout acute hospital medicine.

1 Lassen HCA. A preliminary report on the 1952 epidemic of poliomyelitis in Copenhagen with special reference to the treatment of acute respiratory insufficiency. *Lancet* 1953;i:37–41.
2 Halpern NA, Bettes L, Greenstein R. Federal and nationwide intensive care units and healthcare costs: 1986–1992. *Crit Care Med* 1994;22:2001–7.
3 Bion J. Cost containment: Europe. The United Kingdom. *New Horiz* 1994;2:341–4.
4 Metcalfe MA, Sloggett A, McPherson K. Mortality among appropriately referred patients refused admission to intensive care units. *Lancet* 1997;350:7–11.
5 Sage WM, Rosenthal MH, Silverman JF. Is intensive care worth it? An assessment of input and outcome for the critically ill. *Crit Care Med* 1986;14:777–82.
6 McQuillan P, Pilkington S, Allan A, *et al* Confidential inquiry into quality of care before admission to intensive care. *BMJ* 1998;316:1853–8.
7 Sinclair S, James S, Singer M. Intraoperative intravascular volume optimisation and length of hospital stay after repair of proximal femoral fracture: randomised controlled trial. *BMJ* 1997;315:909–12.
8 Older P, Smith R, Courtney P, Hone R. Preoperative evaluation of cardiac failure and ischemia in elderly patients by cardiopulmonary exercise. *Chest* 1993;104:701–4.
9 Boyd O, Grounds RM, Bennett ED. A randomised clinical trial of the effect of deliberate perioperative increase of oxygen delivery on mortality in high-risk surgical patients. *JAMA* 1993;270:2699–707.
10 Aarons EJ, Beeching NJ. Survey of "do not resuscitate" orders in a district general hospital. *BMJ* 1991;303:1504–6.
11 Murphy DJ, Burrows D, Santilli S, *et al* The influence of the probability of survival on patients' preferences regarding cardiopulmonary resuscitation. *N Engl J Med* 1994;330:545–9.
12 Knaus WA, Harrell FE Jr, Lynn J, *et al* The SUPPORT prognostic model. Objective estimates of survival for seriously ill hospitalized adults. Study to understand prognoses and preferences for outcomes and risks of treatments. *Ann Intern Med* 1995;122:191–203.
13 Department of Health. *Guidelines on admission to and discharge from intensive care and high dependency units.* London: NHS Executive, 1996.

14 Bion JF, Ramsay G, Roussos C, Burchardi H. Intensive care training and speciality status in Europe: international comparisons. *Intensive Care Med* 1998;**24**:372–7.

# 2: Severity scoring and audit

J F BION and K ROWAN

The privilege of self-regulation enjoyed by medical and nursing staff in many countries brings with it responsibility for auditing the quality of care provided. Audit essentially consists of defining a standard, measuring whether the service has achieved that standard, taking action to improve or maintain it, and then continuing to monitor it. Standards can be based either on what seems reasonable (such as defining an "acceptable" level of cross-infection in an intensive care unit (ICU) or accuracy of case records), or on measurement of current practice (for example, average mortality rates). Effective audit should be a routine part of clinical practice; it should be conducted in an objective, constructive, and supportive manner, and have clear goals. Ineffective audit is judgmental and coercive, and fails to enhance practice.

The process of audit can be reduced to three questions: what are we doing, could we do it better, and if so how? Many of the daily activities that constitute intensive care practice can be audited without complicated methods of measurement. All medical disciplines, however, face the challenge of having to demonstrate that what they do is effective and efficient. This requires more sophisticated methods to analyse the links of structure, process, and outcomes of care, and to make comparisons while controlling for variations in case mix. Case mix means describing patient populations in terms of diagnoses, past history, demographic factors, and severity of illness. The measurement of severity of illness is essential, because it is the most important determinant of outcome from intensive care, and without a reliable method for measuring it we cannot easily interpret variations in survival rates, for example, between different treatments. The process of controlling for the effect of population characteristics on outcomes is called risk adjustment.

In this chapter we describe the principles of risk adjustment, and examine the practical application of specific methods.

## Principles of risk adjustment and severity measurement

Accurate risk adjustment involves measuring all the factors that affect a given outcome (usually death or survival for intensive care audit). The most important of these is severity of the acute illness, often defined in terms of physiological derangement, for example, hypoxaemia or hypotension. In addition to severity of illness, there are three other important variables: the diagnosis (or diagnoses), the specificity and timing of treatment, and the patient's prior health. Diagnoses are given separate weighting in some scoring systems. This weighting represents the degree of therapeutic susceptibility; for example, in the APACHE system diabetic ketoacidotic coma has a negative weighting, because the pathophysiology is well understood and readily reversible by insulin and supportive treatment. Sepsis, however, has an extra positive weighting because the term encompasses a range of clinical conditions that generally lack specific curative treatments. The degree to which treatment interferes with the relationship between severity and outcome is demonstrated in Figure 2.1 for diabetic keotacidosis, congestive heart failure, and sepsis;[1] for any given level of physiological severity, the outcomes may be very different.

Prior health status can be difficult to measure objectively, because it includes elements such as physiological reserve, genetic susceptibility, immune competence, and biological (as opposed to chronological) age. Physiological scoring systems do not capture the effect of chronic disease

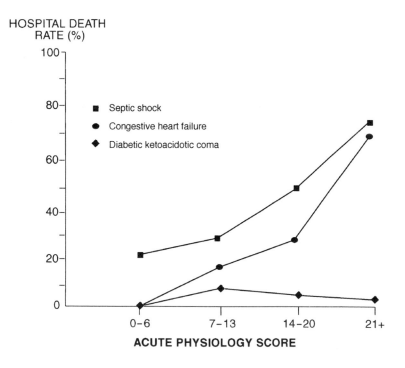

Fig 2.1 Relationship between severity and mortality for three diseases: congestive heart failure, diabetic ketoacidotic coma, and septic shock.

on outcome from critical illness very well, because the physiological response to an acute disease is actually the product of two unmeasured variables – the magnitude of the acute event (trauma, septic shock, etc.), and the extent of the patient's physiological reserve. This may in part explain why individual patients within the same severity band may have very different outcomes. Chronic health limitation has a significant effect on long-term outcomes from intensive care,[2] and on decisions to limit the duration and intensity of care.[3]

Numerical methods for risk adjustment generate a score by processing a number of weighted variables selected for their ability to differentiate between different outcomes. The weights attributed to the component variables are derived either by clinical consensus or by statistical techniques such as logistic regression, or by both. Scoring systems are methods of clinical measurement, and should be thought of as laboratory tests, with a false-positive and a false-negative error rate that depends on the cut-off value (the value of the score at which the test is said to be "positive"). Scoring systems can be compared for their overall accuracy ("discrimination") by plotting the sensitivity (defined for most intensive care scoring systems as the proportion of correctly classified non-survivors) against the specificity (the proportion of correctly classified survivors) at different cut-off values of the score. This plot is called a receiver–operator characteristic curve, from its earlier application during World War II to evaluate radar operators. The greater the area under the curve, the greater the degree of discrimination of survivors from non-survivors. The other technique used to assess scoring systems is to measure calibration; patient scores are grouped into risk bands, and the actual number of deaths (or survivors) is compared with the predicted number in each decile. The predicted number is either based on an earlier cohort of patients or in large studies the population is split, with one half acting as the test population.

It is important not to confuse *measurement*, which is the calculation of a score or an odds ratio, with *prediction*, which is the expression of risk as a binary outcome (death or survival). Scoring systems tell us something about proportionate risk in groups of patients: the patient populations on which they are based contain more patients with a given diagnosis or degree of severity than any clinician is likely to see in a lifetime. However, scoring systems cannot tell us what is going to happen to a specific individual. The obvious case in point is the 50% risk band: as a group, these patients are severely ill, but for any individual within this group the scoring system is maximally uncertain about the outcome.

## Specific risk adjustment methods

A large number of scoring systems are available. Some are generic, whereas others have been designed with a specific purpose or patient group in mind. Some form part of large and growing observational databases containing more than 100 000 patients. The more frequently used methods are described below.

## Acute Physiology, Age, Chronic Health Evaluation (APACHE)

The best known of all intensive care scoring systems is the APACHE method, developed by Knaus and his colleagues. First published in 1981, this has undergone subsequent revisions to the most recent form, APACHE III.[4] This method is based on the principle that critical illness can be described in terms of the extent to which a disease process has affected homeostatic mechanisms, and that the greater the degree of physiological derangement the more severe the disease process. The 34 variables and weights in the original version were selected by clinical consensus, and then refined by statistical techniques to 12 physiological variables for APACHE II, and 17 for APACHE III. Each variable contributes a number of points to the total score depending on the degree of deviation from normal values. There is additional weighting for prior health status, age, urgency, and source of admission. The sum of the weighted values provides the score. This can be converted to a risk of death using a proprietary equation (not in the public domain) which incorporates additional weighting for the primary diagnosis. This is necessary because, although the relationship between score and mortality rate is impressive for large groups of patients, it differs for different diseases (Figure 2.1).

Data for APACHE scoring are derived from the worst values of the variables during the first 24 hours of admission to intensive care. Several factors may influence the accuracy of the method. The more frequently data are recorded (for example, using automated data capture from monitors), the more likely it is that extreme values will be detected, particularly for cardiorespiratory variables. Conversely, certain laboratory variables may be measured only once during the 24-hour period. The Glasgow Coma Scale (GCS) component is heavily weighted, and although this is appropriate for structural cerebral injury for which purpose the scale was originally produced, it is less effective as a measure of severity when influenced by encephalopathies or sedative drugs. Prior treatment (such as tertiary referrals from other ICUs) will reduce physiological abnormalities on admission and produce an underestimation of severity, an effect called lead-time bias for which the compensatory weighting in the APACHE system may be insufficient. Diagnostic labelling requires some experience, and should not be left to untutored or unmotivated staff. Despite these factors, the APACHE system is an impressive system validated in many countries for the stratification of groups of patients. Its main strengths are that it is physiologically based, uses standard clinical and laboratory data, has wide application, and allows time-based analyses.

## Simplified Acute Physiology Score (SAPS)

There are several methods based on the APACHE concept, of which SAPS[5] is the best known. The revised version, SAPS II, incorporates 17 variables, including two (mechanical respiratory support and urine output) that may be affected by therapeutic decisions as much as by severity of illness. It does not include chronic health data or diagnoses. Relatively simple in application, it provides satisfactory risk stratification for groups of patients.

## Mortality Probability Model (MPM)[6]

The Mortality Probability Model II (MPM II) exists as a model on admission and one after 24 hours of intensive care. The admission model (one hour either side of admission) employs 11 categorical variables (requiring "yes/no" responses) selected by multiple logistic regression from a larger number of candidate variables. They include emergency or previous ICU admission, age, coma, previous cardiorespiratory arrest, chronic renal failure, cancer, infection, systolic blood pressure, heart rate, and surgery. MPM is a static measure, and this limits its usefulness in time-based research. It is, however, treatment independent, and could therefore have an application in stratifying patients before ICU admission.

## Organ System Failures (OSFs)

The attraction of OSFs is their simplicity, but there is a price to be paid in terms of loss of precision, and in the variability of the definitions of individual system failures. Knaus and colleagues[1] applied strict definitions which were independent of therapy except for mechanical ventilation; they showed that number and duration of failures were closely related to outcome, as have others.[7] However, the desire for greater precision has resulted in classifications of increasing complexity which incorporate grades of dysfunction, based on deviations in physiology or the level of therapeutic support for each organ system.

## Glasgow Coma Scale[8]

This well known scale was introduced to improve the reliability of clinical descriptions of patients in post-traumatic coma for 6 hours or more from the time of the head injury. The system performs well between different observers. There is an international databank of many thousands of patients relating quality of survival to predicted outcome based on the GCS.[9] The scale is presented as a score, suggesting an equivalence between the various components that may not be valid; the GCS provides non-parametric ordinal data. Its robustness as a descriptor of cerebral trauma has led to its incorporation in other scoring systems, such as the Trauma Score (appropriately) and the APACHE III score, where it has been modified statistically for application to all forms of cerebral dysfunction, not just trauma. For predicting outcome from hypoxic–ischaemic coma, pupillary light reflexes and motor responses are the most powerful predictors. Paediatric versions of the adult GCS have been developed.[10]

### Injury Severity Score (ISS), Trauma Score (TS), and TRISS

The ISS is a score for anatomical severity of injury, which is calculated at death or discharge. Postmortem rates will influence accuracy. It is based on the gradings of the Abbreviated Injury Scale, which it converts into a score by summing the squared values for each of six anatomical areas, thereby producing an almost linear relationship between score and mortality. The revised Trauma Score (rTS) is a simple physiologically based method, which sums coded values for three intervals of the GCS, and five intervals of systolic blood pressure and respiratory rate. Combination of the two gives an anatomical and physiological index of severity of injury, the TRISS (TS + ISS) system,[11] which is being used as the comparative index in multiple trauma outcome studies in the USA and the UK.

### Therapeutic Intervention Scoring System (TISS)

The basis of TISS is that therapeutic intensity equates with severity, but its main application is as a summary measure of cost. The original system awarded one to four points to each of 70 nursing and medical procedures; this has been revised,[12] and there is also a version for high dependency care.[13] Many variants exist, however, which suggests the need for caution when comparing results from different ICUs.

## Applications of risk adjustment methods

Scoring systems have been used in the assessment of quality of care in research, to ensure proper risk stratification or to target a particular risk group, and as aids to clinical decision-making.

### Quality of care assessment

Intensive care presents something of a paradox, because it has contributed more than any other discipline to the theory of severity measurement and risk adjustment, and yet has developed in a somewhat random manner with little objective evidence of its own efficacy or cost-efficiency. The difficulty is that, unlike a comparison of two different but potentially equivalent treatments, it would be considered unethical to submit patients to a randomised controlled trial of intensive care versus lower levels of care, given the existence of a life-threatening illness. An alternative to randomisation would be to use natural variations in clinical practice, such as refused admissions to intensive care because of resource constraints, or apparently random variations between ICUs in terms of risk-adjusted outcomes. The first requires accurate methods for describing patient characteristics (including severity of illness), which have been calibrated for patients before they have received intensive care treatment. All the major methods of risk adjustment have, however, been developed for patients already in receipt of intensive care, and have not been validated for determining prior risk. This approach involves comparison of standardised mortality ratios.

Standardised mortality ratios (SMRs) have been proposed as a method of identifying unexpectedly good or poor outcomes. The SMR is calculated as the observed death rate divided by the expected death rate based on case mix severity. Thus, an ICU with an SMR of 1·25 has a mortality rate that is 25% higher than would have been expected from the average severity of illness of all the patients whom it treats. There are several potential sources of error in this approach. First, the severity scoring method may be inaccurate or poorly adjusted to the patient population being examined. Second, poor quality care could in theory result in more extreme physiological values being identified, a higher score being calculated, and with worse outcomes thus being disguised. Third, there are procedural differences in data collection that could affect the score – accuracy and frequency of data collection, exclusion of certain data items, and lead-time bias. There are certainly substantial differences between ICU mortality rates before and after adjustment for case mix,[14] although one study that examined quality of care and severity-adjusted outcomes independently found no relationship between the two.[15] Few ICUs would, however, like to have their performance assessed *without* adjustment for case mix and, provided that individual units feel empowered and supported in the process of audit, SMRs should be viewed as quality screening tools that still require validation for this purpose.

## Research tools

The efficacy of new treatments cannot be determined without compensating for the main factors that influence outcome. Differences in illness severity between treatment and control groups could exaggerate, reverse, or obscure true treatment differences, and controlling for case mix is therefore essential. Conversely, one might expect a new treatment to have little effect on patients too sick or too well to benefit, and therefore trials may wish to target the mid-severity band where outcome is most uncertain. Observed and expected mortality rates may be inspected for different risk bands in large studies in order to identify possible benefits at different severity levels. Severity scoring can also be used to monitor adverse effects, as was demonstrated in the retrospective use of injury severity scoring to identify a possible adverse effect of etomidate,[16] or to audit the quality of a service such as between-hospital transfers.[17]

15

# Clinical decision-making

This is one of the most contentious aspects of severity measurement. Clinicians vary in their ability to recognise both the severity of illness and the degree to which their patients have responded to treatment, with the result that patients may receive appropriate treatment too late, or may continue to receive inappropriate treatment for too long. However, the SUPPORT study was unable to detect any effect on outcomes of providing clinicians with mortality risk estimates.[18] It is now well understood that, although severity scoring methods provide risk estimates for groups of patients, they do not predict outcome for individuals. The best that a scoring system can do is to place a particular patient within a severity band. Whether medical staff find this sort of information helpful to inform (or substitute for?) clinical judgment is uncertain. It is possible that, with large databases that are made sensitive to local practice and responsive to changes in the patients' condition with treatment, scoring systems may come to have a role in supporting clinical decisions, or – perhaps more importantly – in refuting them.

1 Knaus WA, Draper EA, Wagner DP, Zimmerman JE. Prognosis in acute organ-system failure. *Ann Surg* 1985;202:685–93.
2 Yinnon A, Zimran A, Hershko C. Quality of life and survival following intensive medical care. *Q J Med, New Series 71* 1989;264:347–57.
3 Zimmerman JE, Knaus WA, Sharpe SM, Anderson AS, Draper EA, Wagner DP. The use and implications of Do Not Resuscitate orders in intensive care units. *JAMA* 1986;255:351–6.
4 Knaus WA, Wagner DP, Draper EA, *et al.* The APACHE III prognostic system. Risk prediction of hospital mortality for critically ill hospitalized adults. *Chest* 1991;100:1619–36.
5 Le Gall JR, Lemeshow S, Saulnier F. A new Simplified Acute Physiology Score (SAPS II) based on a European/North American multicentre study. *JAMA* 1993;27:2957–63.
6 Lemeshow S, Teres D, Klar J, *et al.* Mortality probability models (MPA II) based on an international cohort of intensive care unit patients. *JAMA* 1993;270:2478–86.
7 Marshall JC, Cook DJ, Christou NV, Bernard GR, Sprung CL, Sibbald WJ. Multiple organ dysfunction score: a reliable descriptor of a complex clinical outcome. *Crit Care Med* 1995;23:1638–52.
8 Teasdale G, Jennett B. Assessment of coma and impaired consciousness. A practical scale. *Lancet* 1974;ii; 81–4.
9 Murray GD. Use of an international data bank to compare outcome following severe head injury in different centres. *Statistics in Medicine* 1986;5:103–12.
10 Reilly PL, Simpson DA, Thomas L. Assessing the conscious level in infants and young children: a paediatric version of the Glasgow Coma Scale. *Childs Nerv Syst* 1988;4:30–3.
11 Boyd CR, Tolson MA, Copes WS. Evaluating trauma care: the TRISS method. *J Trauma* 1987;27:370–8.
12 Keene AR, Cullen DJ. Therapeutic Intervention Scoring System: update 1983. *Crit Care Med* 1983;11:1–3.
13 Cullen DJ, Nemeskal AR, Zaslavsky AM. Intermediate TISS: a new Therapeutic Intervention Scoring System for non-ICU patients. *Crit Care Med* 1994;22:1406–11.
14 Rowan KM, Kerr JH, Major E, McPherson K, Short A, Vessey MP. Intensive Care Society's Acute Physiology and Chronic Health Evaluation (APACHE II) study in Britain

and Ireland: a prospective, multicenter, cohort study comparing two methods for predicting outcome for adult intensive care patients. *Crit Care Med* 1994;**22**:1392–401.

15 Zimmerman JE, Shortell SM, Rousseau DM, *et al.* Improving intensive care: observations based on organisational case studies in nine intensive care units: A prospective, multicentre study. *Crit Care Med* 1993;**21**:1443–51.

16 Watt I, Ledingham IMcA. Mortality amongst multiple trauma patients admitted to an intensive therapy unit. *Anaesthesia* 1984;**39**:973–81.

17 Bion JF, Edlin SA, Ramsay G, McCabe S, Ledingham IMcA. Validation of a prognostic score in critically ill patients undergoing transport. *BMJ* 1985;**291**:432–4.

18 Teno J, Lynn J, Wenger N, *et al.* Advance directives for seriously ill hospitalized patients: effectiveness with the patient self-determination act and the SUPPORT intervention. SUPPORT Investigators. Study to Understand Prognoses and Preferences for Outcomes and Risks of Treatment. *J Am Geriatr Soc* 1997;**45**:500–7.

# 3: Ethical and legal issues in intensive care

M A BRANTHWAITE

Patients requiring intensive care are often "incompetent" in the sense that they are unable to give rational thought to their own predicament and preferences. This alone poses an ethical dilemma which is compounded by the conflict created when expensive, possibly futile treatments are sought from limited resources. The ethical principles of beneficence, non-maleficence, respect for autonomy, and justice (taken here to mean distributive justice) provide some basis for rational decision-making but the conclusions reached must lie within the law. Transgressing legal rules lays the practitioner open to civil suit or even criminal prosecution, no matter how laudable the motives for action taken. Legal input may also be needed to resolve particular issues pertaining to individual patients. This chapter will address the ethical and legal issues raised by consent to treatment, withholding or withdrawing intensive care, rationing, and research in intensive care.

## Consent

Non-consensual touching of another can provide the basis for an action in tort or even battery. Consent is usually assumed for simple measures such as physical examination, venepuncture, or plain radiograph but it is customary to obtain written consent for surgery, or any major procedure associated with risk or requiring general anaesthesia. Consent is only valid if it is informed, competent, and given freely, criteria that cannot be fulfilled by patients who present for intensive care unconscious or with their understanding compromised by illness, accident, or antecedent drug therapy. Yet the complex, invasive, and often disagreeable nature of the treatments involved is such that formal consent would normally be sought. It is a common misconception that a relative can give consent for incompetent adult patients but such consent has no legal validity. It is courteous to enquire how family members view the proposed treatment and, in particular, whether they have any knowledge of opinions held by the patient. However, the *legal* validity of consent to life-saving treatment relies on the doctrine of necessity – the assumption that most patients would wish to have the benefit of treatment considered to be in their best interests. The doctrine does not justify treatments other than the immediately life-saving, even if convenience would be served by undertaking these at the same time as the urgent measures. Furthermore, the doctrine does not permit treatment of incompetent patients who have expressed a specific wish to avoid particular measures. This has been recognised in the context of adult Jehovah's Witnesses for many years but received additional emphasis in 1992 when criteria which must be fulfilled before prior refusal of life-saving treatment is to be accepted as valid were set out by the Court of Appeal:

• the decision was taken when the subject was legally competent;
• the patient anticipated and intended the decision to apply to the circumstances which now pertain;
• the decision was reached without undue influence.

These recommendations were upheld in 1994 in the case of a schizophrenic patient who refused consent to amputation of his gangrenous leg. Despite his mental illness, it was held that he was competent to evaluate the implications of amputation and his application for an injunction to prevent surgeons amputating his leg then or at any time in the future succeeded. In the event the patient survived after débridement of the leg but the authority of the "living will" at Common Law had been endorsed. It is all too easy to envisage predicaments where those responsible for an incompetent adult would seek to transgress such an advance directive – for example, it was made a long time ago, the patient's circumstances have changed, or he no longer holds such views but has not rescinded his earlier declaration. However, the general rule remains: the living will is to be respected provided it fulfils the criteria set out above.[1]

## Consent to treat children[2]

The difficulties created by legal "incompetence" in the case of adult patients have been noted already. The Family Law Reform Act 1969 entitles children above the age of 16 years to consent to medical treatment without the intervention of their parents. Below that age parental consent is required unless the individual child is considered to have sufficient understanding of the matter in question. Children between the ages of 16 and 18 cannot consent to take part in research nor can they refuse their consent to medical treatment recommended as in their best interests. In these circumstances, consent should be sought from the parent or guardian. If a parent or guardian withholds consent for treatment that is considered necessary for the child, application can be made for the child to become a ward of court. Recourse to the law should be a measure of last resort, not least because, if treatment is given which would be refused by parents on their own behalf, they may reject the child who has received that treatment against their wishes.

# Withholding intensive care

The possibility of withholding intensive care at the behest of a patient, either in response to a wish expressed competently or on the basis of an advance directive, has been explored in the context of consent, but what of the patient who seeks intensive care which the physician believes is not in that patient's best interest? There is no legal or moral compulsion on any physician to act other than in what he or she believes to be the best interests of that patient, but such a view must be held honestly and for valid reasons, and must be capable of explanation and justification if challenged. Thus, in *Re J* a mother sought a court order to compel medical staff to provide mechanical ventilation for her child who suffered from repetitive, uncontrollable, and life-threatening convulsions. Her application failed, the court maintaining that a practitioner would not be required to adopt a course of treatment which *in the bona fide clinical judgment of that practitioner* was not in the patient's best interests. The matter is more difficult to resolve when the practitioner is aware that valid medical opinion is divided on what constitutes "best interests". Here it is wise to seek independent comment on the individual case from practitioners experienced in the relevant field (*R v Cambridge Health Authority* 1995), or at least the views of colleagues within the same hospital. If a consensus cannot be reached, it is sensible to adopt the aphorism "when in doubt, continue". The dynamic nature of intensive care is such that the decision may do no more than change the time course of illness.

# Withdrawing treatment

Intensive therapy is an effective means of supporting body systems but is rarely specifically therapeutic in its own right. Should heroic treatment be continued, often at exceptional cost, when death is anticipated as the final outcome?

Beneficence and non-maleficence can be seen as two sides of the same principle: that which is done should be in the best interests of the individual; but is it in the best interests of any individual to be kept "alive", for death to be prolonged by mechanical measures with consequent loss of dignity, autonomy, or consciousness, quite apart from the pain and discomfort of specific procedures? Many would answer that it is not, but opinions differ on where the balance between benefit and harm should be drawn. Few practitioners have personal experience of the rigours of intensive care and may regard it as more onerous than patients who have – or at least those who have experienced and survived to recount their feelings. We can never know the attitude of those who have experienced intensive care but not survived. The best that can be assumed is that there probably is some point where all would agree that intensive care has moved beyond the realm of beneficence but there is a wide grey area where opinion is bound to differ.

Respect for patient autonomy may be invaluable as a guide where opinion has been clearly stated before the life-threatening illness occurred. Unfortunately few patients have prepared advance directives and there is, as yet, no legal basis for decision-making by a designated proxy. This is where sensitive discussion with family members will help to resolve conflict. Often families have agreed among themselves that they wish treatment could be terminated "so that he doesn't suffer any more". Equally often they are reluctant to broach the subject with professional staff for fear of being considered unduly pessimistic or lacking concern for the afflicted relative. Once the subject is broached with them, they may express their feelings with both conviction and relief. It is commonplace in intensive care units the world over for treatment-limiting or treatment-withdrawing decisions to be made after careful deliberation by professional staff of all grades and disciplines between themselves and with the family. Rarely will dispute follow such an approach and, provided the family can be spared the lonely belief that they were responsible for the decision, the death can be foreseen, accepted, and allowed to occur in surroundings of tranquillity and dignity. The atmosphere of the hospice is not out of place in the intensive care unit and it is far preferable for families to experience death in such circumstances, usually in their presence, than to be ushered from the room while there are heroic, last-minute, and often disfiguring attempts to resuscitate.

Unfortunately such a gentle scene cannot always be achieved, the most common reason being that the patient is stable while the fully panoply of intensive care continues, but deteriorates as soon as it is discontinued. The proximity in time between act and outcome and the causal relationship between them are disturbing and raise questions of law as well as ethics. Resolution of this conflict lies in the distinction between causation in fact and that in law. Causation in fact can be expressed as the "but for" test. But for the act in question, would death have occurred when it did? The answer may well be "no" but causation in law seeks to go beyond the mere immediate antecedent event and identify the cause of the mortal process. Thus, the courts in New Zealand acceded to an application to discontinue mechanical ventilation in a patient suffering from profound and prolonged Guillain–Barré syndrome in whom there was no evidence of sentience or any means of communication or personal expression (*Auckland Area Health Trust v Attorney-General* 1993). It was held that the death was caused by the disease, not by the cessation of treatment for which there was no medical justification, and that there was no duty to provide "necessary life" if no medical benefit ensued. Similar views were expressed in the English case of *Airedale NHS Trust v Bland* 1993 where the House of Lords sanctioned the cessation of nasogastric feeding in a patient in a persistent vegetative state. Their Lordships stated explicitly that their decision was not to be regarded as a precedent and advocated that application be made to the courts for authority to discontinue life-sustaining treatment in such circumstances. The distinction between persistent vegetative state and critically ill patients in intensive care is that the latter are physiologically unstable and the natural progression of their disease is expected to end in death – it is merely the timing of the death that can be influenced by continuing treatment. Such an argument presupposes that prediction of outcome is an accurate science and this of course is far from true. To what extent then can prediction be used as a basis for clinical decision-making? It is done every day of the week in wards and clinics of all hospitals when criteria established by experience are applied to common situations to determine diagnosis, diagnostic category, or recommended best treatment. Attempts to do likewise for intensive care by scoring systems such as those discussed in Chapter 2 have met with a barrage of criticism – for example, "the criteria are no more than self-fulfilling prophesies" and "patients' lives are being determined by computer". Strict adherence to predictive criteria, which are based on statistical analysis of cohorts of patients, is no more justified in intensive care than in any other branch of medicine. Nevertheless, accurate assessment provides a firmer foundation for decision-making than instinct or personal experience. The important point is that the scoring system merely creates the foundation – individual decision-making requires consideration of the personal factors that may apply in specific cases.

## Active intervention

Does active intervention differ from failing to act or treatment withdrawal? The law does not allow one man to kill another, even if the motive for killing is high-principled and beneficent (*R v Cox* 1992). But is there really a distinction between the administration of potassium chloride intravenously and the withdrawal of oxygen or mechanical ventilation from a patient dependent upon them? Although criminal prosecution for murder or manslaughter usually relies on a culpable act, conviction can follow failure to act if a duty of care has already been accepted. However, a distinction can be drawn between the active administration of a drug with the sole, specific intention of causing death and the withdrawal of medication or treatment. Thereafter the patient dies from the disease process; treatment is no longer effective, hence its use is not in the best interests of the patient and therefore it can be withdrawn lawfully. There is often a distinction too in terms of timescale in that measures designed specifically to kill, for example, the administration of potassium chloride, do so in a matter of seconds whereas death after treatment withdrawal is usually – although not always – less abrupt. These principles have been endorsed in the recent past by both medical[3] and judicial[4] opinion and provide welcome guidance in an area where decision-making is peculiarly difficult.

# Rationing resources

This emotive issue figures prominently in dicussions concerning intensive care. Costs are very high and patients who do not survive have on average a far higher unit cost than those who do.[5] This is not an argument for basing clinical decisions on financial priorities. It is, however, a powerful incentive to evaluate results, to refine prediction so that those who are most likely to benefit can be identified accurately, to adopt realistic measures for within-hospital and between-hospital rationalisation of facilities, and to set up agreed protocols for decision-making when triage is inevitable. The need to consider these issues is a measure of the success of modern medicine rather than an index of impoverished resources; practitioners have no right to demand facilities with which to treat patients but they do have a responsibility to use as wisely as possible resources that are allocated. Corporately agreed policies involving lay opinion when possible help to minimise friction but must be kept under regular review. Similarly, systems are needed to ensure that the well-argued case for a trial of new treatments is not compromised by procedural rigidity. Such constraints interfere with clinical freedom but are an inevitable consequence of high-cost, complex interventions.

# Research in intensive care

It is customary to divide clinical research into therapeutic and non-therapeutic. The former involves trial of an agent or procedure which may be of benefit to the individual whereas non-therapeutic research seeks knowledge which will benefit others. Respect for individual autonomy requires that participation in a trial is both informed and consensual, criteria that can be fulfilled reliably only for intensive care patients admitted electively. This should not preclude the reseach worker from including patients unable to consent if the research is therapeutic and can be justified on logical grounds as likely to provide a significant advance over existing methods. However, particularly careful scrutiny by Hospital Research Ethics Committees is a prerequisite and the reasons for recruiting individual subjects should be recorded. Non-therapeutic research should, as a general rule, be carried out only on subjects able to provide fully informed consent although the British Medical Association[2] advises that for the incompetent adult:

> . . . measures which are not contrary to their interests, involve only minimal risk and may potentially benefit others in the same category are not unethical but must be carefully scrutinised by Local Research Ethics Committees.

Research on children is even more difficult. Parental consent should be sought but, even then, it is doubtful whether a parent can give legally valid consent to any treatment or procedure that is contrary to the child's best interest.

The conflict for both adults and children lies between protecting the interests of the individual and ensuring that valid research is carried out on subjects with the relevant characteristics and conditions. A number of national and international guidelines have been drawn up and should be followed as carefully as possible. Above all, clinical research should be considered and approved by Local Research Ethics Committees. The higher the risk, the more marginal the postulated benefit, and the greater the need to recruit subjects incapable of giving fully informed consent, the more essential it is to seek stringent external scrutiny. The practice of intensive care is particularly likely to generate ethical conflict in research as in so many other areas. The discipline is challenging but resolution of these conflicts brings its own reward.

1 British Medical Association. *Advance statements about medical treatment.* London: BMJ Publishing Group, 1995.
2 British Medical Association. *Medical ethics today: its practice and philosophy.* London: BMJ Publishing Group, 1993.
3 Black DAK. Medical management of terminal illness. A statement of the Committee on Ethical Issues in Medicine of the Royal College of Physicians. *J R Coll Physicians Lond* 1993;27:397–8.
4 SCME. *Select Committee on Medical Ethics, House of Lords Report.* London: HMSO, 1994.
5 Atkinson S, Bihari D, Smithies M, Daly K, Mason R, McColl I. Identification of futility in intensive care. *Lancet* 1994;344:1203–6.

## Table of cases

Re J (a minor) – child in care: Medical Treatment [1992] 3 WLR 507.
R v. Cambridge Health Authority, Ex parte B (a Minor) [1995] Med LR 250.
Auckland Area Health Trust v Attorney-General [1993] 1 NZLR 235.
Airedale NHS Trust v Bland [1993] AC 789.
R v Cox. Unreported, 18 September 1992; Ognall J.

# PART TWO

# PATHOGENESIS OF CRITICAL ILLNESS

# 4: Multiple organ failure: clinical features and pathogenesis

J TAKALA

Simultaneou or sequential dysfunction or failure of vital organs (multiple organ failure or MOF) is the most common cause of prolonged intensive care.[1-3] MOF is the most important cause of death after apparently successful primary resuscitation; in those who ultimately survive from MOF, the need for intensive care is always prolonged, often up to several weeks. MOF may develop as a complication and final common pathway of any severe acute disorder of vital functions, including severe infections and especially septic shock, and many clinical conditions without a verified infection, such as acute pancreatitis, major trauma, severe hypovolemic shock, visceral ischemia, and the acute respiratory distress syndrome.[1-7]

Multiple organ failure may be considered a consequence of advanced life support and intensive care: patients, who in the past would have died during the most acute phase of respiratory or circulatory failure, now survive longer and often die in MOF after prolonged intensive care. A systemic inflammatory response (systemic inflammatory response syndrome, SIRS), indistinguishable from that characteristic of a severe infection, usually precedes and accompanies MOF. Even though MOF is often accompanied by infection, it is clear that the inflammatory response and MOF can develop without concomitant infection.[1,2,5,6]

Organ dysfunction should be defined according to objective criteria.[1] Definitions based on an arbitrary limit between "normal" and "abnormal" values of a functional indicator do not sufficiently take into account the dynamic nature of the changes in organ function. The dysfunction of an organ may be better defined as the inability of the organ to maintain homeostasis without therapeutic interventions. In order to emphasise the dynamic changes in organ function and the common pathogenic pathways, the term "multiple organ dysfunction syndrome" (MODS) has been proposed to replace MOF. At present, various scoring systems are used to describe organ dysfunctions and their severity.[1,5,8] Representative examples of variables used to define organ dysfunctions are given in Table 4.1. The variation between definitions should be considered in the assessment of the incidence and prognosis of MOF, and the effects of potential therapeutic interventions.

Table 4.1 Variables used to assess the presence and severity of organ dysfunction in MOF

| Organ system | Variable |
| --- | --- |
| Central nervous system | Level of consciousness in the absence of sedation (usually assessed by the Glasgow Coma Score) |
| Respiratory system | Ventilator dependency, arterial $P_{O_2}/F_{IO_2}$ |
| Cardiovascular system | Hypotension; need for inotropic or vasopressor drugs |
| Kidney | Oliguria or increased serum creatinine without a pre- or postrenal cause; need for renal replacement therapy |
| Liver | Hyperbilirubinaemia and increased transaminase levels |
| Gastrointestinal system | Macroscopic bleeding, ileus |
| Haematological system | Thrombocytopenia, leukopenia, coagulopathy |

## Predisposing factors, incidence, and prognosis

Multiple organ failure is a relatively common complication of multiple injury, protracted hypovolaemia, severe circulatory failure, acute respiratory failure, and septic infection (Box 4.1). Approximately 10% of all intensive care patients require intensive care for more than one week, and MOF is involved in most cases. The care of these patients accounts for about half of all the intensive care days. MOF develops in up to 50% of all patients with severe intra-abdominal infections, in 80% of patients with the acute respiratory distress syndrome (ARDS) or septic shock, and in 7–22% of patients undergoing emergency surgery. In multiple injuries MOF develops in approximately 10% and in major burns in about 25–30% of patients.[1–5,7,9]

MOF increases substantially the risk of mortality. The duration of MOF (that is, the response to intensive care and the number of failing organ

---

**Box 4.1** *Clinical conditions predisposing to multiple organ failure*

- Severe or protracted circulatory failure: septic, cardiogenic, or hypovolemic shock

- Severe infections: sepsis, intra-abdominal infections

- Acute pancreatitis

- Major trauma: multiple injury, burns

- Acute respiratory failure

- Visceral ischaemia

- Major surgery + limited physiological reserves/chronic organ dysfunction

---

systems), and the age of the patient all have a major impact on the prognosis. If MOF progresses for several days despite adequate intensive care, and at least four organ systems are involved, the prognosis is usually poor. Other factors that are associated with a poor prognosis are an inadequately eradicated focus of infection, advanced age, and severe circulatory failure. The mortality is highly dependent on the definition of MOF, and reported mortality rates range from 25% to 100%. Failure of three or more organ systems is associated with a mortality rate of 50% or more.[1]

## Aetiology and pathogenesis

Multiple organ failure can develop as a direct result of a clearly defined event (primary MOF), such as massive transfusion or thoracic contusion. In primary MOF organ dysfunction develops early as the direct consequence of the insult itself. Secondary MOF develops usually following a latent, clinically relatively stable period, after the primary derangement of homeostasis. It is likely that the host response, the systemic inflammatory response, has a central role in the pathogenesis of secondary MOF. Secondary MOF is common particularly in severe infections.[1]

It is evident that the pathogenesis of MOF is multifactorial, and no distinct chain or cascade of pathophysiological events has been proven as the cause of MOF. Whilst the cytokine network and other mediators are essential for appropriate host defence, an excessive inflammatory response is counterproductive and contributes to the pathogenesis of MOF, although the precise mechanisms remain poorly understood. An excessive cell-mediated inflammatory response with activation of neutrophils and macrophages results in the release of mediators, which can cause local tissue damage and perfusion abnormalities. An uncontrolled infection and humoral mediators may interfere with oxidative metabolism in the tissues and contribute to the development of organ function abnormalities.[1-5]

Regardless of the exact pathogenesis of MOF, insufficient tissue perfusion and shock both increase the risk of MOF and may further worsen existing organ failures. When MOF develops as the consequence of severe hypovolaemic shock, the link between insufficient tissue perfusion or tissue hypoxia and organ failures is self-evident: "shock kidney", "shock liver", and "shock lung" are typical manifestations of primary MOF, and were recognised long before MOF as a syndrome was first described. The role of insufficient tissue perfusion in secondary MOF is less well established and somewhat controversial. In secondary MOF, the metabolic demands of the body are increased due to the associated systemic inflammatory response.[1,2] On the other hand, the patient's ability to respond to the increased oxygen demand by increasing tissue perfusion or oxygen extraction is often limited due to hypovolaemia, poor cardiac performance, impaired oxygen extraction capability, and abnormal vasoregulation. In addition, arterial hypoxaemia from concomitant respiratory failure and anaemia may further reduce the oxygen supply to the tissues. The combination of increased metabolic demands and limited ability to increase blood flow make those regions with high metabolic demands susceptible to tissue hypoxia, if any deterioration of haemodynamics occurs. The hepatosplanchnic region appears to be particularly vulnerable because of its high metabolic demand in SIRS, and the heterogeneity of hepatosplanchnic blood flow.[10-13]

It has been suggested that tissue hypoxia secondary to inadequate tissue perfusion may have a pivotal role in the development of organ damage in intensive care patients. Indeed, the role of tissue hypoxia in the pathogenesis of MOF has been the subject of extensive debate during the last few years. Outcome from intensive care is better and MOF occurs less frequently in those high-risk surgical and septic patients who maintain normal haemodynamics and oxygen supply to the tissues, either spontaneously or as the result of therapy.[14-16] Use of supranormal values of cardiac output and oxygen delivery as goals of haemodynamic management has resulted in improved outcome, when they are used peri- and postoperatively in high-risk surgical patients.[15,16] In contrast, the unselective use of supranormal oxygen transport as a haemodynamic goal after admission to intensive care does not improve outcome or the incidence of MOF.[14,17] Whilst aiming at higher than normal oxygen transport may not offer any benefit and can even be counterproductive in some patients, it is clear that failure to achieve even normal haemodynamics in response to therapy carries a very grim prognosis.

Tissue hypoxia alone is unlikely to explain the pathogenesis of MOF in most cases. It is more likely that the combination of SIRS, insufficient tissue perfusion, and episodes of tissue hypoxia acts to produce the progressive organ dysfunctions characteristic of MOF. The gastrointestinal tract is closely involved in this process, although its precise role is presently poorly understood.[3,18,19] The splanchnic region can produce large amounts of cytokines and other mediators of inflammation. During SIRS, the splanchnic tissue macrophages produce cytokines that may modify blood flow and metabolism both locally and in remote organs, and influence the function of extrasplanchnic organs and whole body vasoregulation. Sepsis and circulatory shock increase intestinal permeability and may lead to translocation of intraluminal bacteria and toxins. These may contribute to the activation of mediator cascades, and lead to further perfusion defects and tissue injury. Moreover, a systemic inflammatory response to an extrasplanchnic focus may increase splanchnic metabolic demand and indirectly modify splanchnic perfusion via changes in systemic blood flow. Thus the hepatosplanchnic region can be both the target and the source of the inflammatory, cardiovascular, and metabolic responses that precede and accompany MOF.

Inadequate splanchnic tissue perfusion at any time during intensive care may contribute to the development of organ dysfunction and modify the clinical course. Tissue perfusion and oxygen supply may become inadequate due to insufficient or inadequately distributed blood flow, impaired tissue oxygen extraction or oxygen use, or increased oxygen demand in the tissues. Absolute reduction of splanchnic blood flow is rare, except in hypovolaemia or low cardiac output from other causes.[20] Reduction of splanchnic blood flow due to hypovolaemia may persist after restoration of the circulating blood volume.[13] The increased splanchnic metabolic demand in inflammation and sepsis is not fully compensated by an increase in blood flow.[10–12] Consequently, tissue oxygenation can be preserved only by increased splanchnic oxygen extraction both in low flow states and in hyperdynamic sepsis. Even minor changes in cardiac output and splanchnic blood flow may under these circumstances precipitate tissue hypoxia in the splanchnic region.

Inadequate splanchnic tissue perfusion can be detected before the clinical development of MOF. With the use of tonometry to measure gastric intramucosal acidosis, inadequate gastrointestinal perfusion has been associated with an increased risk of sepsis, MOF, postoperative complications, and death in various categories of intensive care patients.[21–24] Despite this, a cause–effect relationship between inadequate splanchnic tissue perfusion and the pathogenesis or worsening of organ failures has not been confirmed. Nevertheless, prevention of gastric intramucosal acidosis by haemodynamic support improved outcome in intensive care patients, supporting the view that the prevention of splanchnic tissue hypoxia may prevent organ damage.[22]

## Prevention and treatment

Considering the multifactorial pathogenesis of MOF, it is not surprising that no single, specific, preventive measure or treatment is currently available or can be foreseen in the near future. Prevention of MOF is based on prevention and prompt treatment of acute haemodynamic and cardio-respiratory catastrophes, and on control of infections. Most of these measures can be regarded as "good practice of intensive care".

The factors that predispose to MOF usually develop well before admission to intensive care. Since the dynamic process leading to MOF is difficult to stop once started, it is extremely important to recognise patients at risk, to monitor vital functions carefully, and to start supportive therapy early. In this respect, high-risk patients undergoing major surgery are a specific group, where preventive measures are possible before the triggering event. Use of fluid and inotropic agents in order to maintain higher than normal oxygen delivery in high-risk surgical patients has improved postoperative outcome in controlled studies.[15,16] Whether the success of these therapeutic approaches is based on the achievement of supranormal oxygen transport or the maintenance of sufficient blood volume is still an open question. Nevertheless, it emphasises the importance of pre-, peri-, and postoperative haemodynamic assessment, monitoring, and support in the prevention of postoperative organ dysfunction in patients at high risk.

Use of fluid and inotropic agents in order to maintain higher than normal oxygen delivery after admission to intensive care has not been successful in improving outcome and preventing MOF.[14,17] Whilst higher than normal cardiac output or oxygen transport offered no benefit, those patients who failed to achieve normal haemodynamics despite these attempts to increase cardiac output and oxygen transport had a very high mortality. Also, in order to achieve normal haemodynamics, fluid resuscitation alone or together with inotropic drugs was needed in a large group of patients.[14] These observations emphasise the importance of maintaining adequate haemodynamics, with the help of invasive monitoring, in patients at risk of MOF.

In addition to monitoring and supporting vital functions, and prompt treatment of acute haemodynamic and respiratory dysfunction, infection control has an important role in the prevention and treatment of MOF. Whilst infection may not necessarily be a requisite for MOF, it is nevertheless very common.[4,6,9] Every effort should be made to identify possible foci of infection, and eradicate them with appropriate antibiotics and other specific measures.

Once organ dysfunction and failure have developed, appropriate supportive therapy should be started without delay. Acute respiratory failure requiring mechanical ventilatory support is the rule in MOF, and it is usually the last to recover. Cardiovascular failure will require the use of vasoactive drugs, especially inotropes and, in case of septic shock, vasopressors as well. For renal support, continuous filtration techniques, especially venovenous haemodiafiltration, are preferable to intermittent hemodialysis because of superior haemodynamic stability and continuous control of fluid and electrolyte balance. The main role of all the supportive therapies in MOF is to buy time for the underlying clinical condition to be treated and for organ function to recover.

## Conclusions

- MOF is the most common cause of prolonged intensive care and the most important cause of death after apparently successful primary resuscitation of an acute haemodynamic or respiratory disorder or severe infection.
- A systemic inflammatory response usually precedes and accompanies MOF. Even though MOF is often accompanied by infection, the

inflammatory response and MOF also develop without concomitant infection.

- The pathogenesis is multifactorial: inadequate tissue perfusion, excessive inflammation, and activation of cytokine and other mediator networks all contribute.
- Prevention is based on the early identification of patients at risk, monitoring and supporting vital functions, prompt treatment of acute haemodynamic and respiratory dysfunction, and control of infection.
- Once organ dysfunction and failure have developed, therapy involves supporting and replacing failing organ functions while the underlying cause is identified and treated.

1 ACCP/SCCM Consensus Conference 1992. Definitions for sepsis and multiple organ failure and guidelines for the use of innovative therapies in sepsis. *Crit Care Med* 1992;**20**:864–74.
2 Beal AL, Cerra FB. Multiple organ failure syndrome in the 1990s. Systemic inflammatory response and organ dysfunction. *JAMA* 1994;**271**:226–33.
3 Carrico CJ, Meakins JL, Marshall JC, Fry D, Maier RV. Multiple-organ-failure syndrome. *Arch Surg* 1986;**121**:196–208.
4 Fry DE, Pearlstein L, Fulton RL, Polk HC. Multiple system organ failure. The role of uncontrolled infection. *Arch Surg* 1980;**115**:136–40.
5 Goris PJA, te Boekhorst TPA, Nuytinck JKS, Gimbère JSF. Multiple-organ failure. Generalized autodestructive inflammation? *Arch Surg* 1985;**120**:1109–15.
6 Rangel-Frausto MS, Pittet D, Costigan M, Hwang T, Davis CS, Wenzel RP. The natural history of the systemic inflammatory response syndrome (SIRS). *JAMA* 1995; **273**:117–56.
7 Ruokonen E, Takala J, Kari A, Alhava E. Septic shock and multiple organ failure. *Crit Care Med* 1991;**19**:1146.
8 Marshall JC, Cook DJ, Christou NV, Bernard GR, Sprung CL, Sibbald WJ. Multiple organ dysfunction score: a reliable descriptor of a complex clinical outcome. *Crit Care Med* 1995;**23**:1638–52.
9 Bell RC, Coalson JJ, Smith JD, Johanson WG Jr. Multiple system organ failure and infection in adult respiratory distress syndrome. *Ann Intern Med* 1983;**99**:293–8.
10 Dahn MS, Lange P, Lobdell K, Hans B, Jacobs LA, Mitchell RA. Splanchnic and total body oxygen consumption differences in septic and injured patients. *Surgery* 1987;**101**:69–80.
11 Wilmore DW, Goodwin CW, Aulick LH, Powanda MC, Mason AD, Pruitt BA. Effect of injury and infection on visceral metabolism and circulation. *Ann Surg* 1980;**192**:491–500.
12 Ruokonen E, Takala J, Kari A, Saxén H, Mertsola J, Hansen EJ. Regional blood flow and oxygen transport in septic shock. *Crit Care Med* 1993;**21**:1296–303.
13 Edouard AR, Degrémont A-C, Duranteau J, Pussard E, Berdeaux A, Samii K. Heterogeneous regional vascular responses to simulated transient hypovolemia in man. *Intens Care Med* 1994;**20**:414–20.
14 Gattinoni L, Brazzi L, Pelosi P, *et al.* A trial of goal-oriented hemodynamic therapy in critically ill patients. *N Engl J Med* 1995;**333**:1025–32.
15 Boyd O, Grounds RM, Bennett ED. A randomized clinical trial of the effect of deliberate perioperative increase of oxygen delivery on mortality in high-risk surgical patients. *JAMA* 1993;**270**:2699–707.
16 Shoemaker WC, Appel PL, Kram HB, Waxman K, Lee T-S. Prospective trial of supranormal values of survivors as therapeutic goals in high-risk surgical patients. *Chest* 1988;**94**:1176–86.

33

17  Hayes MA, Timmins AC, Yau EHS, Palazzo M, Hinds CJ, Watson D. Elevation of systemic oxygen delivery in the treatment of critically ill patients. *N Engl J Med* 1994;**330**:1717–22.
18  Deitch EA, Berg RA, Specian R. Endotoxin promotes the translocation of bacteria from the gut. *Arch Surg* 1987;**122**:185–90.
19  Baue AE. The role of the gut in the development of multiple organ dysfunction in cardiothoracic patients. *Ann Thorac Surg* 1993;**55**:822–9.
20  Parviainen I, Ruokonen E, Takala J. Dobutamine-induced dissociation between changes in splanchnic blood flow and gastric intramucosal pH after cardiac surgery. *Br J Anaesth* 1995;**74**:277–82.
21  Gys T, Hubens A, Neels H, Lauwers LF, Peeters R. Prognostic value of gastric intramural pH in surgical intensive care patients. *Crit Care Med* 1988;**16**:122–4.
22  Gutierrez G, Palizas F, Doglio G, *et al.* Gastric intramucosal pH as a therapeutic index of tissue oxygenation in critically ill patients. *Lancet* 1992;**339**:195–9.
23  Maynard N, Bihari D, Beale R, *et al.* Assessment of splanchnic oxygenation by gastric tonometry in patients with acute circulatory failure. *JAMA* 1993;**270**:1203–10.
24  Doglio GR, Pusajo JF, Egurrola MA, *et al.* Gastric mucosal pH as a prognostic index of mortality in critically ill patients. *Crit Care Med* 1991;**19**:1037–40.

# 5: Microvascular control and dysfunction

M INTAGLIETTA and K MESSMER

Most critically ill patients share common pathophysiological changes in the microvasculature, caused by either direct damage to cellular components within the microcirculation or interference with physiological control mechanisms. This may result in tissue injury. In general terms, the main aim of therapy should be to establish high rates of blood flow to restore oxygen supply, and clear the tissues of the byproducts of anaerobic metabolism and cellular damage. To achieve this involves opening capillaries, increasing capillary blood flow, restoring normal endothelial function, and re-establishing arteriolar autoregulation which controls spatial and temporal distribution of blood flow through the tissues, via the process of vasomotion. These aims must be achieved concurrently and in conjunction with systemic haemodynamics.

Blood flow regulation, capillary perfusion, and metabolite exchange are closely related. The tissues of the body have widely varying requirements for nutrients and oxygen, and control mechanisms have not only to ensure an adequate oxygen supply, but also to prevent superperfusion. These mechanisms may become overwhelmed in critical illness and become self-perpetuating. For example, hyperoxygenation following ischaemia increases inflammatory injury, vasodilatation in response to hypoxaemia reduces perfusion pressure and capillary flow, and increased microvascular permeability as a means of facilitating nutrient exchange results in oedema.

## Capillary perfusion and recruitment

Although the number of capillaries is very large their small intrinsic oxygen-carrying capacity and low intravascular $Po_2$ mean that cessation of capillary flow may result in anoxic injury to the cells supplied by that capillary. There are several factors that determine the available number of perfused capillaries, that is, the functional capillary density. Whilst mechanical factors such as capillary lumen narrowing, obstruction by leukocytes, microthrombi, and rigid red blood cells are important, it is now accepted that perfusion pressure plays a critical part in maintaining capillary patency. It used to be assumed that a reduction in perfusion pressure resulted in reduced microvascular flow without a reduction in functional capillary density. However, experimental studies in the microcirculation of skeletal muscle[1] have demonstrated a reversible reduction in functional capillary density with reduction in perfusion pressure. Pressure–flow studies in isolated organs have also demonstrated increased flow resistance as perfusion pressure decreases, and a reduction in functional capillary density in low flow states associated with ischaemia–reperfusion injury.[2-4] Indeed, capillary perfusion pressure appears to be the primary factor in determining functional capillary density. Several mechanisms contribute to this:

- The reduction in hydrostatic capillary pressure reduces capillary diameter, and the intravascular pressure gradient becomes insufficient to produce the normal deformation of red blood cells as they cross the capillary.
- Ischaemia and haemorrhagic shock result in endothelial cell swelling which also contributes to the reduction in capillary diameter.[3,4]
- In shock states the endothelial changes tend to be uniform, whereas in ischaemia swollen cells are interspersed between more normal cells.[5]

Capillaries possess mechanical properties which may be compared to those of tunnels in a mountain, that is, their dimensions are in part determined by the volumetric properties of the surrounding tissue.[6] In health, tissue volume is regulated by the Starling forces: when the endothelium is intact, blood and tissue compartments are in a mechanical balance which favours absorption of fluid from the tissue space into blood. Endothelial dysfunction results in increased filtration of fluid into the tissues together with macromolecules, resulting in oedema. This process has a variable effect on functional capillary density depending upon the nature of the tissues enclosing the vessels. Enclosed tissues (muscle, brain) will demonstrate compression of low pressure capillaries by oedema. Tissues without a mechanical boundary, such as the skin and subcutaneous tissues, expand with oedema, and this also increases the capillary lumen and functional capillary density.

In summary, lower perfusion pressure combined with endothelial cell dysfunction will reduce capillary blood flow through three mechanisms:

- reduced elastic recoil
- endothelial oedema
- tissue oedema.

Re-establishing tissue perfusion is primarily dependent upon restoring capillary perfusion pressure.[7]

## Microvascular blood flow

Under normal physiological conditions, microvascular flow is regulated by the interplay of endothelium-derived nitric oxide producing a state of

continuous vasodilatation, various vasoconstrictor stimuli, the flow properties of blood, and tissue metabolism including oxygen consumption and
carbon dioxide generation. The control mechanisms that determine
arteriolar tone, and hence flow, include a pressure-dependent response (the
myogenic response), the autonomic nervous system, endocrine and
metabolic signals, and viscosity. Arteriolar tone is the major mechanism for
controlling capillary perfusion pressure, fluid flux, and tissue metabolism,
and is a complex function of the many variables described above. The result
is that differing physiological and pathophysiological processes produce
varied biological effects through the simple mechanism of varying arteriolar
tone. When taken in conjunction with the differing metabolic requirements
of different tissues and organs, it becomes easier to understand why
therapeutic interventions, such as vasoactive drugs or nitric oxide antagonists, should at times have unpredictable clinical effects depending on
clinical circumstances and the patient population to which these interventions have been applied.

## Autoregulation

Autoregulation is the phenomenon by which blood flow is kept constant
in the presence of varying arterial blood pressure. It is present to varying
degrees in virtually all tissues and organs, keeping the blood flow constant
over a range of perfusion pressures from 50 to 150 mm Hg in health.
Autoregulation is mediated by metabolic and myogenic factors. Metabolic
control is exerted through changes in blood flow altering the concentration
of vasoactive materials which secondarily affect vascular tone. Myogenic
control is the process whereby vascular smooth muscle responds directly to
changes in intraluminal pressure,[8,9] and can be demonstrated experimentally by reducing ambient pressure around a limb, resulting in
vasoconstriction.[10] In hypertension the autoregulatory limits are set higher,
and it is important to remember this when modifying vasoactive drug
therapy to predetermined blood pressure goals: normal values may
represent significant hypotension in a normally hypertensive patient.
Autoregulation may also fail in acutely injured organs, for example, in acute
renal failure, where blood flow becomes linearly related to perfusion
pressure. Autoregulation is also overridden by centrally mediated sympathetic overactivity in conditions such as haemorrhagic shock.

## Blood viscosity

Tissue viability depends on both the provision of nutrients and the
removal of metabolites. Oxygen supply and perfusion are therefore
independent, though related, processes. This can be demonstrated by
experiments showing that hypoxic tissue injury is less severe if flow is

maintained, despite the use of deoxygenated fluid. Thus, therapeutic manoeuvres in critically ill patients must be aimed at supporting flow as well as oxygenation. One of the main determinants of flow is blood viscosity and, in health, a reduction in haematocrit (and hence viscosity) by means of haemodilution results in no net change in oxygen supply because of an increase in cardiac output and reduction in vascular resistance.[11] Indeed, a reduction in red cell numbers may reduce viscosity more markedly than oxygen-carrying capacity and, at a haematocrit of 33% oxygen delivery, viscosity may actually increase by about 10%. This is the reason why many critical care practitioners do not transfuse patients whose haemoglobin is above 9 g/dl.

Maintaining high circulatory flow rates may also improve tissue oxygenation by reducing leakage of oxygen from the cardiovascular system before reaching the microcirculation.[12,13] The juxtaposition of venules and arterioles in a countercurrent configuration is of particular importance in the renal medulla and the gut mucosa, where it allows arteriovenous shunting of oxygen from arteriole to venule, with a consequent distal hypoxia. The increase in blood flow velocity diminishes the transit time and therefore leakage and shunting, allowing more oxygen to reach the capillaries and thereby improve tissue oxygenation.[14]

These factors should influence decisions about resuscitation fluids. Although blood may be the most effective plasma expander, its use may be associated with a reduction in tissue oxygenation because of low levels of 2,3-diphosphoglycerate(2,3-DPG), old, and inflexible red cells, together with microaggregates obstructing capillaries, and the effect on blood viscosity described above. Blood transfusions also have undesirable immunosuppressant effects. Synthetic colloidal solutions are more appropriate for initial resuscitation in conjunction with other standard measures, and the two overriding therapeutic goals must be to restore both flow and perfusion pressure simultaneously. Hyperosmolar solutions may also be of value for the acute phase of resuscitation[15,16] by drawing fluid back from the tissues into the circulation, a process that may also reduce endothelial swelling.[4] This effect is particularly beneficial in shock and conditions of sodium pump dysfunction that result in endothelial swelling and a reduction in functional capillary density. Hyperosmolar sodium chloride solutions (7·5%) also improve cardiac contractility and cardiac output independent of the effects of haemodilution.

This rheological approach to perfusion improvement may not necessarily be beneficial in all circumstances. The production of the vasodilator nitric oxide[17] and of prostacyclin by the endothelium is a direct function of the shear stress generated by blood at the vascular wall.[18,19] Lower blood viscosity will be beneficial only if blood flow velocity increases in proportion so that the shear stress at the wall remains constant or is greater. If this does not occur, vasoconstriction might result. This might be relevant in patients with impaired myocardial function, or those receiving nitric oxide antagonists or prostaglandin inhibitors.

## Vasomotion

Vasomotion is the rhythmic contraction and relaxation of arterioles; this oscillation is necessary for the efficient management and regulation of blood flow. It is characterised by periodic and random fluctuations in arteriolar diameter, and can be seen in most vascular beds. Vasomotion reduces fluid filtration from intravascular compartments, since arteriolar closure will lower distal pressure and promote fluid uptake. It also promotes more uniform oxygen delivery to tissues by increasing spatial diffusion and causing a continuous interdependent adjustment of capillary haematocrit and flow velocity.[20] Haemorrhagic shock and hypoxia stimulate vasomotion in skeletal muscle and the visceral circulation,[21,22] which is an indication that the tissue and the microcirculation are actively attempting to maintain homeostasis. The phenomenon is most marked when blood pressure in the major vessels falls to around 50 mm Hg, indicating the presence of both precarious perfusion and a responsive microvascular system. Vasomotion disappears when perfusion pressures fall below 40 mm Hg,[23] and in the presence of lipopolysaccharide.[24]

## Consequences of shock and ischaemia

Two forms of cell injury occur in ischaemia. The first is anoxic cell death, characteristic of total vascular occlusion. The second is a consequence of reperfusion injury, as described in Chapter 6. The microvasculature suffers both functional and biochemical changes in reperfusion injury,[3] and the degree of injury is related to the severity of shock and its duration, the presence of agents that may reduce oxygen consumption and dependence such as general anaesthesia, and the organ and tissues that are affected. Some organs are more tolerant than others to the consequences of impaired perfusion, and tolerance to reperfusion injury can develop following repeated brief ischaemic episodes.

## Conclusion

Normal organ system function is critically dependent upon adequate tissue perfusion for oxygen supply and drainage of toxic materials. Inadequate perfusion is the consequence of mechanical events including obstruction to flow, reduced functional capillary density, blood hypo-viscosity, and hypotension. The relationship between hypotension and perfusion is non-linear because the distribution of pressure within the microcirculation ensures the availability of a sufficient number of patent capillaries, and therefore of surfaces, for metabolic exchange. In terms of the microcirculation, an adequate perfusion pressure is essential for the maintenance of flow.

1 Lindbom L, Arfors KE. Mechanism and site of control for variation in the number of perfused capillaries in skeletal muscle. *Int J Microcirc Clin Exp* 1985;4:121–7.

2 Messmer K, Sack FU, Menger MD, Bartlett R, Barker JH, Hammersen F. White cell-endothelium interaction during postischaemic reperfusion of skin and skeletal muscle. In *Advances in experimental medicine and biology. Vascular endothelium in health and disease* (Shu Chien, ed.), Vol. 242, 1988.

3 Menger MD, Steiner D, Messsmer K. Microvascular ischaemia–reperfusion injury in striated muscle: significance of "no-reflow". *Am J Physiol* 1992;263:H1892–1900.

4 Mazzoni MC, Borgstrom P, Intaglietta M, Arfors KE. Luminal narrowing and endothelial cell swelling in skeletal muscle capillaries during hemorrhagic shock. *Circ Shock* 1989;29:27–39.

5 Gidlof A, Lewis DH, Hammersen F. The effect of total ischaemia on the ultrastructure of human skeletal muscle capillaries. A morphometric analysis. *Int J Microcirc Clin Exp* 1987;7:67–86.

6 Fung YC, Zweifach BW, Intaglietta M. Elastic environment of the capillary bed. *Circ Res* 1966;19:441–61.

7 Tsai AG, Friesenecker B, Intaglietta M. Capillary flow impairment and functional capillary density. *Int J Microcirc Clin Exp* 1996;15:238–43.

8 Bayliss WM. On the local reaction of the arterial wall to changes in internal pressure. *J Physiol Lond* 1902;28:220–321.

9 Johnson PC. The myogenic response. In *Handbook of physiology. The cardiovascular system. Vascular smooth muscle* (Bohr DF, Somlyo AP, Sparks HV Jr, eds), Vol. II, 15. Bethesda, MD: *America Physiologic Society*, 1988.

10 Johnson PC, Intaglietta M. Contribution of pressure and flow sensitivity to autoregulation in mesenteric arterioles. *Am J Physiol* 1976;231:1686–98.

11 Messmer K, Sunder-Plasmann L, Klovekorn WP, Holper K. Circulatory significance of hemodilution: Rheological changes and limitations. In *Advances in microcirculation*, Vol. 4. Basel: Karger, 1972:1–77.

12 Mirhashemi S, Ertefai S, Messmer K, Intaglietta M. Model analysis of the enhancement of tissue oxygenation by hemodilution due to increased microvascular flow velocity. *Microvasc Res* 1987;34:290–301.

13 Duling BR, Berne RM. Longitudinal gradients of perivascular oxygen tension. *Circ Res* 1973;27:669–78.

14 Kerger H, Torres Filho IP, Rivas M, Winslow RM, Intaglietta M. Systemic and subcutaneous microvascular oxygen tension in conscious Syrian golden hamsters. *Am J Physiol.* 1995;267 *(Heart Circ Physiol* 37): H802–10.

15 Messmer K, Kreimeier U. Microcirculatory therapy in shock. *Resuscitation* 1989;18:51–61.

16 Rocha-e-Silva M, Negraes GA, Soares AM, Pontieri Loppnow L. Hypertonic resuscitation from severe hemorrhagic shock: patterns of regional circulation. *Circ Shock* 1986;19:165–73.

17 Doss DN, Estafanous FG, Ferrario CM, Brum JM, Murray PA. Mechanism of systemic vasodilation during normovolemic hemodilution. *Anesth Analg* 1995;81:30–4.

18 Frangos JA, Eskin SG, McIntire LV, Ives CL. Flow effect on prostacyclin production in cultured human endothelial cells. *Science* 1985;227:1477–9.

19 Grabowski EF, Jaffe EA, Weksler BB. Prostacyclin production by cultured endothelial cell monolayers exposed to step increases in shear stress. *J Lab Clin Med* 1985; **103:** 1774–7.

20 Fagrell B, Intaglietta M, Ostergren J. Relative hematocrit in human skin capillaries and its relation to capillary blood flow velocity. *Microvasc Res* 1980;20:327–35.

21 Weiner RM, Borgstrom P, Intaglietta M. Induction of vasomotion by hemorrhagic hypotension in rabbit tenissimus muscle. *Progr Appl Microcirc* 1989;15:93–9.

22  Zweifach BW, Lee RE, Hyman C, Chambers R. Omental microcirculation in morphinized dogs subjected to graded hemorrhage. *Ann Surg* 1944;**120**:250–73.

23  Schmidt JA, Intaglietta M, Borgstrom P. Periodic hemodynamics of skeletal muscle during local arterial pressure reduction. *J Appl Physiol* 1992:**73**:1077–83.

24  Bouskela E, Rubanyi GM. Effects of $N_W$-nitro-L-arginine (L-NAG) and dexamethasone on early events following LPS injection. Observations in the hamster cheek pouch microcirculation. *Shock* 1994;**1**:347–53.

# 6: Tissue hypoxia and ischaemia–reperfusion injury

J PINCEMAIL and J O DEFRAIGNE

Increased free radical formation derived from abnormal metabolism of oxygen and leading to oxidative damage has been implicated in over 100 different human diseases. Preoxygenation injury or ischaemia–reperfusion makes a major contribution to organ dysfunction in trauma, shock, sepsis, cardiovascular diseases, and organ transplantation. Ischaemia or hypoperfusion will trigger a cascade of biochemical events resulting, at reperfusion, in a heightened production of toxic and oxidant radical species which can mediate tissue injury. Preventing their formation by appropriate therapy should provide beneficial clinical consequences. The development of drugs with antioxidant properties is an important challenge for the future.

## Normal circulatory system and disorders

The purpose of the circulatory system is transportation. Each major segment of this system has a specialised structure and function to effect nutrient delivery and removal of metabolic byproducts. Control and distribution are mainly accomplished by resistance changes at the arteriolar and precapillary sphincter level. This is regulated by a complex interaction of myogenic and metabolic effects, neural control (primarily sympathetic), and humoral control (accomplished through circulating vasoactive hormones). These mechanisms provide strict autoregulation of blood flow in some tissues, whilst allowing major activity-related increases in others. The capillary distribution network accomplishes efficient exchange of oxygen, nutrients, and metabolic waste, whilst the venous system returns blood to the heart, adjusts volume to accommodate different flow requirements, and regulates transcapillary perfusion pressure via postcapillary sphincter mechanisms.

Unfortunately, these control mechanisms can be severely compromised by acute disease processes resulting in inadequate blood flow and cellular ischaemia. In this situation, oxygen delivery to and metabolite removal from tissues is reduced or virtually absent. Hypoxia is defined as an oxygen deficiency at the tissue level and is a more appropriate term than anoxia, since it is rare to have no oxygen in the whole tissue. Hypoxia may be classified by the following pathophysiological mechanisms:

- hypoxic hypoxia (reduction of arterial blood $Po_2$);
- anaemic hypoxia (arterial $Po_2$ is normal but the amount of haemoglobin is reduced);
- stagnant or ischaemic hypoxia (arterial $Po_2$ and amount of haemoglobin are normal, but blood flow is reduced so that oxygen supply is inadequate); and
- histotoxic hypoxia (oxygen supply is adequate, but cells cannot use it because of the action of a toxic agent).

When partial or total arterial occlusion occurs acutely in any organ, tissue ischaemia, acidosis, and subsequent cell death are most probably produced by a combination of oxygen deficiency and accumulation of $CO_2$ and acidic metabolites (with a corresponding failure of cellular metabolism). The intestinal mucosa, for example, loses its integrity and allows access to the circulation of micro-organisms, toxins, and powerful digestive enzymes, which leads to secondary infections. However, tissue injury only becomes clearly evident at reperfusion, when oxygen-derived free radicals, together with enzymes and mediators, are produced and released from damaged cells, attracting and activating macrophages and granulocytes and leading to membrane injury.

## Oxygen radical and non-radical species

A free radical is defined as any species capable of independent existence that contains one or more unpaired electrons. This confers high reactivity to the molecule, and therefore allows it to damage multiple biological substrates (proteins, lipoproteins, deoxyribonucleic acid, carbohydrates, and polyunsaturated fatty acids), leading to tissue injury.[1]

Abnormal increased oxygen metabolism during ischaemia–reperfusion results in free radical production. Oxygen reduction, electron by electron, gives rise to the formation of a cascade of activated oxygen species including the superoxide anion $O_2^-$ radical. By dismutation, the superoxide anion generates the non-free radical species hydrogen peroxide ($H_2O_2$) and singlet oxygen, both possessing strong oxidant activity. Moreover, iron catalyses the interreaction of superoxide anion and hydrogen peroxide (Fenton reaction) to generate the hydroxyl radical ($OH^.$), one of the most harmful oxidant species. Peroxidation of polyunsaturated fatty acids induced by the hydroxyl radical results in loss of membrane integrity and merging of intracellular and extracellular environments, with the destruction of membrane-associated enzymic and transport functions.

43

# Biochemical changes during ischaemia (Figure 6.1)

### Inhibition of ATP synthesis

The maintenance of normal adenosine triphosphate (ATP) is important for cell and organ function. A variety of redox reactions take place in the respiratory chain of mitochondria, allowing the flow of electrons from NADH to oxygen to produce water and the phosphorylation of adenosine diphosphate (ADP) for the synthesis of ATP (oxidative phosphorylation). During ischaemia, when oxygen levels are diminished, the ATP cannot be formed from ADP at the normal rate, and the ADP that accumulates degrades to purine end products (inosine, hypoxanthine, xanthine, uric acid). Moreover, as the cell's energy charge drops, it is no longer able to maintain normal ion gradients across its membranes with consequent failure of ATP-dependent sodium, potassium, and calcium pumps. This precipitates a massive entry of calcium ions into the cell, leading to swelling, cellular oedema, and activation of deleterious processes. Calcium can activate phospholipases, resulting in cell membrane de-esterification with release of arachidonic acid that is synthesised into prostaglandins and leukotrienes. These possess potent chemotactic activity leading to activation and recruitment of polymorphonuclear (PMN) cells into ischaemic tissue.

### Xanthine oxidase activation

Elevated cytosolic calcium concentration within ischaemic cells can also activate proteases that are capable of converting xanthine dehydrogenase (XDH) to xanthine oxidase (XO); both enzymes play an important role in the catabolism of purine bases such as hypoxanthine. The conversion of XDH, widely distributed among tissues (particularly in the endothelial cell), to XO is dependent on the type of tissue and the duration of ischaemia.[2]

# Biochemical changes during reperfusion (Figure 6.1)

During ischaemia, several mechanisms have been set up so that reoxygenation results in massive production of activated oxygen species, including free radicals.

### Mitochondria

Because of the decrease in ATP production, electron transport is disturbed in mitochondria at the moment of reperfusion. Instead of being transformed into water by cytochrome oxidase, oxygen is reduced to the superoxide anion, hydrogen peroxide, and hydroxyl radical at the

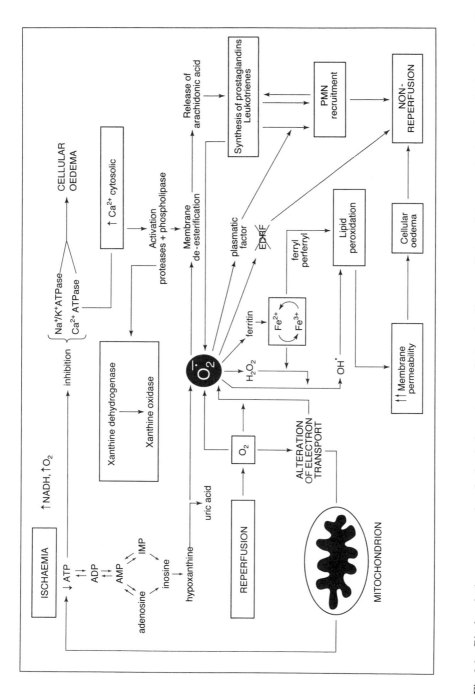

Fig 6.1  Biochemical events occurring during ischaemia–reperfusion, leading to cellular calcium overload and to the formation of a cascade of activated oxygen species, particularly the superoxide anion $O_2^{\cdot-}$. ATP: adenosine triphosphate; ADP: adenosine diphosphate; AMP: adenosine monophosphate; IMP: inosine monophosphate; EDRF: endothelial-derived relaxing factor or nitric oxide NO.

ubiquinone site, and at the level of the first component of the respiratory chain, the enzyme NADH dehydrogenase.[3]

## Xanthine oxidase

In contrast with XDH, which never uses molecular oxygen as an electron acceptor, XO transfers electrons to oxygen with consequent reduction to the anion ($O_2^-$) radical.[2]

## Iron release

Iron is by far the most biologically relevant and extensively studied transition metal capable of promoting superoxide-driven oxidations and it readily catalyses the Fenton reaction.[4] More important, in the presence of an $O_2^-$ generating system or low-molecular-weight reductants (for example, thiols or ascorbate), iron undergoes reactions that result in the generation of other oxidants capable of initiating lipid peroxidation.

In normal conditions, the amount of free iron is negligible since almost all iron is physiologically stored in ferritin, lactoferrin, and transferrin. However, under the action of the superoxide anion, iron can be released as free or low-molecular-weight complexes from stored proteins and then be able to participate in free radical reactions.[5] In vivo, it has been shown that post-ischaemic reperfusion is accompanied by a net increase in low-molecular-weight iron complexes and accumulation of lipid peroxidation byproducts. Moreover, iron is also involved in the formation of ferryl or perferryl ion complexes (ferrous dioxygen), which can directly induce lipid peroxidation processes.

## Polymorphonuclear cells

Oxygen-derived free radicals are also produced in the extracellular medium by activated PMNs, which infiltrate the ischaemic and reperfused tissue and constitute an important component of the inflammatory response.[6] During PMN activation, myeloperoxidase (MPO), specifically located in the azurophilic granules, is also released from cells with consequent production of highly oxidant species such as hypochlorous acid (HOCl).[7] Leukocyte and endothelial cell interaction is, of course, essential for leukocyte migration across the endothelial cell surface. Superoxide anions, generated by endothelial cells through XO activity, have been demonstrated to increase the adhesion of neutrophils to the endothelium.

A large variety of neutrophil chemotactic agents is formed at the site of ischaemic tissue. Components of the complement cascade, biomolecules related to the coagulation system (fibrinogen, fibrinopeptide B), derivatives of arachidonic acid (leukotrienes, platelet-aggregating factor, PAF), and cytokines are among the important participants that serve to amplify the reponse to injury and attract inflammatory cells to the reperfused region. Complement fragment C5a, but also interleukins secreted by activated PMNs, can also stimulate superoxide anion production by PMNs and increase the adherence of neutrophils to the vascular wall.

The accumulation of the neutrophils within the vascular space results not only in the destruction caused by neutrophil-derived products and proteolytic enzymes, but also in the formation of cellular aggregates that can physically impair blood flow to the capillary bed and thereby exacerbate ischaemic injury.

### Nitric oxide

During ischaemia–reperfusion, inflammatory and endothelial cells release increased amounts of nitric oxide (NO), recognised as the endothelial-derived relaxing factor (EDRF). This vasoactive metabolite, which at physiological concentrations plays a key role in regulating blood flow, becomes toxic when produced in large amounts. It can injure cells, accelerate intracellular iron release, or inhibit mitochondrial function. Toxicity of NO, which is a free radical species, can be partially attributed to its reaction with the superoxide anion leading to the formation of oxidant peroxynitrites (ONOOH) with subsequent generation of hydroxyl radicals.[8]

# Antioxidant interventions (ESR)

Electron spin resonance, spectroscopy in ischaemia–reperfusion experiments has shown, as directly as possible, that free radical formation is rapidly followed by a decrease in endogenous antioxidant defences such as glutathione (GSH) and vitamin E within the first minutes after reperfusion.[9][10] Although the toxicological role of radicals is firmly established from in vitro studies, data obtained from clinical investigations are, however, unable to inform us whether free radicals are really participating in the production of tissue injury. The prevalent idea is that an initial insult induces a secondary increase in the rate of free radical production, and that oxidative stress exacerbates the primary tissue injury. If true, free radical ablation by substances able to scavenge free radicals or to limit their production should offer significant protection against ischaemia–reperfusion injury. Figure 6.2 shows where the process of oxidation-mediated injury can potentially be reduced by antioxidant intervention.

Each antioxidant has its own specificity and may act at different stages in inhibiting free radical formation. They can prevent tissue injury by directly scavenging free radicals in an enzymatic way or not, by increasing

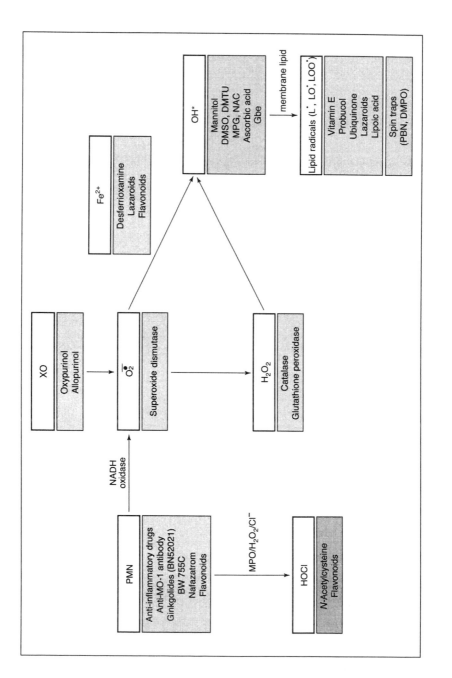

Fig 6.2 Antioxidant approaches for limiting postischaemic tissue injury. NAC: *N*-acetylcysteine; Gbe: *Ginkgo biloba* extract; HOCl: hypochlorous acid; XO: xanthine oxidase; PMN: polymorphonuclear cell; MPG: $N^2$- mercaptopropionylglycine; DMSO: dimethysulphoxide; DMTU: dimethylthiourea; PBV and DMPO: see text.

antioxidant status, by chelating iron, by blocking free radical-generating enzymes, and by inhibiting neutrophil activity.[11]

## Free radical scavengers

Among enzyme scavengers are superoxide dismutase (SOD), which reduces the half-life of superoxide anion, and catalase or glutathione peroxidase, which degrades hydrogen peroxide or lipid peroxides. Both enzymes have been studied in animal models of brain and heart ischaemia–reperfusion, but their real effectiveness is, however, a controversial matter. This is mainly because of their short circulatory half-life (for example, six minutes for SOD). This problem has been solved to some extent with the use of polyethylene glycol (PEG) conjugation or liposomal entrapment, which extend the circulatory half-life of SOD to four hours and contribute to a significant increase in the intracellular transport of both enzymes.

Other antioxidants are molecules that directly interact with free radicals to form oxidation products normally devoid of toxicity. Mannitol, dimethylsulphoxide (DMSO), and dimethylthiourea (DMTU) have been proposed as appropriate drugs since they are able to scavenge hydroxyl radical. However, the concentrations required for such activity are extremely high and can, therefore, be responsible for toxic effects. Vitamin E (or $\alpha$-tocopherol) which strongly interacts with lipid free radicals is a safer molecule. Many animal studies have indicated that supplementation with vitamin E before ischaemia–reperfusion can significantly reduce the size of the myocardial infarct.[12] Vitamin E is often associated with vitamin C (or ascorbic acid), an hydroxyl radical scavenger, at concentration of 1 mmol/l, since both vitamins can act in a synergistic way. Recently, 21-aminosteroids ("lazaroids") devoid of glucocorticoid activity, but possessing free radical scavenging activity similar to that of vitamin E, have been found to protect the brain against ischaemia–reperfusion injury.[13] Many other free radical scavengers have been tested, such as probucol, ubiquinone, lipoic acid, captopril, $N^2$-mercaptopropionylglycine (MPG), carvedilol (antihypertensive drug), [$N^5$-(thioxo-L-prolyl-L-cysteine] known as P 1507, and *Ginkgo biloba* extract (Gbe) containing flavonoids. Administration of MPG to open-chest dogs undergoing a 15-minute coronary occlusion followed by 4 hours of reperfusion resulted in a marked reduction of free radical production, which was associated with a better recovery of contractile function.

For detecting in vivo free radical formation, electron spin resonance (ESR) spectroscopy is the method of choice. The technique of spin trapping agents is often required for increasing the half-life of free radicals generated in vivo. These cyclic nitroxides, such as 5,5-dimethyl-l-pyrroline-1-oxide (DMPO) or $\alpha$-phenyl-N-tert-butyl nitrone (PBN), react with transient radicals to form more stable radicals that can be detected by ESR. Recent studies have revealed that PBN and a novel series of PBN analogue compounds, acting as free radical scavengers, were able significantly to reduce in vivo neuronal damage and central nervous system (CNS) oxidative damage.[14] However, toxic side effects prevent the clinical use of these agents.

### Increasing antioxidant status

Thiol-containing compounds such as N-acetylcysteine (NAC) are rapidly deacylated and increase the intracellular pool of GSH, considered as the first defence against the toxicity of free radicals. Moreover, NAC is able to interact directly with free radicals and with toxic hypochlorous acid generated by the MPO of PMNs. In experimental animal models and in patients undergoing elective coronary artery bypass grafting, NAC has been shown to exert significant cardioprotective effects.

### Chelators of iron

Iron, ubiquitously present in living organisms, plays a key catalytic role in free radical reactions. During ischaemia–reperfusion, it can be released as free iron from storage proteins (ferritin, lactoferrin, transferrin) by the superoxide anion. Desferrioxamine, a trihydroxamate hexadentate drug, is a powerful chelator of iron, making it unavailable for participating in free radical reactions. Many animal studies have shown that desferrioxamine can reduce postischaemic tissue injury but with limited efficacy, because of its poor ability to cross cell membranes. New drugs (monohydroxamate compounds, hydroxypyridin-4-ones CP20 and CP94, desferrioxamine-linked starch plasma expanders) with greater efficacy and less toxicity than desferrioxamine are now being examined.

### Inhibition of enzymes

Free radical production during ischaemia–reperfusion, particularly at the level of the endothelial cell, occurs with activation of xanthine oxidase which generates the superoxide anion. In many animal models, and recently in a clinical study of coronary artery bypass patients,[15] xanthine oxidase inhibitors (allopurinol and oxypurinol) have been shown to improve postischaemic myocardial function. When administered at the moment of reperfusion, allopurinol also significantly reduces the incidence of early renal dysfunction after renal transplantation from human cadavers.[16]

During ischaemia–reperfusion, PMNs are another important source of activated oxygen species through the increased activity of their membrane-bound NADPH oxidase, which is stimulated by complement activation and neutrophil adherence to endothelium. Non-steroidal anti-inflammatory agents, diphenylene iodonium, adenosine, or flavonoids can inhibit NADPH oxidase non-specifically. Recently a monoclonal antibody (anti-

Mo-1 antibody) has been developed against NADPH oxidase which significantly reduces infarct size[17] in animals. Neutrophil infiltration can be reduced by BW 755 C or nafazatrom, inhibitors of lipoxygenase activity, which are responsible for increased production of powerful chemotactic agents, the leukotrienes. Inhibiting neutrophil adherence to endothelial cells by ginkgolides (BN 52021) can also reduce reperfusion injury. PMN MPO produces highly oxidant hypochlorous acid or chloramines, and can be inhibited by flavonoids (quercetin, rutin, *Ginkgo biloba* extract).

## Antioxidant paradox

Despite encouraging results, firm evidence of the efficacy of antioxidants in vivo is difficult to obtain in animal experiments and even more so in humans. Possible explanations for this include difficulties in site delivery of the drug (for example, SOD), drug concentration, secondary free radical-mediated reactions, and measures of outcome.

The protection against reperfusion injury is dose dependent, as is well illustrated with the use of SOD in myocardium. In isolated rabbit heart, the manganese form of SOD, MnSOD, offers maximum protection at 10 mg/kg; a lower dose of 1 mg/kg is without any marked effect whilst a larger dose of 100 mg/kg significantly increases the infarct size.[18] Antioxidants themselves can produce toxic antioxidant-derived free radicals. Moreover, the reaction of antioxidants with free iron can confer significant pro-oxidant activity as demonstrated in vitro for vitamin C, *N*-acetylcysteine, flavonoids, and even for vitamin E.[19]

End-points for studying antioxidant efficacy vary from one study to another. They include recovery of organ function, lipid peroxidation, protein oxidation, and histological analysis. However, these methods are indirect and do not directly measure the effect of free radical formation on tissues. By its ability to provide an integrated measure of free radical production over a given interval of time, studies using ESR spectroscopy (the methodology of choice for detecting in vivo free radical formation) associated with spin trapping techniques are better at evaluating the impact of free radical ablation by antioxidants on tissue injury, and may help to define the therapeutic window for antioxidant therapy during ischaemia–reperfusion.[20]

## Conclusion

There is growing evidence that free radicals play a key role in mediating tissue injury during ischaemia–reperfusion. Many antioxidants able to scavenge or inhibit free radicals may be organ specific. Each antioxidant acts at different stages of free radical production which complicates the design of clinical studies. Moreover, it should be kept in mind that any antioxidant can be associated with a pro-oxidant activity, the consequences of which are difficult to measure in vivo. Improved in vivo measurement techniques and long-term studies are required to clarify our understanding of the link between free radical ablation and the prevention of tissue injury by antioxidants during ischaemia–reperfusion.

1 Roberfroid M, Calderon PB. *Free radicals and oxidation phenomena in biological systems.* New York: Marcel Dekker Inc, 1995.
2 McCord JM. Oxygen-derived free radicals in postischaemic tissue injury. *N Engl J Med* 1985;**312**:159–63.
3 Cadenas E, Boveris A, Ragan CI, Stoppani AOM. Production of superoxide anion and hydrogen peroxide by NADH-ubiquinone reductase and ubiquinol-cytochrome c reductase from beef heart mitochondria. *Arch Biochem Biophys* 1977;**180**:248–57.
4 Walling G. Fenton's reagent revisited. *Acc Chem Res* 1975,**8**:125–31.
5 Thomas CE, Morehouse LA, Aust SD. Ferritin and superoxide-dependent lipid peroxidation. *J Biol Chem* 1985;**260**:3275–80.
6 Engler R. Consequences of activation and adenosine-mediated inhibition of granulocytes during myocardial ischaemia. *Fed Proc* 1987;**46**:2407–12.
7 Clark RA. Extracellular effects of the myeloperoxidase hydrogen peroxide-halide system. In *Advances in inflammation research* (Wesmann G, ed.), Vol. 5. New York: Raven Press, 1983:107–46.
8 Grisham MB. *Reactive metabolites of oxygen and nitrogen in biology and medicine.* Medical Intelligence Unit, RG Landes Co, 1992.
9 Bolli R, Patel BS, Jeroudi MO, Lai EK, McCay PB. Demonstration of free radical generation in "stunned" myocardium of intact dogs with the use of the spin trap α-thenyl-N-tert-butyl-nitrone. *J Clin Invest* 1988;**82**:476–85.
10 Pincemail J, Defraigne JO, Franssen C, *et al.* Evidence for free radical formation during human kidney transplantation. *Free Rad Biol Med* 1993; **15**:343–8.
11 Rice-Evans C, Diplock AT. Current status of antioxidant therapy. *Free Rad Biol Med* 1993;**15**:77–96.
12 Axford-Gately RA, Wilson GJ. Myocardial infarct size reduction by single high dose or repeated low dose vitamin E supplementation in rabbits. *Can J Cardiol* 1993;**9**:94–8.
13 Truelove D, Shuaib A, Richardson JS, Kalra J. Superoxide dismutase, catalase and U-78517F attenuate neuronal damage in gerbils with repeated brief ischaemic insults. *Neurochem Res* 1994;**19**:665–71.
14 Thomas CE, Carney JM, Bernotas RC, Hay DA, Carr AA. In vitro and in vivo activity of a novel series of radical trapping agents in model systems of CNS oxidative damage. *Ann NY Acad Sci* 1994;**738**:243–9.
15 Gimpel JAG, Lahpor JR, Van der Molen A-J, Damen J, Hitchcock JF. Reduction of reperfusion injury of human myocardium by allopurinol: a clinical study. *Free Rad Biol Med* 1995;**19**:251–5.
16 Rangan U, Bulkley GB. Prospects for treatment of free radical-mediated tissue injury. *Br Med Bull* 1993;**49**:700–18.
17 Arfors KE, Lundberg C, Lindbom, L. A monoclonal antibody to the membrane glycoprotein complex CD18 inhibits polymorphonuclear leucocyte accumulation and plasma leakage in vivo. *Blood* 1987;**254**:5564–8.
18 Omar B, McCord J, Downey J. Ischaemia-reperfusion. In *Oxidative stress* (Sies H, ed.). London: Academic Press, 1991:493–527.
19 Bowry VW, Stocker R. Tocopherol-mediated peroxidation. The prooxidant effect of vitamin E on the radical-initiated oxidation of human low-density lipoprotein. *J Am Chem Soc* 1993;**115**:6029–44.
20 Schiller HJ, Reilly PM, Bulkley GB. Antioxidant therapy. *Crit Care Med* 1993;**21**:S92–102.

# 7: Cytokines and the inflammatory response in sepsis

S J H van DEVENTER

Sepsis is a generalised inflammatory state, frequently complicated by tissue injury, organ failure, and death in critically ill patients. This systemic inflammatory reaction can be induced by a wide range of noxious stimuli, including invasive micro-organisms, toxins, trauma, and thermal injury, and is characterised by recruitment of inflammatory cells from the circulation to local sites of injury, fever, induction of the acute phase response, and activation of the complement, coagulation, and fibrinolytic cascades.

Previously thought to be a direct result of toxic injury, inflammatory responses are now known to be tightly regulated by a network of endogenous proteins called cytokines. Cytokines were first discovered as endogenous pyrogens produced by leukocytes that were able to alter the function of other leukocytes (hence the classification as *interleukins*), and were thought to have predominantly *pro*-inflammatory biological effects. Subsequently, the notion emerged that many other cell types, including endothelial cells, epithelial cells, fibroblasts, smooth muscle cells, and keratinocytes, are capable of cytokine production (hence the term "cytokines"), and that some cytokines have potent anti-inflammatory effects. Virtually all inflammatory stimuli simultaneously elicit pro- *and* anti-inflammatory cytokine responses, and clinical outcome may depend more on maintenance of this delicate balance than on the severity of the causative stimulus. In this respect sepsis bears some resemblance to the anaphylactic reaction, where an insignificant insult may cause severe systemic illness. This brief overview examines cytokine responses in sepsis, with particular emphasis on reciprocal effects (*cytokine networks*) and interactions with other inflammatory cascades.

## Pro-inflammatory cytokines in sepsis

Tumour necrosis factor-$\alpha$ (TNF$\alpha$) and interleukin-1$\alpha$ (IL-1) are the two archetypal pro-inflammatory cytokines.[1,2] These cytokines were initially discovered as secretory products from monocytes, but the spectrum of

53

source cells has subsequently been extensively expanded. IL-1, for example, is, among many other types of cells, produced by endothelial cells, keratinocytes, mucosal cells, smooth muscle cells, and T lymphocytes. Both TNFα and IL-1 have pleiotropic effects, which include the induction of endothelial cell adhesion molecules,[3] activation of neutrophils,[4-6] activation of the extrinsic pathway of blood coagulation,[7] and elaboration of a wide range of secondary cytokines.

It should be noted that, apart from their effects on the non-specific immune response, both TNFα and IL-1 have an important function in the cellular immune reaction. In many experimental systems of acute intravenous challenge with either live Gram-negative or Gram-positive bacteria or endotoxin (lipopolysaccharide, LPS), circulating levels of IL-1 and TNFα become *transiently* increased. In general, blood levels of TNFα in these models exceed IL-1 levels by several orders of magnitude. Administration of low amounts of endotoxin to healthy volunteers also induces a marked increase of circulating TNFα levels, but in this setting IL-1 usually remains undetectable in blood.[8-10] It should be noted that these cytokines have potent autocrine and paracrine effects, which are important at the tissue level, and hence the failure of detection of circulating cytokines does not exclude a potential biological function. For example, in experimental peritonitis TNFα circulates at a low concentration, but blockade of TNFα bioactivity using neutralising antibodies results in a dramatic *increase* of mortality.[11] Therefore, in this condition, *local* expression of TNFα is necessary in order to mobilise a sufficient protective immunological response.

There are many other examples of localised cytokine responses in experimental sepsis,[12] and even in endotoxaemia in humans.[13,14] It is likely that tissue cytokine production is of major importance in the pathogenesis of organ damage, for example, adult respiratory distress syndrome (ARDS),[15] but the same cytokines may be necessary for successful clearance of bacterial infections. If this hypothesis were confirmed, it could explain the relative inefficacy of *systemic* neutralisation of particular pro-inflammatory cytokines.

In most cases of clinical sepsis, with the notable exception of meningococcal septic shock,[16] blood TNFα levels are much lower than in experimental models. Furthermore, in septic patients low concentrations of circulating TNFα may remain detectable for many days or weeks. In endotoxin-challenged volunteers, TNFα is produced within the splanchnic circulation (presumably in the liver), but the exact source of TNFα in clinical sepsis remains unknown. In fact, monocytes isolated from blood of septic patients (or endotoxin-challenged volunteers) respond to endotoxin stimulation with a reduced TNFα production,[17,18] and even in meningococcal septic shock peripheral blood mononuclear cells predominantly release anti-inflammatory cytokines after stimulation in vitro.[19]

54

The effects of TNF$\alpha$ and IL-1 are mediated by two specific receptors: TNFR-I and TNFR-II, IL-1RI, and IL-1RII, respectively. TNFR-1 is thought to be responsible for mediating TNF$\alpha$ toxicity in sepsis, and IL-1RI for mediating the effects of IL-1$\alpha$. Because IL-1RII binds IL-1 but does not cause signal transduction, this receptor may act as a "decoy" for IL-1, by interference with IL-1R1 binding. Monocytes can produce a cytokine, IL-1 receptor antagonist (IL-1RA), that binds to IL-1RI, without causing cell activation. High circulating IL-1RA levels (exceeding IL-1 levels by several orders of magnitude) are induced by endotoxin in volunteers, and in experimental and clinical sepsis.[20] IL-1RA has been shown to be a pure antagonist of the biological effects of IL-1[21] but, in order to be effective, a very high percentage of all IL-1 receptors need to be blocked. Therefore, therapeutic use of recombinant IL-1RA requires continuous infusion of high doses of protein. Both TNF$\alpha$ and IL-1 receptors can be proteolytically cleaved for the cell membrane, and the circulating forms retain the capacity to bind their natural ligands. Soluble IL-1 receptors therefore act as natural antagonists, and could potentially be used therapeutically to block IL-1 in inflammation and sepsis.[22]

In healthy individuals, TNFR-1 and TNFR-II are easily detected in the circulation, and in sepsis circulating levels become dramatically increased.[23] Because soluble TNF$\alpha$ receptors retain the ability to bind TNF$\alpha$, the high circulating TNFR levels in sepsis in part explain the observation that, in septic serum, TNF$\alpha$ antigen levels (as measured by enzyme-linked immunosorbent assay) are generally much higher than TNF$\alpha$ bioactivity (with the use of TNF$\alpha$-responsive cells). In addition, soluble TNFR has been shown to interfere with the biological activity of TNF$\alpha$ in vivo, thus being one of the endogenous anti-inflammatory mechanisms.[24] The TNF$\alpha$-binding domains of both TNF$\alpha$ receptors have been identified, and proteins have been engineered that consist of two TNF$\alpha$ receptors coupled by an IgG tail or by polyethylene glycol. Interestingly, administration of sTNFR-I, but not sTNFR-II-based dimers was shown to be protective in acute overwhelming sepsis.[25] Similar results have been obtained by specifically blocking both receptors using monoclonal antibodies.[26] The most likely explanation for this observation is that TNF$\alpha$ bound to TNFR-II forms a reservoir that prolongs TNF$\alpha$'s biological activity.

## Interindividual differences in cytokine responses

Animal models of sepsis are designed to control for variables that may confound morbidity and mortality. Nevertheless, it is clear that animals differ widely in their susceptibility to endotoxin and various cytokines. In mice, rats, and baboons, very large doses of endotoxin are required to induce mortality, whereas rabbits, chimpanzees, and humans are rather sensitive to endotoxin. Various factors, including previous exposure to low doses of endotoxin, may decrease the cytokine response to endotoxin, whilst the presence of growing tumours or bacterial infections sensitise for endotoxin.[27] Finally, the TNF$\alpha$ response of healthy humans may differ more than 10-fold following a standardised endotoxin injection, and these differences have been correlated to genetic factors, such as HLA class II haplotypes and DNA polymorphism within the vicinity of the TNF$\alpha$ gene.[28] These genetic and environmental factors provide an explanation for the absence of dose–response interrelationships of circulating levels of endotoxin, cytokine levels, and clinical outcome. In fact such correlations have only been convincingly demonstrated in acute fulminant infections such as overwhelming meningococcal septic shock.[29,30]

## Cytokine networks

Cytokines may have additive, synergistic, or antagonistic effects. For example, in mice, TNF$\alpha$ and IL-1 display marked synergism in inducing mortality.[31,32] This synergism may explain why, in animal models of sepsis blocking just one of the pro-inflammatory cytokines may result in improved outcome. Interferon-$\gamma$ is a cytokine that appears rather late in experimental endotoxaemia, but high IFN-$\gamma$ levels can be detected in many patients in the acute stages of sepsis. Recently, IL-12 has been identified as a major stimulus of IFN-$\gamma$ induction in sepsis.[33] IFN-$\gamma$ is a major inducer of the inducible form of NO synthase, and increases endotoxin-induced mortality. However, because neutralisation of IFN-$\gamma$ by administration of antibodies results in improved outcome without decreasing TNF$\alpha$ release, it is possible that IFN-$\gamma$ sensitises for TNF$\alpha$ rather than for endotoxin directly.[34,35]

Despite these apparent adverse effects of IFN-$\gamma$ in acute systemic bacterial challenge, in some conditions IFN-$\gamma$ may be beneficial. Most patients with extensive trauma, sepsis, or burn injury have a marked defect in the capacity to present antigen, which is probably related to downregulation of HLA class II molecule expression on antigen-presenting cells.[36] This observation has prompted some investigators to speculate that administration of IFN-$\gamma$ to selected patients with sepsis might improve outcome.

The normal host immune response consists of tightly controlled networks of cytokines and other mediator systems that prevent extensive tissue damage. Apart from the soluble cytokine receptors and IL-1RA the "anti-inflammatory" response also involves induction of IL-10. IL-10 is a potent inhibitor of the production of pro-inflammatory cytokines by monocytes, downregulates expression of HLA class II molecules on monocytes, and is a growth factor for B lymphocytes. In experimental sepsis, IL-10 downregulates the release of TNF$\alpha$ and IFN-$\gamma$.[37] Interestingly, in primate endotoxaemia, the induction of IL-10 in part *depends* on

TNF$\alpha$ and, in contrast to the in vitro situation, occurs early.[38] Neutral-isation of IL-10 markedly increases mortality in experimental sepsis[39] and, conversely, administration of IL-10 protects against lethal endotoxaemia in mice.[40] Increased levels of IL-10 can be demonstrated in most patients with sepsis, in particular those in septic shock, and extremely high IL-10 levels have been reported in patients with meningococcal septic shock.[41]

Granulocyte colony-stimulating factor (G-CSF) is mainly known as a growth factor for neutrophils, which also has neutrophil-stimulating effects. Increased circulating G-CSF concentrations can be demonstrated in the early stages of sepsis but, in a surprisingly large fraction of septic patients admitted to the ICU, circulating G-CSF levels are low or undetectable. Administration of G-CSF to normal volunteers caused a significant reduction in the release of pro-inflammatory cytokines following in vitro stimulation of blood samples when various stimuli including endotoxin were used, whereas release of IL-1RA and TNFR-I and -II were increased by G-CSF treatment. Hence, G-CSF may be considered as yet another anti-inflammatory cytokine and indeed, in several non-neutropenic animal models of sepsis, G-CSF protected against mortality induced by Gram-negative bacteria and endotoxin.

## Chemokines

Chemokines are low-molecular-weight cytokines, which have chem-otactic properties and the ability to activate target cells. Probably the most important chemokine in sepsis is IL-8. IL-8 is produced by T cells, monocytes, endothelial cells, neutrophils, fibroblasts, and endothelial cells, and appears early in endotoxaemia and sepsis.[42,43] Together with platelet-activating factor (PAF), IL-8 is necessary for transmigration of neutrophils through the endothelial monolayer, necessary for recruitment to sites of inflammation. Because in this process IL-8 in part functions as a chemotactic factor, the presence of a concentration gradient is important. Endothelial cells express IL-8 at the luminal surface, bound by heparan sulphate, but secrete most of the IL-8 basally, thus causing the necessary chemotactic gradient. Very high circulating levels of IL-8 may interfere with neutrophil recruitment by reversing the chemotactic gradient, and by causing shedding of L-selectin by neutrophils, which is necessary for the initial tethering to endothelial cells. Hence, although the role of IL-8 as a neutrophil–chemotactic and stimulating protein has been well established, intravenous administration of large amounts of IL-8 does not induce neutrophils to egress the circulation, or result in organ damage.[44] It should be noted that many other endotoxin-inducible chemokines have been identified[45] including monocyte-chemoattractant protein-1, which specifi-cally targets monocytes, and RANTES which acts on T cells, but their importance in sepsis remains to be characterised.

## Interactions with other inflammatory cascades

Cytokines interact with virtually all other endogenous (inflammatory) mediator systems.[46] For example, TNF$\alpha$ causes upregulation of tissue factor, resulting in activation of the extrinsic pathway of blood coagulation,[47] and has complex effects on the fibrinolytic system.[48] Administration of TNF$\alpha$ to healthy volunteers causes early release of tissue plasminogen activator (tPA), causing fibrinolysis, but later blocks this response by inducing plasminogen activator inhibitor I (PAI-I). The net effect of blockade of TNF$\alpha$ in experimental endotoxaemia is a complete inhibition of the release of tPA (fibrinolytic response), while thrombin formation continues, hence resulting in a procoagulant state.[49] The latter effect is mediated by IL-6, which has no effects on the fibrinolytic system.[50] Hence, TNF$\alpha$ and IL-6 have opposing effects on haemostasis in endotoxaemia. Other examples are the interactions of cytokines, glucocorticoids, and eicosanoids.[51] TNF$\alpha$ is known as a stimulus for the production of the pro-inflammatory phospholipid mediator PAF, and conversely PAF may induce IL-1, IL-8, and TNF$\alpha$. In primate endotoxaemia, administration of a specific PAF antagonist significantly reduces the release of TNF$\alpha$, IL-6, and IL-8. These data underscore the notion that various inflammatory mediator cascades interact in a complex manner. It is therefore inappropriate to consider the inflammatory response in sepsis as a pyramid, in which the pro-inflammatory cytokines induce cascades of "secondary" inflammatory mediators. Rather, an interactive and at times redundant network of mediators is simultaneously activated.

## Why is neutralisation of pro-inflammatory cytokines in sepsis ineffective?

The recognition of the importance of pro-inflammatory cytokines as endogenous mediators of sepsis, and the successful development of specific inhibitors, caused considerable optimism that "immunotherapy" would significantly decrease the mortality in sepsis. However, several large and well-designed clinical studies using TNF$\alpha$-neutralising antibodies and recombinant IL-1RA have failed to improve survival in sepsis. Because there is sufficient evidence to indicate that these reagents effectively block the targeted cytokine, these findings indicate that the concept that pro-inflammatory cytokines cause mortality in sepsis should be revised. In addition, there is now little doubt that sepsis is a heterogeneous syndrome, in which a single therapy would not be likely to show overall benefit. Even in controlled animal models of invasive infectious disease, the outcome of neutralisation of a single cytokine may result in different outcomes. The complex role of TNF$\alpha$ in the pathophysiology of sepsis is well illustrated by data obtained in mice where the TNFR-I was silenced by genetic engineering. Whilst these animals are strikingly resistant to the effects of endotoxin, they display a severe defect in bacterial clearance, and frequently die from infections.[52] Likewise, blockade of the TNFR-I by specific antibodies protects against endotoxin shock, but interferes with successful clearance of bacteria.[27] Hence, neutralisation of certain pro-inflammatory cytokines may have decreased bacterial clearance as a trade-off. Many experimental studies have been performed in models of acute overwhelming sepsis, and would seem to have most relevance for sepsis induced by meningococci, *Haemophilus*, or *Aeromonas*. Most "septic" patients have a very different clinical picture which is characterised by low-level bacteraemia and, with the exception of IL-6 and IL-8, relatively *low* levels of circulating pro-inflammatory cytokines.

## Conclusion

No doubt cytokines are of utmost importance for initiation, control, *and* termination of inflammatory processes. Acute and overwhelming bacterial infections, such as meningococcal septic shock, are characterised by release of large amounts of pro-inflammatory cytokines. However, in many patients with clinical features of sepsis, circulating cytokine levels are much lower, although the release of pro-inflammatory cytokines may be inappropriately prolonged. Even in patients with overwhelming sepsis, anti-inflammatory cytokine responses are rapidly aroused, and the induction of certain pro-inflammatory cytokines can be compartmentalised, in particular within the peritoneal cavity of the lungs. Certain pro-inflammatory cytokines are thought to induce a cascade of other inflammatory mechanisms, and this has led to the hypothesis that blockade of these cytokines would improve survival of patients with sepsis. Although such approaches have been successful in certain experimental models of sepsis, their clinical efficacy has not been proved. In fact, there is reason to assume that a complete blockade of specific pro-inflammatory cytokines may interfere with necessary host defence responses, thereby increasing mortality. Clearly, the cytokine response in sepsis is a complex network of *simultaneously* induced pro- and anti-inflammatory cytokines. The mechanisms controlling the multiple delicate equilibria within this network remain to be determined.

1 Beutler B, Grau GE. Tumor necrosis factor in the pathogenesis of infectious diseases. *Crit Care Med* 1993;21:S423–35.
2 Dinarello CA. The biological properties of interleukin-1. *Eur Cytokine Netw* 1994;5:517–31.
3 Carlos TM, Harlan JM. Leukocyte-endothelial adhesion molecules. *Blood* 1994; 84:2068–101.
4 Chignard M, Renesto P. Proteinases and cytokines in neutrophil and platelet interactions in vitro. Possible relevance to the adult respiratory distress syndrome. *Ann N Y Acad Sci* 1994;725:309–22.
5 Fujishima S, Aikawa N. Neutrophil-mediated tissue injury and its modulation. *Intensive Care Med* 1995;21:277–85.

6 Fujishima S, Hoffman AR, Vu T, *et al.* Regulation of neutrophil interleukin 8 gene expression and protein secretion by LPS, TNF-alpha, and IL-1 beta. *J Cell Physiol* 1993;**154**:478–85.

7 Levi M, ten Cate H, van der Poll T, van Deventer SJ. Pathogenesis of disseminated intravascular coagulation in sepsis (see comments). *JAMA* 1993;**270**:975–9.

8 van Deventer SJH, Buller HR, ten Cate JW, Aarden LA, Hack E, Sturk A. Experimental endotoxaemia in humans. Analysis of cytokine release and coagulation, fibrinolytic and complement pathways. *Blood* 1990;**76**:2520–6.

9 van der Poll T, Levi M, ten Cate H, van Deventer SJ. The role of tumor necrosis factor in systematic inflammatory responses in primate endotoxemia. *Prog Clin Biol Res* 1994;**388**:425–33.

10 Kuhns DB, Alvord WG, Gallin JI. Increased circulating cytokines, cytokine antagonists, and E-selectin after intravenous administration of endotoxin in humans. *J Infect Dis* 1995;**171**:145–52.

11 Bagby GJ, Plessala KJ, Wilson LA, Thompson JJ, Nelson S. Divergent efficacy of antibody to tumor necrosis factor-alpha in intravascular and peritonitis models of sepsis. *J Infect Dis* 1991;**163**:83–8.

12 Feuerstein GZ, Neville LF, Rabinovici R. Pulmonary TNFα is a critical mediator in adult respiratory distress syndrome. *J Endotox Res* 1995;**2**:189–93.

13 Christman JW, Blackwell TR, Cowan HB, Shepherd VL, Rinaldo JE. Endotoxin induces the macrophage inflammatory protein 1 alpha mRNA by rat alveolar and bone marrow-derived macrophages. *Am J Respir Cell Mol Biol* 1992;**7**:455–61.

14 Boujoukos AJ, Matich GD, Supinski E, Suffrendini AF. Compartmentalisation of the acute cytokine response in humans after intravenous endotoxin administration. *J Appl Physiol* 1993;**74**:3027–33.

15 Suter PM, Suter S, Giradin E, Roux-Lombard P, Grau GE, Dayer JM. High bronchoalveolar levels of tumor necrosis factor and its inhibitors, interleukin-1, interferon, and elastase, in patients with adult respiratory distress syndrome after trauma, shock, or sepsis. *Am Rev Respir Dis* 1992;**145**:1016–22.

16 Waage A, Brandtzaeg P, Halstensen A, Kierulf P, Espevik T. The complex pattern of cytokines in serum from patients with meningococcal septic shock. *J Exp Med* 1989;**169**:333.

17 Ertel W, Kremer JP, Kenney J, *et al.* Downregulation of proinflammatory cytokine release in whole blood from septic patients. *Blood* 1995;**85**:1341–7.

18 Granowitz EV, Porat R, Mier JW, *et al.* Intravenous endotoxin suppresses the cytokine response of peripheral blood monocular cells of healthy humans. *J Immunol* 1993;**151**:1637–45.

19 van Deuren M, van der Ven-Jongekrijg J, Demacker PN, *et al.* Differential expression of proinflammatory cytokines and their inhibitors during the course of meningococcal infections. *J Infect Dis* 1994;**169**:157–61.

20 Granowitz EV, Santos AA, Poutiaska DD, *et al.* Production of interleukin-1 receptor antagonist during experimental endotoxaemia. *Lancet* 1991;**338**:1423–4.

21 Arend WP. Interleukin-1 receptor antagonist. *Adv Immunol* 1993;**54**:167–227.

22 Dower SK, Fanslow W, Jacobs C, Waugh S, Sims JE, Widmer MB. Interleukin-1 antagonists. *Ther Immunol* 1994;**1**:113–22.

23 van der Poll T, Jansen J, van Leenen D, *et al.* Release of soluble receptors for tumor necrosis factor in clinical sepsis and experimental endotoxemia. *J Infect Dis* 1993;**168**:955–60.

24 Van Zee KJ, Kohno T, Fischer E, Rock CS, Moldawer LL, Lowry SF. Tumor necrosis factor soluble receptors circulate during experimental and clinical inflammation and can protect against excessive tumor necrosis factor alpha in vitro and in vivo. *Proc Natl Acad Sci USA* 1992;**89**:4845–9.

25 Evans TJ, Moyes D, Carpenter A, *et al.* Protective effect of 55- but not 75-kd soluble tumor necrosis factor receptor-immunoglobulin G fusion proteins in an animal model of Gram negative sepsis. *J Exp Med* 1994;**180**:2173–9.

26 Sheehan KC, Pinckard JK, Arthur CD, *et al.* Monoclonal antibodies specific for murine p55 and p75 tumor necrosis factor receptors: identification of a novel in vivo role for p75. *J Exp Med* 1995;**181**:607–17.

27 van Deventer SJH. Tolerence and susceptibility to bacterial endotoxins. In *Organ metabolism and nutrition: Ideas for future critical care* (Kinney J, ed.). New York: Raven Press, 1994:149–63.

28 Derkx BHF, Bruin KF, Jongeneel V, *et al.* Familial differences in endotoxin-induced TNF release in whole blood and peripheral blood monocular cells in vitro: relationship to HLA-haplotype and TNF gene polymorphism. *J Endotox Res* 1995;2:19–25.

29 Girardin E, Grau GE, Dayer JM, Roux-Lombard P, Lambert PH. Tumor necrosis factor and interleukin-1 in the serum of children with severe infectious purpura. *N Engl J Med* 1988;319:397–400.

30 Waage A, Halstensen A, Espervik T. Association between tumour necrosis factor in serum and fatal outcome in patients with meningococcal disease. *Lancet* 1987;i:355–7.

31 Okusawa S, Gelfand JA, Ikejima T, Connolly RJ, Dinarello CA. Interleukin-1 induces a shock-like state in rabbits. Synergism with tumor necrosis factor and the effect of cyclooxygenase inhibition. *J Clin Invest* 1988;81:1162–72.

32 Waage A, Espevik T. Interleukin 1 potentiates the lethal effect of tumor necrosis factor alpha/cachectin in mice. *J Exp Med* 1988;167:1987–92.

33 Heinzel FP, Rerko RM, Ling P, Hakimi J, Schoenhaut DS. Interleukin 12 is produced in vivo during endotoxemia and stimulates synthesis of gamma interferon. *Infect Immun* 1994;62:4244–9.

34 Doherty GM, Lange JR, Langstein HN, *et al.* Evidence for IFN-gamma as a mediator of the lethality of endotoxin and tumor necrosis factor-alpha. *J Immunol* 1992;149:1666–70.

35 Silva AT, Cohen J. Role of interferon-gamma in experimental Gram-negative sepsis. *J Infect Dis* 1992;166:331–5.

36 Volk HD, Thieme M, Heym S, *et al.* Alterations in function and phenotype of monocytes from patients with septic disease – predictive value and new therapeutic strategies. *Behring Inst Mitt* 1991;208–15.

37 Matchant A, Bruyns C, Vandenabeele P, *et al.* Interleukin-10 controls interferon-gamma and tumor necrosis factor production during experimental endotoxemia. *Eur J Immunol* 1994;24:167–71.

38 van der Poll T, Jansen J, Levi M, *et al.* Regulation of interleukin 10 release by tumor necrosis factor in humans and chimpanzees. *J Exp Med* 1994;180:1985–8.

39 Marchant A, Bruyns C, Vanderabeele P, *et al.* The protective role of interleukin-10 in endotoxin shock. *Prog Clin Biol Res* 1994;388:417–23.

40 Howard M, Muchamuel T, Andrade S, Menon S. Interleukin 10 protects mice from lethal endotoxemia. *J Exp Med* 1993;177:1205–8.

41 Derkx H, Marchand A, Goldman M, van Deventer SJH. Release of high levels of IL-10 in meningococcal septic shock. *J Infect Dis*, 1995;171:229–32.

42 Redl H, Schlag G, Bahrami S, Schade U, Ceska M, Stutz P. Plasma neutrophil-activating peptide-1/interleukin-8 and neutrophil elastase in a primate bacteremia model. *J Infect Dis* 1991;164:383–8.

43 van Deventer SJH, van der Poll T, Hack CE, *et al.* Endotoxin and TNF-induced IL-8 in human volunteers. *J Infect Dis* 1993;167:461–4.

44 van Zee KJ, Fischer E, Hawes AS, *et al.* Effects of intravenous Il-8 administration in nonhuman primates. *J Immunol* 1992;148:1746–52.

45 van Deventer SJH, Cerami A. Novel endotoxin-induced *cytokines.* In *Bacterial endotoxic lipopolysaccharides* (Ryan JL, Morrison DC, eds). Boca Raton, FL: CRC Press, 1992.

46 van der Poll T, Levi H, ten Cate H, van Deventer SJH. The role of tumor necrosis factor in systematic inflammation responses in primate endotoxemia. *Prog Clin Biol Res* 1994; 388:425–33.

47 Levi M, ten Cate H, Bauer KA, *et al.* Inhibition of endotoxin-induced activation of coagulation and fibrinolysis by pentoxifylline or by a monoclonal anti-tissue factor antibody in chimpanzees. *J Clin Invest* 1994;93:144–20.

48 van der Poll T, Levi M, Buller HR, *et al.* Fibrinolytic response to tumor necrosis factor in healthy subjects. *J Exp Med*, 1991;174:729–32.

49 van der Poll T, Levi M, van Deventer SJH, *et al.* Differential effects of anti-tumor necrosis factor monoclonal antibodies on systematic inflammatory responses in experimental endotoxemia in chimpanzees. *Blood* 1994;83:446–50.

50 van der Poll T, Levi M, Hack CE, ten Cate JW, Aarden LA. Elimination of interleukin-6

attenuates coagulation activation in experimental endotoxemia in chimpanzees. *J Exp Med* 1994;**179**:1253–9.

51 Barber AE, Coyle SM, Marano MA, *et al.* Glucocorticoid therapy alters hormonal and cytokine responses to endotoxin in man. *J Immunol* 1993;**150**:1999–2006.

52 Pfeffer K, Matsuyana T, Kundig T, *et al.* Mice deficient for the 55kd tumor necrosis receptor are resistant to endotoxic shock, yet succumb to L-monocytogenes infection. *Cell* 1993;**73**:457–67.

# PART THREE

# CLINICAL MANAGEMENT

# 8: Assessment and prevention of critical illness

K HILLMAN, G BISHOP and P BRISTOW

Intensive care units (ICUs) initially evolved from the concept of operating theatre recovery rooms as an extension of anaesthetic care.[1] Specialised areas were then established where the seriously ill, especially those being artificially ventilated, could be managed in one area. Nurses and doctors have come to practise full time in intensive care, specific training programmes have been established, and ICUs are now an integral part of most acute hospitals, providing an area where the monitoring, equipment, and expertise necessary to support critically ill patients can be concentrated. For many years the geographical boundaries of the ICU defined those who were critically ill in a hospital. However, many patients are admitted to the ICU as a result of clinical deterioration in other areas of the hospital. Delayed recognition and treatment of cellular ischaemia and hypoxia play a crucial role in determining admission to the ICU and eventual outcome. The irony is that, because ICUs are an expensive and limited resource, patients are often not admitted to them until they have severe multi-organ failure as a result of delayed or inappropriate resuscitation. These patients have a poor outcome and consume enormous resources. Now that high standards of care within the ICU have been developed, the challenge is to develop systems that operate at all times within all areas of the hospital, the aim of which is to recognise and prevent critical illness early in its course.

This chapter will cover how to assess seriously ill patients. Details of treatment are covered in other sections of this book. Rather than examine specific diagnoses or diseases, we will instead outline a generic framework to use when approaching patients with life-threatening illness.

## Assessment of the critically ill patient

We are all familiar with the traditional approach to disease, based on history, examination, provisional diagnosis, investigations, final diagnosis, and treatment. This does not work in the critically ill. Some parts of the conventional approach are incorporated, but the order and emphasis is different. Diagnosis, investigations, and treatment must occur simultaneously. The assessment process is not fixed. It changes continuously as a result of the course of the underlying disease and the patient's response to your interventions. Assessment in the critically ill is based more on the response to your interventions than on initial impressions. The key to good practice is to be comfortable with watching and reassessing this interaction of disease and interventions.

You need to understand the immediate functional impairment and threat to the patient's life rather than simply making a diagnosis. The degree of functional impairment depends on a combination of the underlying disease process, the acute physiological reserves of the patient, and their chronic state of health. For example, in acute life-threatening cardiogenic pulmonary oedema, the initial assessment should determine how sick the patient is and what interventions are immediately necessary to prevent deterioration and death. This will be affected by the patient's age and other co-morbidities such as the extent of underlying ischaemic heart disease or lung disorders. These chronic factors will influence your assessment in many ways. The cardiorespiratory system will not have the same reserves as in a younger patient, and the heart and brain will probably be accustomed to higher systemic blood pressures. Indeed, is active resuscitation appropriate at all? The initial assessment of illness severity is important, in that it will determine the type of intervention and the rapidity with which it needs to be delivered. Conventional medicine such as the management of hypertension usually involves simple interventions without urgency, but assessment and decision-making in acute medicine are compressed in time, and involve the simultaneous interaction of acute pathophysiological disturbances, the underlying state of health, and interventions such as drugs and artificial ventilation.

When acute cardiogenic pulmonary oedema is used as a general example, the severity of the illness must be ascertained rapidly and management instituted at the same time. The general approach for any life-threatening disease is *airway, breathing, and circulation*. The level of consciousness and state of the airway are rapidly assessed and the need for airway protection determined. Next the rate and nature of breathing are rapidly assessed and an appropriate level of assistance chosen, such as facemask with high flow oxygen, continuous positive airway pressure (CPAP), or artificial ventilation. Structured assessment of the circulation is similarly followed by preliminary support with, for example, fluid or inotropes. The response to each intervention must be observed minute by minute, and further treatment modified accordingly. Further deterioration should prompt early intubation and ventilation in preference to waiting for imminent cardio-respiratory arrest. If there is an improvement with initial treatment, this then allows time for investigation of the underlying cause.

Outlined below is a framework for assessing seriously ill patients, first for acute life-threatening situations, and then for more stable circumstances in an ICU.

# Assessment of life-threatening conditions

As described above, the assessment process is based on airway, breathing, and circulation. Always use it as your framework to assess critically ill patients and for correcting life-threatening situations. It includes:

- initial and rapid examination of the airway, breathing, and circulation;
- simultaneous correction of the most life-threatening abnormalities of the airway, breathing, and circulation;
- continual reassessment of the patient in the light of response to initial resuscitation and further management;
- simultaneous integration of a brief current and past history as well as initial investigations (chest radiograph, electrolytes, urea, arterial blood gases, haematology);
- monitoring of vital signs – continuous where possible (systemic blood pressure, ECG, and pulse oximetry);
- more detailed history, examination, and investigation when the patient is stable;
- if the patient deteriorates, going back to assessment and correction of airway, breathing, and circulation problems.

## Airway

It is crucial to guarantee a clear airway and protect the lungs from aspiration. Hoarseness and stridor are good indicators of a narrowed airway. The patient will also demonstrate a high workload of breathing in an attempt to overcome increasing resistance as the diameter of the airway decreases. This will be seen as increased use of accessory muscles as well as obvious distress and sweating.

*Patients at risk of airway problems*
Patients at risk are those who:

- are unconsciousness (GCS < 8);
- are at risk of obstructed airway (tracheobronchitis, epiglottitis, post-operative bleeding into the neck, and oedema secondary to conditions such as upper airway burns and anaphylaxis;
- have potentially blocked artificial airways (tracheostomies, endotracheal tubes);
- are having seizures.

*Major immediate interventions*
Depending on the type of problem and the degree of obstruction, the following may be urgently required:

- oxygen and airway suction;
- left lateral position, chin lift, and jaw thrust;

- Guedel airway;
- nebulised adrenaline;
- changing artificial airway;
- intubation;
- emergency cricothyroidotomy.

---

**Special note**
**Intubating a patient**

Intubating a patient with an obstructed airway requires special skills and experienced operators. Expert assistance must be sought urgently. Trainees should never undertake an emergency intubation without informing a senior colleague. A long angled-tip introducer facilitates passage of an endotracheal tube if intubation is difficult.

---

## Breathing

*Patients at risk of major respiratory problems*
Patients at risk are those:

- with increased resistance in the smaller airways, such as in acute severe asthma;
- with a large shunt, usually accompanied by increased lung stiffness, such as in severe pneumonia, aspiration, lung collapse, and pulmonary oedema;
- who are victims of chest trauma (flail, contusion, pneumothorax, haemothorax)
- with muscle weakness (for example, in neuromuscular disorders or as a result of drugs such as neuromuscular blocking agents);
- with underlying chronic lung impairment (for example, chronic airway limitation (CAL)).

*Rapid assessment*
- *Respiratory rate*
  - tachypnoea: good indicator of severity of disease;
  - bradypnoea: usually drugs (for example, opioids) or preterminal event.
- *Symmetry* – the side that moves less on respiration is the side with the pathology.
- *Work of breathing* – the effort a patient needs to maintain adequate respiration correlates well with the severity of the illness; look for tachypnoea and signs of distress, such as sweating, exhaustion, and the use of accessory muscles; do not forget to expose the abdomen in order to evaluate accessory muscle use.
- *Cyanosis* – unreliable sign in the acute situation; pulse oximetry is readily

available in many areas of the hospital as a rapid guide to adequacy of oxygenation.

*Major immediate intervention*

- *High-flow oxygen mask* – remember oxygen rarely depresses breathing and, even when it does, the depression does not occur suddenly and can be monitored.
- *CPAP* – especially in pulmonary oedema and at low levels in resistance problems such as asthma and CAL.
- *Drugs* – bronchodilators, steroids, antibiotics, diuretics.
- *Artificial ventilation.*
- *Intercostal catheter insertion* for pneumothorax and haemopneumothorax.

## Circulation

*Patients at risk of major circulatory problems*

Major circulatory problems include dysrhythmias, and the various forms of shock:

- *Hypovolaemia*: haemorrhage, burns, and excessive gastrointestinal tract losses.
- *Primary cardiac failure*: tamponade, myocardial infarction, valvular dysfunction.
- *Circulatory vasodilatation*: sepsis, anaphylaxis.
- *Obstructive shock*: pulmonary embolism, aortic dissection.

*Rapid assessment*

- Feel for the presence or otherwise of a central pulse.
- Count the pulse rate, and note the rhythm and whether it is chronic or new.
- Review the ECG and monitor patient if needed.
- Take the blood pressure.
- Inspect less well perfused part of the body such as hands, feet, knees, and anterior abdominal wall. They may be mottled and feel cold in a severely compromised patient.
- Review hourly urine output.
- There is little or no place in this phase of the resuscitation period for more complex assessment such as central venous pressure (CVP), cardiac output, or pulmonary artery wedge pressure (PAWP) measurement.

*Major immediate interventions*

- Intravenous cannulation.
- Rapid intravenous fluid replacement.
- Inotropes – adrenaline or noradrenaline are effective first-line adjuncts to therapy for hypotension after lack of response to intravenous fluids.

- Vasodilators for heart failure.
- Emergency pacemaker.

---

**Special note**
**Pulmonary oedema**

Pulmonary oedema as a result of excess fluid administration is a relatively rare and easily reversible condition compared with the devastating effects of systemic underperfusion and ischaemia.[2]

---

## Assessment of the stable, critically ill patient in the ICU

This section will provide you with a framework for assessment, rather than focusing on specific diseases and how they should be managed. It differs from the conventional approach to a patient on a general ward, with whom you can easily communicate and who usually has a single diagnosis and simple management plan. Once the acute resuscitation has been completed the patient needs a thorough secondary assessment.

### History

A critically ill patient in the ICU is unlikely to be able to give you a clear history, either because of the underlying disease or as a result of interventions such as sedation or intubation. A member of the managing team becomes the patient's spokesperson starting with the patient's name, age, and other demographic information. A background history should be given at each ward round, even though the managing team may be familiar with it. Owing to shift work and junior medical staff rotations, there is often a different team of doctors and nurses at the bedside. A summary of the patient's history is an important ritual for focusing attention on both the current problems and the patient's progress.

### Examination

*The patient's surroundings*
Information obtained from an inspection of the patient's immediate environment (Figure 8.1) will complement a conventional physical examination. For example, the bank of syringe pumps, the drugs they contain, and the rate of delivery provide information about the underlying disease and its severity. Ventilator settings such as the inspired oxygen concentration and airway pressures will tell you about the severity of the underlying lung disease. More information can be gained rapidly from the monitor, from the presence of enteral or parenteral nutrition, the type and rate of intravenous fluids, surgical drains, or other devices.

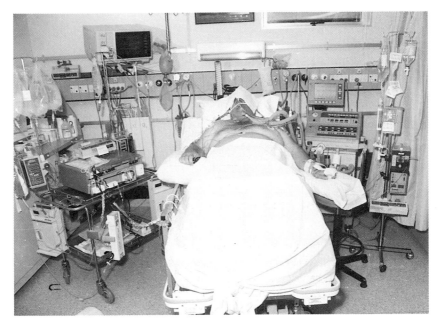

Fig 8.1    Sources of information for assessing patients in the ICU.

*Physical examination and standard investigations*

Introduce yourself, even if the patient is sedated. This reminds you that the patient is a human being and not just a physiological preparation. While you are talking to the patient, begin your neurological assessment.

*Neurology*
- Does the patient obey commands?
- What response is there to pain?
- Ask the nurse whether the patient has been moving all limbs and whether there are any fluctuations in the level of consciousness.

*Airway*
- Is the airway adequate?
- Endotracheal tube (ETT):
    - type
    - cuff pressure
    - does it need changing?
    - does it need converting to a tracheostomy?
- Cough:
    - is the patient coughing adequately?
    - what are the type and colour of the sputum?

71

*Breathing*
- Check $F_{IO_2}$.
- Check saturation.
- Check respiratory rate and pattern.
- If ventilated:
  - check mode
  - levels of positive end-expiratory pressure
  - inspiratory pressures
  - level of pressure support
  - patient–ventilator interaction.
- Chest:
  - inspection
  - percussion
  - auscultation.
- Arterial blood gases.
- Review the chest radiograph.

*Circulation*
- Is the patient warm, pink, and well perfused?
- Heart rate and rhythm.
- Blood pressure – is this adequate or inadequate?
- Cardiac output – is this adequate or inadequate?
- Oedema, jugular venous pressure.
- Heart sounds – murmurs.
- Peripheral circulation.
- ECG.
- Pulmonary artery catheter measurements.
- Results of latest echocardiography.

*Fluids, electrolytes, and renal function*
- State of circulatory volume – is this adequate or inadequate?
- Peripheral oedema, sacral oedema.
- Fluid requirements.
- Urine output.
- Other outputs: nasogastric, fistula, temperature, diarrhoea.
- Biochemistry: urea, creatinine, and electrolytes.
- Serum sodium – as guide to total body water requirements.

*Gastrointestinal tract/liver/nutrition*
- Is the gastrointestinal tract working: nasogastric aspirate, ileus.
- Nutrition status: nutrition type, route, volumes; if not being fed, why not?
- Liver function: albumin, prothrombin time, transaminases, bilirubin.
- Examine the mouth.

- Palpate/auscultate abdomen.
- Check intra-abdominal pressure if relevant.
- Check perineum/per rectum/per vagina if required.
- Check the back for pressure areas, rashes, etc.
- Check blood glucose.
- Is prophylaxis for stress ulceration required?

*Haematology*
- Haemoglobin levels, coagulation tests, platelet count.
- Anticoagulation/prophylaxis against deep vein thrombosis (DVT).

*Infection*
- Are there any signs of systemic sepsis?
- Temperature, white cell count, and differential.
- Latest microbiology results.
- Background surveillance.
- What are the likely sites of a source of infection?
- Antibiotics – what sort, how long have they been prescribed, and do they need to be continued?

*Cannulae and tubes*
- Are they necessary?
- Do they need changing?
- Are the sites clean?

*Medication*
- Are they all necessary?
- Can the antibiotics be stopped?
- Are routine medications properly charted?

## Summarise information and make an action plan

- Check the results of most recent tests and investigations.
- Summarise the existing problems.
- Focus on and list major unsolved problems.
- Devise a management plan – this is an overall plan for the next 24 hours. As with all aspects of acute medicine, the assessment and management are interdependent and need to be continually reassessed according to changes in the patient's underlying condition and response to treatment.
- Agree among medical and nursing staff what common message needs to be conveyed to the family in order to avoid confusion and mixed messages.

• Finally, ask yourself why the patient is in the ICU. Could he or she be transferred to a general ward? Is continuing active management warranted?

## Prevention of critical illness

In the last decade, the number of acute hospital beds all over the world has decreased, partly for economic reasons but also because of the recognition that patients can often be managed in more appropriate environments.[3] For example, almost 50% of surgery is now conducted on a day-only basis; many patients are being investigated on an outpatient basis; those requiring palliation or rehabilitation are being managed in the community. Acute hospitals are increasingly managing patients who are sicker, resulting in pressure to provide appropriate care for them outside the ICU. The challenge is to provide a system to manage the critically ill early in the course of their illness, limiting multi-organ dysfunction and their requirement for support in the ICU.[4]

Unfortunately, the general wards of acute hospitals are not always ideal places for dealing with patients with life-threatening conditions.[5] Traditionally, patient management in hospitals has been based on separate islands of care, such as the general wards, departments, and specialised areas. Patients are usually cared for by an individual clinician's team. This assumes that the managing team has the expertise and training to recognise life-threatening situations at all times.

In reality, what often happens is that a nurse in the general wards, who is concerned about a patient, alerts the most junior member of the admitting team, who may in turn seek advice from the next in line and so on. There are often long delays when a response within minutes is required. Often the only systematic and immediate response to serious illness occurs after the patient has died, when the cardiac arrest team is called. Moreover, even the most senior doctor in that team may not be trained or skilled in advanced resuscitation techniques, such as intubation, central line insertion, artificial ventilation, and use of inotropes. Whilst the specialties of emergency medicine and intensive care medicine guarantee training in procedural skills and theoretical knowledge about critical illness, this is not necessarily the case with other medical specialties. Apart from basic cardiopulmonary resuscitation (CPR), there is little in the way of training in advanced resuscitation skills in the medical undergraduate curriculum.[6] Even though trainees may be able to recognise life-threatening illness, for some reason they graduate from medical school remembering that oxygen stops patients breathing and intravenous fluid infusions can cause pulmonary oedema. For these reasons, acute care physicians need to be more involved in changing the culture of resuscitating the seriously ill.

# A systematic approach to critical illness

## Severe multitrauma – a model for standardised care

It is generally accepted that early recognition and resuscitation of the critically ill patient improves outcome – the so-called "golden hour". Delays may cause renal failure, acute lung injury (ALI), multiple organ failure (MOF), and a high mortality rate.[7] When blood flow is restored early, complications are minimised. The importance of early restoration of the circulation may be related to gut dysfunction:[8] hypovolaemic vasoconstriction may result in gut mucosal ischaemia with consequent translocation or release of mediators followed by MOF.[9] Once MOF has occurred, intensive care may increase costs merely by prolonging the dying process, whilst opportunities to prevent deterioration at an earlier stage are lost.[4]

The one area of acute medicine that has recognised the value of a systematic and standardised approach to early resuscitation is trauma.[10,11] The framework of this system is a patient-focused multidisciplinary approach (Box 8.1) where all the necessary skills are rapidly available to the seriously injured patient. This involves assessment at the site of trauma, triage to the most appropriate centre, and a rapid, structured, multidisciplinary approach to resuscitation in the emergency department using the Advanced Trauma Life Support (ATLS) system.[12] Data collection and audit are an essential part of maintaining quality of care.[13]

## A systematic approach for all at-risk patients

Apart from patients who have suffered a cardiorespiratory arrest, a systematic approach to medical emergencies other than trauma is rare. It is 30 years since the concept of CPR was introduced and survival rates remain very low.[14] In almost 60% of cases of arrest, antecedent factors occur hours before the terminal event,[5] usually cardiorespiratory abnormalities such as hypotension, tachycardia, tachypnoea, and bradycardia. This has led to changing the concept of a cardiac arrest team to a medical emergency team (MET) in order to achieve earlier recognition and

---

**Box 8.1** *Elements of an effective system for dealing with severe multitrauma*

- Triage to the most appropriate centre
- Calling criteria to identify serious trauma
- Rapid response by multidisciplinary team trained in advanced resuscitation
- Standardised approach to resuscitation
- Outcome indicators
- Audit cycle

---

Table 8.1  Medical emergency team (MET) calling criteria

| Acute changes in | Physiology |
| --- | --- |
| Airway | Threatened |
| Breathing | All respiratory arrests:<br>• Respiratory rate <5<br>• Respiratory rate >36 |
| Circulation | All cardiac arrests:<br>• Pulse rate <50<br>• Pulse rate >140<br>• Systolic blood pressure <90 mm Hg |
| Neurology | • Sudden fall in level of consciousness (fall in GCS of >2 points)<br>• Repeated or prolonged seizures |
| Other | • Any patient who does not fit the criteria above about whom you are seriously worried |

resuscitation of life-threatening conditions and so improve patient outcomes.[15] The criteria for calling the MET are based on abnormalities of the airway, breathing, and circulation (Table 8.1) and apply to all cardiac and respiratory arrests as well as those in the table. The team is multidisciplinary and all are skilled in advanced resuscitation. Hospital medical and nursing staff are encouraged to call the team when they are concerned about a patient. The emphasis is changed from waiting until serious organ damage or death has occurred to early resuscitation and restoration of normal cardiorespiratory function.

Other measures that have been shown to reduce mortality and provide better patient care within hospitals include the establishment of high dependency or intermediate care units.[16] These are areas where at-risk patients can be monitored and cared for in an environment more appropriate than a general ward but with a lower staff ratio than an ICU. It is a cost-effective solution for improving patient care. It is important that both nursing and medical staff working in these areas are appropriately trained and experienced in the care of the critically ill.

## Conclusion

When you are assessing the critically ill patient, diagnosis and management go hand in hand. The priority is to resuscitate the patient and if necessary diagnosis needs to be addressed after the patient is stable. The "ABC" of resuscitation remains the basis for physiological management. All acute hospitals should ensure that a system is in place that provides appropriate skills and expertise for early recognition and management of

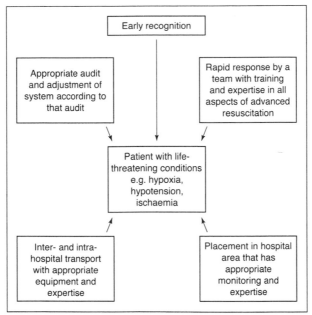

Fig 8.2    A systems approach to critically ill patients.

patients at risk of critical illness, and which will rationalise existing resources.[17] This will include the establishment of intermediate care areas, integration of services caring for high-risk populations, the provision of an intra- and interhospital transport team, and resources for audit. The efficacy of this approach must be assessed by analysing outcome indicators such as preventable deaths and unanticipated admissions to intensive care, and identifying those parts of the system responsible for poor or unexpected outcomes.[18] Thus the management of the acutely ill shifts from the traditional individual patient–doctor relationship to teamwork (Figure 8.2)

---

**Box 8.2**    *Key elements of a hospital-wide system for caring for the critically ill*

• Standardised guidelines for recognising at-risk patients
• Multidisciplinary team rapidly responding 24 hours a day
• Training of team in all aspects of advanced resuscitation
• Standardised guidelines for resuscitation
• Managing at-risk patients in an appropriate environment
• Measurement of outcome indicators to measure effectiveness of system
• Audit cycle

and problem sharing. A multidisciplinary team using a standardised approach and being made accountable by measuring outcomes and allowing adjustments and improvements to the system is the key to improved care of seriously ill patients (Box 8.2).

1 Lassen HCA. A preliminary report on the 1952 epidemic of poliomyelitis in Copenhagen. *Lancet* 1953;i:37–41.
2 Hillman KM, Bishop G, Bristow P. Fluid resuscitation. *Curr Anaesth Crit Care* 1996; 7:187–91.
3 Braithwaite J, Vining RF, Lazarus L. The boundaryless hospital. *Aust NZ J Med* 1994; 24:565–71.
4 Bion J. Rationing intensive care. *BMJ* 1995;310:682–3.
5 Schein RMH, Hazday N, Pena M, Ruben BH, Sprung CL. Clinical antecedents to in-hospital cardiopulmonary arrest. *Chest* 1990;98:1388–92.
6 Buchman TG, Dellinger RP, Raphaely RC, Todres ID. Undergraduate education in critical care medicine. *Crit Care Med* 1992;20:1595–603.
7 Henao FJ, Daes JE, Dennis RJ. Risk factors for multiorgan failure: a case-control study. *J Trauma* 1991;31:74–80.
8 Mythen MG, Webb AR. The role of gut mucosal hypoperfusion in the pathogenesis of postoperative organ dysfunction. *Intensive Care Med* 1994;20:203–9.
9 Rush BF Jr. The bacterial factor in hemorrhagic shock. *Surg Gynecol Obstet* 1992; 175:285–92.
10 Shackford SR, Mackersie RC, Hoyt DB, *et al.* Impact of a trauma system on outcome of severely injured patients. *Arch Surg* 1987;122:523–7.
11 Deane SA, Gaudry PL, Pearson I, Misra S, McNeil RJ, Read C. The hospital trauma team: a model for trauma management. *J Trauma* 1990;30:806–12.
12 *Advanced Trauma Life Support Program for Physicians. Instructors manual*, 5th edn. Chicago: American College of Surgery, Chicago: 1993.
13 Nayduch D, Moylan J, Snyder BL, Andrews L, Rutledge R, Cunningham P. American College of Surgeons trauma quality indicators: an analysis of outcome in a statewide trauma registry. *J Trauma* 1994;37:565–75.
14 McGrath RB. In-house cardiopulmonary resuscitation – after a quarter of a century. *Ann Emerg Med* 1987;16:1365–8.
15 Lee A, Bishop G, Hillman KM, Daffurn K. The medical emergency team. *Anaesth Intensive Care* 1995;23:183–6.
16 Franklin CM, Rackow EC, Mamdani B, Nightingale S, Burke G, Weil MH. Decreases in mortality on a large urban medical service by facilitating access to critical care. *Arch Intern Med* 1988;148;1403–5.
17 Thompson DR, Clemmer YTP, Applefield JJ, *et al.* Regionalization of critical care medicine. *Crit Care Med* 1994;22:1306–13.
18 Runciman WB, Webb RK, Lee R, Holland R. System failure: an analysis of 2000 incident reports. *Anaesth Intensive Care* 1993;21:684–94.

# 9:  Drug handling in critical illness

P E HERSCH and G R PARK

Many drugs are used in the critically ill. It is important that these are used properly and safely in this group of patients, because even the limited normal tolerance of humans to misuse of drugs is reduced further in critically ill patients. Not only should drugs be used as safely as possible, but also the number of drugs prescribed should be kept to a minimum. It is therefore important that, when a drug is first prescribed, its stop or review date is also clearly written on the chart. If this is not done, then drugs may be inadvertently continued for a long time. Furthermore, it may be useful to write on a prescription chart why a drug was started. For example, the infection that led to the prescription of an antibiotic.

Drugs do not always behave in the way that they are described in textbooks, papers in journals, and package inserts. This is because of the extreme changes that these patients may have in drug elimination, distribution, and sensitivity. Thus the following may occur:

- *Exaggerated effects*, such as the production of profound coma in patients with hepatic encephalopathy, given normal doses of sedative or analgesic drugs.
- *Prolonged effects*, such as that seen when morphine is prescribed in patients with renal failure who can remain narcotised because of failure to excrete the metabolite.
- *Reduced effects*: catecholamines, such as adrenaline, may need to be given in large amounts to patients with chronic cardiac failure because of the down-regulation of the adrenergic receptors.
- *Toxic effects*: aminoglycosides given in large amounts may be nephrotoxic and cause renal failure.
- *Unexpected effects*: these usually occur when an organ other than the one the drug is given for is affected by the drug; one example of this is the effect of some colloid solutions on the coagulation cascade, making blood hypocoagulable.

## Drug interactions

These are common when several drugs are given to patients and need to be carefully watched for. There are several ways in which interactions may occur.

*Pharmaceutical interactions*

These usually result in a drug being made insoluble and this results in precipitation of the drug; midazolam, for example, will precipitate out of solution if mixed in an infusion line with an amino acid solution – not only does precipitation render the drug inactive, it will also result in micro-embolisation of the lungs. The precipitate will eventually be cleared by the reticuloendothelial system.

*Drug–drug interactions at the receptor*

Three types of interaction may be seen when two drugs are given:
- "additive" – in this instance, if the effect of each drug is represented by 1, then $1 + 1 = 2$; the mixture of propofol and alfentanil is an example of this;
- synergy – this occurs when $1 + 1 > 2$; an example of this is the use of midazolam and propofol together;
- antagonism $(1 + 1 < 1)$ is exemplified by the use of naloxone and opioids.

*Drug interaction and protein binding*

Most drugs are transported in the blood bound to some extent to protein. Some drugs are highly protein bound. Warfarin is one of these and is 99% bound. If another drug is given that displaces even a small amount of this drug, say 1%, then the amount of free drug will be greatly increased. In the example of warfarin, if an extra 1% is displaced by, for example, phenylbutazone, then the amount of free drug will be doubled to 2%. As only the free drug can exert an effect, the effect will be greatly increased. Only those drugs that are largely protein bound will be affected by this. It should be remembered that many of these changes are short lived. The increased amount of free drug is quickly redistributed and metabolised.

*Drug–drug interactions at the enzyme level*

Two types of interaction are possible: inhibition and induction. These are discussed below.

# Enzymes

Drugs are metabolised by enzymes to change them from lipophilic compounds able to cross membranes, to polar, water-soluble, inactive substances that can be excreted by the liver and kidney. For most drugs there are two phases. The first, phase I, commonly, but not exclusively, involves the cytochrome P450 superfamily. Enzymes performing phase I reactions are shown in Box 9.1.

There are about 25 cytochromes P450 so far described in the human body. Between them these enzymes metabolise many thousands of

---

**Box 9.1** *Enzymes performing phase I reactions*

- Cytochromes P450
- Alcohol dehydrogenase
- Aldehyde dehydrogenase
- Alkylhydrazine oxidase
- Amine oxidases
- Aromatases
- Xanthine oxidase

---

compounds. Drugs are but one group of these substances. The cytochromes P450 are identified by an Arabic number that describes the family, a capital letter that describes the sub-family, and a further Arabic number that describes the gene product. These enzymes undertake reactions that mostly add oxygen to the molecule, such as oxidation and hydroxylation. Occasionally, they perform other reactions such as reduction. The metabolites of a phase I reaction are sometimes highly reactive. They therefore need further metabolism and this is called phase II. These reactions conjugate the phase I metabolite with a group such as glutathione or a sulphate. Examples of phase II reactions are shown in Box 9.2.

Phase I metabolism takes place in the endoplasmic reticulum and mitochondrion which contain small amounts of these phase I enzymes. Phase II reactions take place mostly in the cytoplasm where there is a large amount of these enzymes. Because of the difference in quantity of enzymes, phase I reactions are more affected by disease processes than phase II reactions. In addition, if there is a reduction in the phase I metabolic ability, then phase II metabolism cannot occur. It should be noted that a few drugs such as propofol, morphine, and lorazepam undergo predominantly phase II metabolism.

Many of the drugs used in the critically ill are metabolised by phase I and phase II metabolism. The phase I enzyme present in the largest amount in the body is cytochrome P450 3A4. This metabolises many of the drugs that are used in the critically ill, some of which are shown in Box 9.3.

---

**Box 9.2** *Examples of phase II reactions*

- Glucuronidation
- Sulphation
- Methylation
- Acetylation
- Amino acid conjugation
- Glutathione conjugation

---

---

**Box 9.3**  *Commonly used drugs that are substrates for cytochrome P450 3A4*

- Alfentanil
- Bupivacaine
- Cyclosporin
- Diazepam
- Digoxin

- Fentanyl
- Lignocaine
- Midazolam
- Nifedipine
- Pethidine

- Phenytoin
- Prednisolone
- Theophylline
- Verapamil

---

Many things affect the expression and function of cytochromes P450 in the cell. Some are described below.

### Induction

Some drugs may increase the expression of enzymes in the cell. Thus, rifampicin increases the amount of cytochrome P450 3A4. It does this by increasing its production. Alternative ways of inducing an enzyme are to reduce its breakdown.

### Inhibition

This generally occurs quickly and may be seen after only one or two doses of a drug are given. The inhibition may be caused by *substrate inhibition* when two drugs compete for the same enzyme. Erythromycin is metabolised by cytochrome P450 3A4 which also metabolises midazolam. Alternatively, there may be *direct inhibition of the enzyme itself*. Propofol binds to the haem part of the cytochromes P450 and inactivates them. Finally, there may be *metabolite inhibition*. This occurs when a metabolite of the parent drug inhibits further metabolism of the parent drug. This occurs with nortriptyline.

### Hypoxia

Tissue hypoxia is common in the critically ill. The liver is particularly prone to hypoxia as its dual blood supply is predominantly venous (70%). The cells in the liver most susceptible to hypoxia are those surrounding the central vein of each hexagonal lobule. The cells closer to the portal triads receive a higher concentration of oxygen because of the contribution from branches of the hepatic artery. Hypoxia reduces both the amount of cytochromes P450 and phase II enzymes in the liver and possibly elsewhere.

### Inflammatory mediators

During many acute conditions such as sepsis and trauma, inflammatory mediators are released. These include interleukins 1, 4, and 6. In addition, there is release of substances such as tumour necrosis factor $\alpha$ and interferon. All of these have been shown to reduce the amount of messenger RNA for cytochromes. Endotoxin, released from bacteria, has also been shown to do this.

## Diet

High fat diets and starvation, both common in the critically ill, have been shown to induce some of the phase I enzymes in the body. The polyunsaturated fats, especially linoleic and arachidonic acids, are responsible for this increase in metabolising capacity. High glucose intake has been shown to decrease hepatic cytochrome P450 content and inhibit barbiturate metabolism. A low protein diet in humans decreases theophylline metabolism, whilst its effects on phase II drug metabolism are variable.

## Stress

Non-traumatic stress in rats has been shown to reduce the function of phase I enzymes. The mechanism behind this is probably the increased circulating catecholamines which cause a reduction in liver blood flow; this results in a reduction in delivery of the drug to the liver and a reduction in oxygen delivery to the liver, causing tissue hypoxia.

## Age

Age affects metabolic activity. For example, it has been found that the ratio of morphine to its metabolites is higher in neonates than in children. As the phase II glucuronidation enzymes mature with advancing growth, so the ratio becomes normal. In elderly people, there is a decrease in the clearance of drugs metabolised by cytochromes P450.

## Genetic polymorphism

The type of enzyme produced is controlled by the genetic makeup of the individual. Some humans will not have the genes to produce all of the enzymes. In many instances this does not matter since some drugs will go through several enzymes. However, there are some enzymes that do not have this redundancy built into them. One such example is pseudocholinesterase, which metabolises suxamethonium. There are several genes controlling the expression of this enzyme. A spectrum of activity exists from normal to an enzyme that is unable to metabolise suxamethonium at all, resulting in prolonged paralysis.

## Sex

Many of the enzymes are controlled by the sex hormones. For example, cytochrome P450 3A4 is expressed in larger amounts in females than in males. This is because of the difference of excretion of growth hormones in males and females. If a human male liver is transplanted into a female recipient, then the expression of this enzyme increases to that of the female level.

# Prescribing in organ failure

### Brain failure

Coma from whatever cause may reduce the need for sedation. However, injury to the brain causes cerebral oedema. This often results in increased intracranial pressure and reduced intracranial compliance. Procedures that cause episodes of coughing or hypertension may cause a precipitous increase in intracranial pressure. Sedative, analgesic, and neuromuscular blocking drugs are commonly used to prevent the coughing or hypertensive episodes and the accompanying increase in intracranial pressure.

Sedative and analgesic agents have direct effects in reducing intracranial pressure as well as cerebral oxygen consumption. However, they also reduce systemic arterial pressure, which may compromise the cerebral perfusion pressure. This is because cerebral perfusion pressure (CPP) is dependent on intracranial pressure (ICP) and mean arterial pressure (MAP):

$$CPP = MAP - ICP.$$

Short-acting agents are best used to allow for periodic assessment of neurological status. Benzodiazepines may have an unexpectedly long duration of action. Reversal of the effects of these agents with flumazenil may precipitate seizures and an increase in intracranial pressure.

Sedative drugs are also used in the management of seizures. Many of these agents act as both anticonvulsants and sedative agents. Whatever agent is used, respiratory depression should be managed promptly and aspiration of gastric contents avoided. Drugs should also be suspected as the cause of seizures. Management may require withdrawal or substitution of the precipitating drug.

Sedation may also be required for patients who are disorientated or agitated. Pain may worsen these states and should be treated first.

### Liver failure

The liver is the principal site of drug metabolism. The effects of one dose of a sedative or analgesic drug may be prolonged in liver disease. Since both the sensitivity and number of receptors in the central nervous system are

84

altered in liver disease, the effect of sedative and analgesic agents is increased. Respiratory depression and encephalopathy may be precipitated.

Plasma proteins made by the liver are usually reduced in liver failure. The proportion of free drug for highly protein-bound agents may be increased with a resulting increase in effect.

When you use sedative and analgesic agents, it may be easier to assess the duration of action of a drug using bolus doses, rather than a continuous infusion.

## Kidney failure

The major pharmacological role of the kidney is excretion of water-soluble drugs and their metabolites. The problem with renal failure is therefore one of drug or metabolite accumulation. Most drugs can be safely administered as a single dose. An exception to this is suxamethonium which may cause fatal hyperkalaemia. The loading dose of the drug may be altered because of an increased volume of distribution and changes in plasma protein binding. Uraemia may also potentiate the actions of sedative and analgesic agents. This may be caused by uraemia changing the expression of cytochromes P450.

Drugs with known toxic or active metabolites should be avoided. Norpethidine, a metabolite of pethidine, may cause seizures, and morphine-3-glucuronide, a metabolite of morphine, is possibly antianalgesic. Another metabolite of morphine, morphine-6-glucuronide, is highly active, whilst one of the metabolites of midazolam has a small amount of activity. Atracurium is not contraindicated, as laudanosine, the epileptogenic metabolite, does not appear to accumulate to toxic amounts in humans.

Glomerular function is best estimated by the creatinine clearance. The plasma concentration of urea is dependent on a number of factors, including state of hydration and liver function, and may be misleading. Creatinine concentration is influenced by age and muscle bulk. Drugs, such as the penicillins, that are excreted by tubular mechanisms will be affected only late in the disease process, whereas those excreted by glomerular filtration, such as the aminoglycosides, are affected earlier.

Continuous haemodiafiltration incorporates a filter that is freely permeable to substances with a molecular weight of below approximately 20 000 daltons. This includes most drugs that are not bound to plasma proteins. The amount and effect of filtered drug depend, however, on a number of factors, including blood flow through the filter, size and age of the filter, the amount of protein binding, and the water solubility of the drug.

## Gut failure

Gastric stasis results in pooling of drugs in the stomach. The drugs are therefore usually not absorbed, which renders them ineffective. Their actions may, however, also be delayed and unpredictable. Only as the patient recovers and gastrointestinal function returns to normal, should drugs be given enterally.

**Cardiovascular failure**

Reduced cardiac output initially results in a decreased volume of distribution. This in turn causes a higher concentration of drug for a given dose. With the development of oedema, the volume of distribution will, however, increase for a water-soluble drug. The elimination of the drug is also reduced as a result of decreased liver and kidney perfusion, resulting in a prolonged duration of action.

Sedative and analgesic agents cause a reduction in sympathetic tone. This results in venodilatation and reduced preload, and, to a lesser extent, vasodilatation and reduced afterload. The overall effect is to cause a decrease in blood pressure, which can be profound. This is seen especially in patients in cardiac failure where the high sympathetic drive is needed to maintain blood pressure.

# How to prescribe a drug

## Pharmacokinetic factors

- Intravenous administration is the most reliable route owing to the variable absorption of drugs administered by other routes. The latter should be used only for specific indications, such as sucralfate given enterally to protect the gastric mucosa.
- Consider the altered volumes of distribution and whether the drug is water or fat soluble. This will influence the dose requirement. For example, the volume of distribution for a water-soluble drug is greater in oedematous states and smaller in dehydration.
- Consider the route of elimination. This will determine the dosing interval. Try to avoid using drugs that are metabolised or excreted through failing organ systems.

## Pharmacodynamic factors

- Drugs are usually given to achieve a therapeutic effect, not to attain a blood "therapeutic level". Blood concentration of a drug may be misleading. It may help to avoid toxicity.
- Consider the age of and organ system(s) failure in the patient. These factors may affect patient sensitivity to the drug.
- Decide on the exact therapeutic effect required. Use a single agent to achieve this, if possible. This will minimise unwanted side effects.
- Remember that each patient may react differently to a drug.

- Remember that the same patient may respond differently to the same drug at different times. Doses should therefore be reviewed regularly and adjusted if necessary.

## Safety factors

- Determine the duration of treatment. This should be constantly under review and drugs should be stopped whenever possible.
- Write the generic name of the drug in capital letters and in ink so that it is easily read.
- Make sure the route of administration is clear.
- Doses and dilutions should be clear.
- Look for drug toxicity.

# What to do if a drug does not do what you expected

A systematic evaluation of the pharmacokinetic and pharmacodynamic properties of the drug will help you to come to a logical conclusion. Remember the acronym ADME.

*Absorption*
- Has the drug actually been given in order to be absorbed?!
- Is the dosage, dilution, and rate of administration correct?
- Is the equipment working?
- Is the cannula still in the vein?

*Distribution*
- Is the patient dehydrated or oedematous?
- Is the drug highly water or lipid soluble?
- Is the drug usually highly protein bound?

*Metabolism and Excretion*
- Are the effects those of accumulated toxic amounts of the drug or its metabolites?
- Is the patient going into organ failure?

Pharmacodynamic variation is seen even when blood concentrations of the drug are within the "therapeutic range". A knowledge of the expected effects and side effects of the drug, together with an understanding of the pathophysiology of critically ill patients, is required to interpret unusual responses. For example, denervation injuries result in an increase in the number of muscle acetylcholine receptors. Suxamethonium will activate these receptors and fatal hyperkalaemia may result from the simultaneous contraction of these denervated muscles. If a drug does not work, have you waited long enough to let it work fully? It may be useful even to reconsider whether the drug is the best choice for the particular problem. For example, sedatives and analgesics are often used interchangeably. In infections antibiotic resistance may have developed.

Drug interactions always need to be specifically thought of, as they are easily overlooked. Other interactions also need to be thought of, such as hypokalaemia predisposing to digoxin toxicity.

It is also important to remember that solvents or carriers for drugs may also cause adverse effects. Cremaphor EL, used to dissolve some preparations of vitamin K, can cause anaphylactoid reactions. Soya bean extract, used to solubilise propofol, can be toxic if given in excessive amounts.

## Conclusion

Every critically ill patient gets given drugs. These may behave in an unpredictable way. There may be changes in both the pharmacokinetics and the pharmacodynamics. Many factors cause this, including changes in enzyme function, excretion, and receptors. In addition, there may be changes in the composition of the body, such as alterations in body water and serum proteins, and physiological variations, such as pH, which may produce further abnormalities in drugs. Besides these changes the risk of toxicity is increased, which may be as a result of active metabolites, drug interactions, or accumulation of toxic solvents. Only if clinicians are aware of the potential for these changes will drugs be used safely and efficaciously in critically ill people.

## Further reading

Chernow B. *The pharmacologic approach to the critically ill patient*, 2nd edn. Baltimore: Williams & Wilkins, 1988.

Cholerton S, Daly AK, Idle JR. The role of individual human cytochromes P450 in drug metabolism and clinical response. *TIPPS* 1992;**13**:434–9.

Dundee JW, Clarke RSJ, McCaughey W. *Clinical anaesthetic pharmacology*. Edinburgh: Churchill & Livingstone, 1991.

Elston A, Bayliss MK, Park GR. Effect of renal failure on drug metabolism by the liver. *Br J Anaesth* 1993;**71**:282–90.

Gibson G, Skett P. *Introduction to drug metabolism*, 2nd edn. London: Chapman & Hall 1994.

Park GR. Pharmacokinetics and pharmacodynamics in the critically ill patient. *Xenobiotica* 1993;**23**:1195–230.

Park GR. Molecular mechanisms of drug metabolism in the critically ill. *Br J Anaesth* 1996;**77**:32–49.

Williams R, Benet LZ. Drug pharmacokinetics in cardiac and hepatic disease. *Annu Rev Pharmacol Toxicol* 1980;**20**:389–413.

Woodrooffe AJM, Bayliss MK, Park GR. The effects of hypoxia on drug metabolising enzymes. *Drug Metab Rev* 1995;**27**:471–95.

# 10: Sedation, analgesia, and paralysis

M P SHELLY

Sedation is more accurately termed comfort care, with the individual components (hypnosis, analgesia, paralysis) considered separately. Attitudes to the sedation of critical patients have changed considerably in the past 15 years. In 1981 Merriman found in a survey of 24 ICUs that 67% preferred their patients to be deeply sedated and wakened only occasionally; 91% used neuromuscular blocking agents frequently.[1] In 1987, Bion and Ledingham surveyed all general ICUs in the UK and found that 69% preferred patients to be easily rousable from light sleep, and only 16% used muscle relaxants frequently.[2] Better drugs, ventilators, nursing care, and understanding of the risks associated with sedative agents have all influenced sedation management in the ICU. However, there are still considerable limitations in all these areas.

## Indications for sedation

Patients recovering from an episode of critical illness have reported factors that they found distressing during their ICU stay. The most consistently unpleasant memories are: anxiety, pain, fatigue, weakness, thirst, the presence of various catheters, and minor procedures such as physiotherapy.[3] These distressing factors need to be minimised to ensure patient comfort. Another way of reducing unpleasant memories is to produce amnesia. Sedative agents may also be necessary to produce respiratory depression and antitussive effects so that ventilation is effective.

It is important to differentiate the particular aspects of comfort that need to be improved for each individual patient. Anxiety is common and is often recognised; depression is also common but less well recognised.[4] It usually occurs as the patient is recovering, and responds to antidepressant treatment. Pain is a common complaint but is generally poorly treated. Each patient will have different requirements which will change as the disease process improves or worsens. The aim of intensive care sedation is to ensure that a patient is comfortable all the time. The appropriate level of sedation will, therefore, vary with the level of stimulus; patients need to be more awake for assessment of conscious level or for visits by family, and more asleep for insertion of lines or physiotherapy. Some patients require deep sedation for specific illnesses, such as critically raised intracranial pressure, or tetanus injection when there is a need to abolish autonomic activity.

The preferred level of sedation will also vary between ICUs. In well-staffed ICUs, more time is available to talk to the patients, whilst deeper sedation levels may be used to compensate for any deficiency in quantity and quality of staff in other ICUs. Patient comfort can be achieved by attention to the ICU environment but may need to be supplemented by drugs.

## Environment

The ICU is frightening to critically ill patients already concerned about their illness and possible death. Reassurance and the presence of relatives or friends will reduce these fears. Pain must be relieved and different types of pain appreciated. Prolonged immobility causes aches from muscles and joints that may be difficult to treat but are helped by regular physiotherapy or massage. The patient's dignity should be maintained and cultural differences respected. Adequate fluids and oral hygiene will help to minimise thirst. Warmth and air-fluidised mattresses will reduce discomfort and ease nursing care. Improvements in ventilator design and early tracheostomy have reduced the need for heavy sedation and muscle relaxation to allow efficient ventilation.

Maintainance of a normal diurnal rhythm may help to orientate the patient, and is best achieved with windows, natural light, and reduced activity and noise at night. Sedative drugs reduce the amount of rapid eye movement sleep, and fatigue during recovery from critical illness may reflect incomplete sleep cycles. Sleep is important to allow tissue regeneration.

## Drug administration

Fixed sedative drug dosage regimens may result in undersedation or insidious oversedation from drug accumulation. The consequences are listed in Box 10.1. Monitoring of the sedation level minimises these risks. Most sedative drugs are given either by continuous intravenous infusion or by bolus. Intermittent bolus will produce alternating undersedation and oversedation, and may cause hypotension from cardiovascular depression or histamine release. Continuous infusion is convenient and produces more stable conditions, but oversedation from drug accumulation is a risk with certain drugs, particularly in the presence of deteriorating renal or hepatic function. Continuous infusions of sedative agents may also prolong mechanical ventilation.[5] A combination of continuous infusion with

90

---

**Box 10.1**  *The effects of undersedation and oversedation*

*Undersedation*
- Agitation
- Pain and discomfort
- Catheter displacement
- Inadequate ventilation
- Hypertension
- Tachycardia

*Oversedation*
- Prolonged sedation
  - respiratory depression
  - hypotension, bradycardia
  - increased protein breakdown
  - ileus
  - immunosuppression
- Renal dysfunction
- Deep venous thrombosis
- Cost

---

intermittent bolus to cover stimuli such as physiotherapy or repositioning may be most effective.

### Drug tolerance and withdrawal

Tolerance means that progressively more drug is needed to produce a given effect. It occurs with sedative, analgesic, or neuromuscular blocking agents, usually when these are given by continuous infusion over several days. It may be caused by altered receptor affinity.[6] Tolerance should be distinguished from a change in the patient's condition causing increased physical distress.

Sudden withdrawal of sedative or analgesic drugs may produce phenomena ranging from mild irritability or anxiety to frank psychosis, particularly if they have been given in high doses for long periods. Withdrawal can also be precipitated by the administration of antagonists such as naloxone and flumazenil; these should always be administered carefully to critically ill patients. Withdrawal should be managed initially by reintroducing the drug at a low dose, changing to the oral route, and then progressively reducing the dose over several days or occasionally weeks.

## Sedation

Communicating with critically ill patients is complicated by tracheal intubation or the severity of illness, and it can be difficult to distinguish between anxiety, depression, and discomfort. Sedative (hypnotic) agents are used to help the patient tolerate these symptoms and to cope with the organ system support. There are many hypnotic agents available. None is ideal, and the choice should be determined by patient needs.

### Benzodiazepines

These are potent amnesic and hypnotic agents. Many of them have active metabolites which will accumulate in patients with impaired renal function.

91

Renal replacement techniques do not clear benzodiazepines adequately. Diazepam given by intermittent bolus is widely used in some countries. Its long half-life and active metabolites demethyldiazepam and oxazepam will result in accumulation, particularly if given by continuous infusion to patients with impaired renal function. Clearance is also reduced in patients with liver disease.[7] Midazolam has a shorter half-life than diazepam, and an active metabolite, $\alpha$-hydroxymidazolam, with a shorter half-life than the parent compound. Delayed clearance has been reported in some critically ill patients and normal volunteers,[8] from altered metabolism.[9] Midazolam is metabolised primarily by the liver, and clearance is impaired when liver blood flow to these areas is reduced, for example, in sepsis.

## Propofol (diisopropylphenol)

Propofol is cleared rapidly by the liver, and patients wake rapidly even after infusions lasting several days. Propofol is presented in a lipid emulsion and with high infusion rates patients receive a significant fat load; the 2% formulation will reduce this. Propofol has been reported to cause convulsions, but these are not associated with abnormal electrical activity and the drug has anticonvulsant activity in other situations. In patients with impaired myocardial function, it can produce significant hypotension from vasodilatation and myocardial depression. It may cause unusual colouration of the urine. Its main limitation is cost.

## Thiopentone

This drug is slowly cleared by the liver and accumulates; it is no longer used for routine sedation. It is occasionally used with EEG monitoring for control of resistant status epilepticus.

## Volatile agents

Nitrous oxide is no longer used for sedating critically ill patients because it produces bone marrow suppression. Isoflurane is an effective agent for short-term sedation,[10] but there are practical problems with vaporisers and the need for scavenging. Only 2% of isoflurane is metabolised but the fluoride ions produced by this metabolic pathway could theoretically be nephrotoxic.

## Ketamine

Ketamine is a dissociative anaesthetic agent which produces not only sedation but also analgesia, bronchodilatation, and an increased blood pressure. Hallucinations limit its use by continuous infusion. It is of value for inducing anaesthesia before tracheal intubation in physiologically unstable patients.

## Chlormethiazole

This has historically been used for managing acute withdrawal from drugs or alcohol. It constitutes a significant fluid load, and has no obvious advantages. Clonidine is a useful alternative for alcohol withdrawal, but should be administered only in the ICU.

## Etomidate

This is an anaesthetic induction agent, which appears to be non-cumulative and has little effect on blood pressure. However, it is also the most potent known inhibitor of adrenocortical function, and should never be used for infusion sedation. It was the association of an increased mortality rate with the unlicensed use of etomidate for long-term sedation of multiple trauma patients that first drew attention to this side effect.[11]

## Antidepressants

These may be valuable during recovery from critical illness. Their effect is delayed. Most must be given enterally. Amitriptyline given at night helps to facilitate sleep.

# Analgesia

Pain is common in critically ill patients and analgesia is the most important component of any sedative regimen. In critical illness even apparently minor procedures such as routine nursing care can be painful. Different analgesic agents act in different ways and are indicated for different types of pain. Opioids affect perception of pain through central opioid receptors. Non-steroidal anti-inflammatory drugs help inflammatory and skeletal pain; local anaesthetics block transmission of pain impulses. Some drugs may be effective for specific conditions, for instance carbamazepine for neurological pain.

## Opioids

Opioids are the most commonly used analgesic agents in the ICU, and are in general effective and safe when properly employed. Accumulation can affect neurological assessment. Delayed gastric emptying or ileus may be worsened by opioids.

### Morphine

Morphine is metabolised in the liver, mainly to morphine-3-glucuronide and morphine-6-glucuronide. Morphine-3-glucuronide has no apparent analgesic effects. Morphine-6-glucuronide, however, is a potent analgesic, and accumulates in renal impairment.[12] Morphine should be used with caution, or avoided, in patients with impaired hepatic or renal function. It is otherwise effective and cheap, and represents the standard analgesic for critically ill patients.

### Fentanyl

This is a lipid-soluble synthetic opioid with a short duration of action determined by redistribution rather than clearance of the drug. Its clearance is prolonged during long-term administration because of the large volume of distribution, and the pharmacokinetics vary unpredictably in individual patients.

### Alfentanil

This is less lipid soluble than fentanyl, more highly protein bound, and has a shorter duration of action Its pharmacokinetics are also unpredictable, but its action is terminated by drug clearance and accumulation is less likely. Alfentanil has inactive metabolites and is the agent of choice for patients with impaired renal or hepatic function.

### Pethidine

Pethidine is an inappropriate drug for use in the ICU. It has anticholinergic side effects, and its metabolite norpethidine accumulates in renal impairment and causes central excitatory effects, which manifest as shaky movements, anxiety, and grand mal convulsions

### Non-steroidal anti-inflammatory drugs

These are commonly used for postoperative analgesia, but in the ICU, and particularly in patients following cardiopulmonary bypass, even a single dose may result in significant renal dysfunction. Other side effects include gastric erosions and platelet abnormalities. They should be reserved for analgesia in high-dependency care patients with normal renal function and adequate splanchnic blood flow.

### Local and regional analgesic techniques

These provide excellent postoperative analgesia and may be useful in critically ill patients with pain from a single well-circumscribed site such as the chest or abdomen. Their use may be limited by a coagulopathy. The pharmacokinetics of local anaesthetic agents have not been fully investigated in critically ill patients and the risks of accumulation should not be ignored.

## Assessment of sedation and analgesia

The simplest method, and the one most often overlooked, is to ask the patient, but obtaining clear responses is often difficult for obvious reasons. Instead, several "observer-operated" methods are employed.

## Physiological responses

Responses such as tachycardia or hypotension are known to be unreliable guides to depth of anaesthesia and in the ICU they have little place for the assessment of adequacy of sedation. However, abolition of normal heart rate variability has been used to assess depth of anaesthesia, and is being studied in the ICU. Sedative agents should not be used routinely to control cardiovascular responses as this may cause oversedation.

## Scoring systems or rating scales

Such systems for sedation assessment use the patient's response to standard stimuli. The first of these was Ramsay's six-point-scale[13] (Box 10.2), which uses three rousable levels of sedation and three asleep. The asleep levels depend upon the patient's response to a light glabellar tap or a loud auditory stimulus. Variations have been used in the evaluation of new sedation techniques.[10] The Addenbrooke's sedation score[14] was designed for regular clinical use and has continued to evolve, currently using seven points. The Glasgow Coma Scale was produced to standardise descriptions of neurological function after trauma, and cannot be used for sedation assessment, but a modification has been devised for this purpose.[15] A comprehensive algorithm has also been developed[16] which combines assessment of sedation, anxiolysis, analgesia, confusion, and neuromuscular blockade with management options. Linear analogue scales are useful for research purposes and allow the combined analysis of several components of sedation. Sedation scores cannot be used when the patient is paralysed The precise scoring system employed is less important than the fact that sedation is being regularly assessed by experienced medical and nursing staff.

## Electroencephalography

The EEG is a record of cortical activity against time taken from a series of scalp electrodes. The amplitude and frequency distribution are affected by changes in conscious level, by disease states and by drugs. The interplay

---

**Box 10.2**  *The Ramsay sedation score*

*Awake levels*
  1 Patient anxious and agitated or restless or both
  2 Patient cooperative, orientated, and tranquil
  3 Patient responds to commands only
*Asleep levels dependent on response to glabellar tap or loud auditory stimulus*
  4 Brisk response
  5 Sluggish response
  6 No response

---

between these factors means that the EEG cannot be used as a reliable measure of sedation, but it can help to discriminate between drug and disease effects given expert interpretation. Various processing techniques have been employed, including two channel plots of amplitude and frequency, power spectral analysis, and auditory or evoked potentials.

## Neuromuscular blockade

The need for therapeutic paralysis of critically ill patients has been reduced by the rational use of sedative drugs, improved ventilator design with patient-triggered modes of ventilation, and the increased use of early tracheostomy. However, a significant proportion of critically ill patients still receive neuromuscular blocking drugs (NMBs) at some point during their intensive care stay. The indications are summarised in Box 10.3. The disadvantages of using NMBs are:

- interference with patient assessment;
- conscious awareness of paralysis by the patient;
- increased risk of apnoea if accidental ventilator disconnection were to occur;
- immobility;
- deep venous thrombosis;
- disuse muscle atrophy;
- myopathy.

### Physiology and mode of action of NMBs

Acetylcholine released by the motor nerve terminal at the neuromuscular junction crosses the junctional cleft, binds to receptors on the motor end-plate, and causes membrane depolarisation. This stimulates muscle contraction. The released acetylcholine is hydrolysed by acetylcholinesterase to avoid restimulation after the membrane has repolarised.

Depolarising NMBs (suxamethonium) mimic acetylcholine and produce depolarisation with characteristic fasciculation, but are cleared relatively slowly so that repolarisation is delayed. Recovery occurs within a few minutes. It is used to facilitate rapid tracheal intubation. Suxamethonium causes hyperkalaemia in paraplegic patients and those with burns. Other

---

**Box 10.3**  *Indications for neuromuscular blocking agents*

- Tracheal intubation
- Stablisation and facilitating procedures
- Ventilatory control
- Critical oxygenation
- Specific disease states, e.g. tetanus, head injury

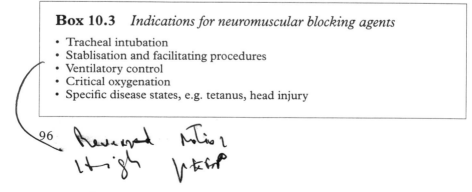

important side effects include bradycardia and increased intraocular pressure. Its effect is markedly prolonged in patients with pseudocholinesterase deficiency who may require ventilatory support for many hours.

Non-depolarising NMBs bind competitively to the receptor on the motor end-plate and effectively prevent access of acetylcholine. Paralysis develops without fasciculation, and lasts for a variable period (10–45 min) depending on factors such as the receptor affinity of the drug. The paralysis can be reversed by inhibiting acetylcholinesterase wih neostigmine, thus increasing the concentration of acetylcholine at the receptor site and displacing the muscle relaxant. The main non-depolarising NMBs are the steroidal relaxants (vecuronium, pancuronium) and the benzylisoquinoliniums (atracurium).

## Specific NMBs

### Atracurium

Atracurium and the single isomer preparation *cis*-atracurium undergo spontaneous hydrolysis in plasma as well as being degraded by esterases. Full recovery of neuromuscular transmission can be expected within 30 minutes even after prolonged administration in the ICU. Its clearance is independent of hepatic or renal function, and the metabolites have no neuromuscular blocking properties. The major metabolite, laudanosine, is degraded in the liver. Laudanosine is associated with cerebral excitation and convulsions in animals but not in humans. Atracurium is best given by continous infusion. It is probably the most appropriate agent to use in patients with multiple organ failure.

### Vecuronium and pancuronium

These are metabolised in the liver to active metabolites which are excreted by the kidneys. They are best avoided in renal or hepatic disease, and both have been associated with prolonged paralysis. Pancuronium has a duration of action of around 40 minutes, and should not be given by continuous infusion; it has vagolytic activity. Vecuronium has no cardiovascular effects and is shorter acting.

## Complications of NMBs

Awareness of paralysis is particularly frightening, and must be avoided by stopping therapeutic paralysis regularly and assessing depth and adequacy of sedation. All staff should be reminded that NMBs have no sedative properties. Immobility, loss of protective reflexes, and complete ventilator dependence all carry their own risks. Prolonged use of NMBs may cause changes in receptor sensitivity and local accumulation of drug metabolites. Multiple organ failure is also associated with altered neural and muscular function, with axonal degeneration and denervation atrophy.[17] The steroidal NMBs in particular have been associated with a specific myopathy, especially when used in conjunction with corticosteroids; key features include elevation in plasma creatine phosphokinase, motor denervation–fibrillation on electromyography, and vacuolation and loss of muscle fibres on biopsy.

### Monitoring the neuromuscular junction

Neuromuscular blockade is monitored by applying a single supramaximal stimulus to a motor nerve and evoking a twitch in the muscle innervated by that nerve. The electrical response can be recorded or the mechanical force of contraction can be measured. The muscle response to single and tetanic stimuli can be quantified with a force transducer or by recording and amplifying the electrical activity of the muscle. In clinical practice, a simple nerve stimulator is applied to the ulnar nerve and the response of the adductor pollicis noted visually. For research purposes in the ICU the accelerometer is the most appropriate method for measuring force of contraction. The main reason for monitoring neuromuscular blockade in critically ill patients is to avoid excessive paralysis from drug overdose or accumulation, and to ensure full recovery before neurological assessments are made, particularly of the brain stem. This is particularly important with the steroidal relaxants.

A non-depolarising block has two main characteristics when the force of contraction is monitored (Figure 10.1).[18] A series of single stimuli or a prolonged or tetanic stimulus produces a weakening response known as fade. After a tetanic stimulus a single twitch stimulus will show an increased response. This is called post-tetanic facilitation and is thought to be due to increased mobilisation of acetylcholine during and after tetanic stimulation. In a depolarising block, the force of contraction is reduced but there is no fade or post-tetanic facilitation. As recovery from block occurs, the number of observed muscle twitches in response to a train of four stimulus increases from 0 to 4. Full clinical recovery of muscle power is indicated by four responses of constant force (Figure 10.2).[18]

## Conclusion

Critically ill patients should be free from pain and, able to sleep if undisturbed, and their comfort facilitated by contact with relatives and compassionate staff. No ideal drug exists for sedation, analgesia, or paralysis. However, an understanding of potential problems allows therapeutic agents to be used safely. The presence and severity of any unwanted drug effects should be reviewed daily. Any changes in a patient's condition which may alter drug kinetics and dynamics, such as impaired renal or hepatic function, should also be noted, and the drug regimen adjusted accordingly. Drug doses should always be kept to the minimum compatible

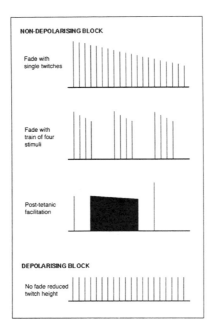

Fig 10.1   Characteristic responses of a non-depolarising neuromuscular block to single twitch, tetanic, and train of four stimuli. A depolarising neuromuscular block does not demonstrate fade or post-tetanic facilitation. The X axis represents time (s) and the Y axis represents force of contraction. (Reproduced with permission from Shelly.[13])

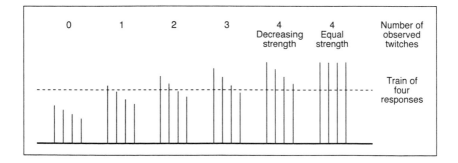

Fig 10.2   The observed response to a train of four stimulus with resolving neuromuscular blockade. The number of observed twitches increases as recovery progresses. Full clinical recovery is indicated by four twitches of constant force. Time (s) is represented on the X axis and force of contraction on the Y axis. (Reproduced with permission from Shelly.[13])

with achievement of the desired effect. Sedation regimens should be tailored to the needs of the individual patient and monitored according to clear guidelines. Each ICU should have a clear sedation policy against which practice can be audited.

1 Merriman HM. The techniques used to sedate ventilated patients. *Intensive Care Med* 1981;7:217–24.
2 Bion JF, Ledingham IMcA. Sedation in intensive care – a postal survey. *Intensive Care Med* 1987;13:215–16.
3 Bion JF. Sedation and analgesia in the intensive care unit. *Hosp Update* 1988;14:1272–86.
4 Bronheim HE, Iberti TJ, Benjamin E, Strain JJ. Depression in the intensive care unit. *Crit Care Med* 1985;13:985–8.
5 Kolley MH, Levy NT, Ahrens TS, Schaill R, Prentice D. The use of continuous IV sedation is associated with prolongation of mechanical ventilation. *Chest* 1998;114:541–8.
6 Mhatre MC, Ticku MK. Chronic ethanol administration alters GABA-A receptor gene expression. *Mol Pharmacol* 1992;42:415–22.
7 Ochs HR, Greenblatt DJ, Eckhardt B, Harmatz JS, Shader RI. Repeated diazepam dosing in cirrhotic patients: cumulation and sedation. *Clin Pharm Ther* 1983;33:471–6.
8 Shelly MP, Mendel L, Park GR. Failure of critically ill patients to metabolise midazolam. *Anaesthesia* 1987;42:619–26.
9 Dundee JW, Collier PS, Carlisle RJT, Harper KW. Prolonged midazolam half life. *Br J Clin Pharmacol* 1986;21:425–9.
10 Kong KL, Willatts SM, Prys-Roberts C. Isoflurane compared with midazolam for sedation in the intensive care unit. *BMJ* 1989;298:1277–9.
11 Ledingham IMcA, Watt I. Influence of sedation on mortality in multiple trauma patients. *Lancet* 1983;i:1270.
12 Shelly MP, Cory EP, Park GR. Pharmacokinetics of morphine in two children before and after liver transplantation. *Br J Anaesth* 1986;58:1218–23.
13 Ramsay MAE, Savage TM, Simpson BRJ, Goodwin R. Controlled sedation with alphaxalone-alphadolone. *BMJ* 1974;2:656–9.
14 O'Sullivan G, Park GR. The assessment of sedation in critically ill patients. *Clin Intensive Care* 1991;2:116–22.
15 Cook S. Technical problems in intensive care. In *Intensive care rounds*. Abingdon, UK: The Medicine Group (Education) Ltd, 1991:20.
16 Armstrong RF, Bullen C, Cohen SL, Singer M, Webb AR. Critical care algorithm. Sedation, analgesia and paralysis. *Clin Intensive Care* 1992;3:284–7.
17 Bolton CF. Neuromuscular complications of sepsis. *Intensive Care Med* 1993;19:S58–63.
18 Shelly MP. Assessment of sedation. In *Intensive care rounds*. Abingdon, UK: The Medicine Group (Education) Ltd, 1994:14–15.

# 11: Cardiovascular and respiratory monitoring

## T CLUTTON-BROCK

Monitoring in intensive care patients has two major roles: first, it warns of potentially life-threatening disasters permitting prompt detection and correction. Examples of this role are ventilator disconnect alarms and ECG arrhythmia detection. Second, it allows us to detect expected deviations from normality; these act as part of a feedback control loop and are essential to maintain physiological stability in sick patients. Examples of this are the continuous measurement of arterial blood pressure to control vasopressor therapy and the use of arterial $CO_2$ tension ($Pa_{CO_2}$) levels to guide weaning from ventilation.

Cardiovascular and respiratory monitoring make up the bulk of intensive care monitoring and as such are a major component of the nursing workload. Although the principles of monitoring have not changed greatly over the last 10 years there are still controversies about interpretation.

## Cardiovascular monitoring

### ECG

Continuous ECG monitoring is used in virtually all patients in an intensive care unit (ICU), with occasional exceptions being made for stable patients with long-term respiratory weaning problems. In addition to displaying the patient's cardiac rhythm and conduction, it also facilitates early detection of myocardial ischaemia. Continuous ECG monitoring does not replace the conventional 12-lead paper ECG record, and this should still be used for accurate diagnosis and to provide a hard copy of arrhythmias for the patient's records.

Modern ECG monitoring usually forms part of a multicomponent system and sophisticated signal processing is employed to reduce movement artefacts and noise. Disposable self-adhesive electrodes are used and are typically placed on the right arm, left arm, and V5 sites. The lead to be monitored can be selected by the user, but it is not always easy to tell which lead is in use, so care should be exercised before interpreting the site of displayed ischaemia. Heart rate is usually calculated from the detected R–R interval and, if the gain is set inappropriately high, then T waves may be detected as well, leading to a doubling of the displayed heart rate. Automated arrhythmia detection and ST segment analysis are available on some ICU monitoring systems. They vary in their usefulness and have not replaced the need for an experienced observer.

# Arterial blood pressure

### Invasive pressure monitoring

The continuous measurement of arterial blood pressure from an indwelling arterial cannula is widely practised in ICUs.[1] Arterial cannulation also provides convenient access for arterial blood gas and other samples. Modern systems that monitor arterial pressure comprise an arterial cannula, a connecting manometer line, a disposable pressure transducer, and a pressure amplifier and display system (usually contained within the multicomponent monitor).

Most peripheral arteries can be cannulated for the purposes of pressure monitoring, although a balance has to be struck between using a large artery that will give a more faithful reproduction of aortic pressure and the potential for disaster if arterial occlusion occurs.

In adults, the radial artery is widely used and combines ease of access with a high margin of safety. Most patients have a dual arterial supply to the hand from the radial and ulnar artery and radial occlusion does not usually lead to serious ischaemia. Allen's test has been popular as an indicator of the adequacy of dual supply, although its exact role is disputed.[2] It is also very difficult to perform in anaesthetised patients. Clearly, attempted cannulation of both the radial and ulnar arteries courts disaster and should not be done.

The brachial artery is readily accessible in the antecubital fossa. It is a larger vessel than the radial and occlusion rarely leads to ischaemia because of collaterals around the elbow. Forearm claudication has been reported after cannulation and the site is inconvenient in patients who are able to flex their forearms.

The femoral artery is widely used in paediatric practice and may be a useful site in very hypotensive and peripherally shut-down patients. The site is difficult to dress and the cannula is likely to become displaced in moving patients. The dorsalis pedis artery is also used in adult patients; this is a small vessel and occlusion may lead to distal ischaemia.

The cannula is connected to a pressure transducer by a length of relatively rigid plastic tubing filled with flush solution. The tubing supplied with modern disposable transducer sets is hydraulically far superior to the fine-bore plastic tubing used for drug infusions. It is important that air bubbles are excluded from the whole of the system, because they will not only affect the quality of the pressure signal recorded but could also be inadvertently flushed into the patient.

Modern transducers are sophisticated disposable devices with a low zero drift and a standardised sensitivity. The transducer should be fixed at the level of the patient's heart and the tap opened to air before pressing the zero button on the monitor. The transducer should be fixed at this level during monitoring; a transducer hanging off the edge of the bed is a common cause of a sudden rise in blood pressure! Transducers are not routinely calibrated for sensitivity any more.

The monitoring system calculates systolic, mean, and diastolic pressures from the signal and these are displayed. There are many causes of errors in the analysis of arterial waveforms, the most common being an excessively damped signal resulting from a kinked cannula. Care should be exercised in the use of systolic pressures in these circumstances, the value of the mean tending to be more accurate. Myocardial contractility, stroke volume, and peripheral vascular resistance all affect the shape of the waveform. These features have been used over the years in attempts to develop continuous cardiac output monitors using pulse contour analysis with only limited success.

## Non-invasive pressure monitoring

Automated non-invasive blood pressure monitoring (NIBP) is widely available on ICUs, again often as part of the multicomponent monitor. NIBP monitoring is useful in the more stable patient not requiring arterial blood samples and is frequently used on admission to the ICU before insertion of an arterial cannula. Measurements should not normally be made more frequently than every five minutes and the measurements are unreliable in low cardiac output states, during rapidly changing pressures, and in the presence of many arrhythmias.

# Central venous pressure

Central venous pressure (CVP) monitoring, together with ECG and arterial pressure monitoring, form the basis of "standard" cardiovascular monitoring in ICU patients.[3] To measure accurately the pressure of venous blood returning to the right atrium, the tip of the catheter must be sited in the superior vena cava (SVC). Placement in the inferior vena cava via the femoral vein has been advocated and with certain provisos gives a reasonable estimate of true CVP.

The common routes used for central venous catheter placement are listed in Table 11.1, together with their important features.

Table 11.1 Comparison of central venous access routes

| Route | Access | Arterial puncture | Success | Pneumo-thorax | Haemo-thorax | Comments |
|---|---|---|---|---|---|---|
| Subclavian | Skilled | Moderate | High | Highest | Highest | Good long term |
| Internal jugular | Skilled | Highest | High | Low | Moderate | |
| External jugular | Moderate | Low | Moderate | Low | Low | Need J-wire |
| Antecubital | Easy | Low | Moderate | Very low | Low | Thrombo-phlebitis |
| Femoral | Easy | Low | Moderate | Very low | Very low | Need long line |

Access to the SVC is usually via the internal jugular or subclavian veins. The internal jugular vein lies lateral to the carotid artery in the neck, with the right side being easier to cannulate for most people and with a direct route into the SVC. The left internal jugular route gains access to the SVC via the innominate vein. The internal jugular route is widely used both during anaesthesia and in the ICU; the route carries a lower risk of pneumothorax than the subclavian, and accidental arterial puncture is more easily controlled.

The subclavian vein lies immediately beneath the clavicle medial to the subclavian artery and just lateral to the first rib. Either side provides excellent access into the SVC and the catheters are easily secured and dressed. The route carries the highest risk of pneumothorax in most series and arterial puncture may be difficult to control with the potential to produce a life-threatening haemothorax.

The SVC may be reached via either the antecubital or the femoral veins. It is more difficult to place catheters successfully into the SVC from these routes and special, long catheters are required. They do, however, carry a very low risk of pneumothorax and still have a place under special circumstances.

Having placed the catheter, its position should be checked with a chest radiograph while, at the same time, excluding a pneumothorax. To measure CVP, the catheter is connected to a monitoring line and transducer system as for arterial pressure monitoring. It is common today to make use of multilumen catheters for pressure measurement and drug/fluid administration. CVP measurements should usually be made from the most distal lumen, making sure first that no drugs or fluids are being administered through that lumen. The position of the transducer is critical because venous pressures are much lower than arterial ones. The transducer should be placed at the level of the right atrium and repeated measurements should be made with the patient in the same position (usually on the back).

The interpretation of the measured CVP is surprisingly complex and the cause of much confusion. The pressure measured is influenced by several factors, including the volume of blood returning to the heart, tricuspid valve function, right ventricular function, and intrathoracic pressures. As a guide, a low CVP is most likely to be the result of inadequate venous return to the heart (hypovolaemia, vasodilatation, etc.), whereas interpretation of a "normal" or elevated CVP requires more care. The CVP may reach normal levels in a patient who is still inadequately volume resuscitated, partly as a result of reduced right ventricular function from the tachycardia and partly as a feature of positive pressure ventilation. The exact influence of intrapulmonary pressures on the cardiac filling pressures is a topic of much debate. It is the pressure difference between the inside and the outside of the atria that determines the true filling pressure, and only a proportion of the intrapulmonary pressure is transmitted to the outside of the heart. In the patient with very stiff lungs, even less intrapulmonary pressure is transmitted. The practice of subtracting the level of positive end-expiratory pressure (PEEP) from the CVP is not logical and causes further confusion. *Changes* in CVP may be more usefully clinically than the absolute level.

## Pulmonary artery and pulmonary artery occlusion pressures[4]

"Floating" a catheter through the right atrium, right ventricle, and into the pulmonary artery (PA) was described in 1968 by Branthwaite and Bradley, but has been popularised with the names of Swan and Ganz after their description of a balloon-tipped catheter in the 1970s. Access to the right atrium is via the SVC using the routes described above. A sheath of 7–8 French gauge (FG) diameter is inserted using a Seldinger technique. These sheaths are supplied with an internal vein dilator, a self-sealing valve on the proximal end, and a sterile protective cover for the catheter. All of the risks of central venous cannulation are present, along with the added complication that an 8 FG hole in an artery may require surgical repair.

After inserting the sheath, the flushed pulmonary artery catheter is passed so that its tip lies just beyond the end of the sheath (about 12 cm). Connecting the distal lumen (yellow connector) to a pressure transducer arranged as for CVP monitoring allows the pressure waveforms to be monitored during insertion. The catheter is inserted smoothly through the heart, while observing the waveform change from atrial to ventricular to pulmonary arterial, and finally to that of a pulmonary capillary wedge pressure (Figure 11.1). Some of the common problems and suggested remedies encountered during insertion are given in Table 11.2.

The pressure in the inflated balloon may exceed 500 mm Hg and it is essential to observe the waveform while slowly inflating the balloon. If the

105

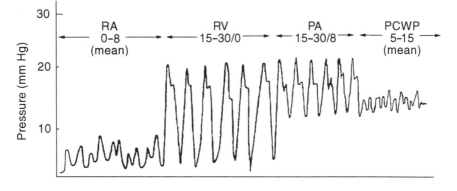

Fig 11.1  Diagram of pressure waveforms seen during insertion of a pulmonary artery flotation catheter. PCWP, partial capillary wedge pressure.

catheter wedges at less than 1·25 ml, then the catheter should be withdrawn slightly. Pulmonary artery rupture is a rare but often fatal complication of catheterisation; it is more common in the presence of pulmonary hypertension and in anticoagulated patients. Pulmonary infarction can occur if the balloon is left inflated or if the catheter is allowed to migrate and wedge spontaneously.

Table 11.2  Common problems encountered during pulmonary artery catheterisation

| Problems | Causes | Solutions |
| --- | --- | --- |
| Unable to pass catheter through sheath | Sheath kinked or against SVC wall | Withdraw sheath carefully |
| Unable to obtain atrial trace | Catheter passing into IVC | Rotate catheter, check balloon inflated |
| Unable to enter ventricle | Low flow states | Check balloon up, advance more slowly |
| | Tricuspid regurgitation | Try with balloon down |
| Ventricular tachycardia | Catheter stimulating ventricle | Check balloon inflated, lignocaine bolus |
| Unable to enter pulmonary artery | Low flow states | Check balloon up, advance more slowly |
| | Catheter looping in ventricle | Try with balloon down |
| Unable to wedge | Catheter looping in ventricle | Withdraw to ventricle and reinsert |
| | Balloon not inflated | |
| | Balloon ruptured | Remove completely, use new catheter |
| Spontaneous wedging | Inserted too far, small PA | Withdraw, reinsert if necessary |

The interpretation of the pulmonary capillary wedge pressure carries all of the complexities associated with CVP measurements discussed above. In addition in the severely diseased lung, there may not be an unobstructed connection between the pulmonary vessel in use and the left atrium.

Pulmonary artery flotation catheters have been developed with the facility for continuous mixed venous saturation monitoring using a fibreoptic channel. Mixed venous saturation is determined by the balance between oxygen delivery and consumption, and is thus affected by a number of changing variables in the sick patient, including: cardiac output, arterial saturation, haemoglobin concentration, and oxygen consumption.

Indications for pulmonary artery catheterisation and the impact on ICU outcomes have become the subject of considerable debate. Pulmonary artery catheterisation is indicated where a measurement of left-sided filling pressures, pulmonary artery pressures, cardiac output (see below), mixed venous saturation, or the direct injection of drugs into the pulmonary vasculature is deemed to be important in the management of a particular patient. Monitoring of physiological variables guides therapy and is not therapeutic as such.

## Cardiac output

The cardiac output is the net forward flow of blood through the aortic valve and is clearly an important determinant of oxygen delivery to the body. Although "normal" cardiac output values are often quoted, usually with a correction for different body size as cardiac index (cardiac output/ body surface area), it is apparent that the "adequate" cardiac output for a given patient at a given time varies greatly. The cardiac output cannot be measured directly in patients and a number of more or less indirect techniques are employed.

### Clinical signs

Although non-specific and impossible to calibrate, clinical signs remain a useful estimate of the adequacy of cardiac output in many ICU patients and should not be overlooked. Typical signs of low and high cardiac output states are listed in Table 11.3.

### Thermodilution

The injection of cold 5% dextrose into the right atrium (via the blue connection of a PA catheter) is a modified indicator dilution technique; this measures the temperature fall with a small thermistor attached to the tip of a pulmonary artery flotation catheter.[5] This has replaced the use of dye dilution techniques in clinical practice. Thermodilution catheters are often inserted as standard and most ICU monitoring systems have the necessary

Table 11.3 Typical clinical signs of low and high cardiac output states

| Low | High |
| --- | --- |
| Hypotension | Strong, bounding pulses |
| Weak pulses | Warm peripheries |
| Cold peripheries | Flushed appearance |
| Reduced urine output | Hypotensive if vasodilated (for example, sepsis) |
| Confusion | |
| Metabolic acidosis | |

cardiac computers built in. Use of cold solutions improves the precision of measurement. Dedicated cold injection sets are available with a coil to place in a bucket of iced water and an insulated multi-use 10 ml injection syringe. An in-line thermistor is attached at the syringe and the cardiac output computer automatically computes injectate to PA temperature changes.

Most cardiac output monitors display the PA temperature, the injectate temperature, and the temperature curve during injection. The size and type of catheter affect the calculation, and it is important to check that either the correct computation constant or the correct catheter details have been entered into the computer before making measurements. The PA and injectate temperatures should also be checked after the first injection to confirm that the connections and injectate probes are correct. As pulmonary blood flow and the specific heat capacity of the lung vary with the phase of ventilation, it is ideal to inject at the same time in the ventilatory cycle, though this is often difficult to perform in practice.

An impressive range of results is presented on the "haemodynamic calculations" page of ICU monitors; the calculated systemic vascular resistance (SVR) is commonly quoted and is calculated from:

$$SVR = (Mean\ PA\ pressure\ - CVP)/Cardiac\ output.$$

The result is usually multiplied by 79.9 to convert to the old units of $dyn \cdot s/cm^5$. The normal range is quoted between 770 and 1500. A common source of confusion is the automated entry of a CVP value even if the transducer is not connected to the patient. It is important to check the calculation if strange results are reported. The calculated SVR is purely a theoretical value and is used for convenience to distinguish between hypotension caused by a low cardiac output state and that caused by arterial vasodilatation.

A number of specially modified thermodilution catheters are available, one of which performs a very fast dilution curve and can calculate the right ventricular ejection fraction. A semi-continuous thermodilution catheter is available which heats a small coil in the right ventricle and measures the temperature changes in the PA. The results from this system are less precise than from conventional thermodilution, but the attractions of an almost continuous reading with a marked reduction in fluid loading are considerable.

## Doppler ultrasonographic cardiac output

The aorta may be reached with a narrow ultrasound beam either in its ascending portion via the trachea and the suprasternal notch, or in its descending intrathoracic portion via the oesophagus. Measurement of the Doppler frequency shift in the returning beam allows the velocity of the insonated blood to be calculated. If the angle of incidence of the beam and the cross-sectional area of the aorta are also measured (or estimated), then the blood flow in the aorta can be calculated. Several systems have been described and marketed; of these only transoesophageal monitoring has become popular in the ICU setting. A single-use or sheathed probe is inserted into the oesophagus and manipulated until a suitable signal is received. The calculations of stroke volume and cardiac output are complicated by the fact that only descending aortic blood is insonated, and the angle of incidence and aortic cross-sectional area are not fixed. It is probably unfortunate that these devices were marketed as cardiac output monitors because there is a great deal of additional information available from the signals received. The active but empty heart can be distinguished from the struggling overfilled one, even though both may produce the same flow figures.

## Non-invasive cardiac output monitoring

Many different systems for the non-invasive monitoring of cardiac output in ICU patients have been described over the years. These include thoracic bioimpedance, indirect Fick (using the uptake of oxygen as an "indicator"), and pulse contour analysis. Most perform poorly in low output states and few have achieved a precision of measurement suitable for routine clinical use.

## Gastric tonometry

The measurement of cardiac output gives an indication of the total flow of blood entering the arterial circulation, but gives no direct information as to the adequacy of organ perfusion. In gastric tonometry, a small gas-permeable balloon filled with saline is passed into the patient's stomach; $CO_2$ diffuses from the lumen of the stomach into the saline and, after aspiration, can be measured using a conventional blood gas analyser. It is assumed that the $CO_2$ in the lumen of the stomach is in equilibrium with the gastric mucosa. A bicarbonate level is derived from an arterial blood gas sample taken at the same time and, using a modified Henderson–

Hasselbach equation, a value for gastric mucosal pH ($pH_i$) is calculated. The $pH_i$ falls in situations when gastric mucosal blood flow is reduced such as hypovolaemia, sepsis, etc. Some studies have shown that $pH_i$ may be a more sensitive indicator of inadequate organ perfusion than measurements of cardiac output or arterial acid–base status. The measurements are, however, full of errors; in particular, the measurement of $P_{CO_2}$ in saline is very imprecise and the exact role of gastric tonometry in clinical practice has yet to be fully defined. More recently, a continuous measuring system has become available using a gas-filled balloon and a modified capnometer.

## Respiratory monitoring

### Monitoring the mechanics of ventilation

Most ICU patients are mechanically ventilated at some point during their stay on the unit. ICU ventilators have become highly sophisticated, microprocessor-controlled devices, although many of the basic functions remain unchanged.

All modern ICU ventilators measure expired tidal volumes and calculate expired minute volume. Most machines use a flow transducer at the expiratory limb of the breathing system for this measurement. Many ventilators also measure inspired tidal volumes as well, a large difference between inspired and expired volumes indicating a leak in the breathing system. An increasing appreciation that excessive tidal volume may be as dangerous as excessive pressure to the lungs makes the monitoring of ventilator volumes important. Respiratory rate is easily measured by the ventilator and is particularly useful when split into the patient's own (spontaneous) and mechanical breath rates.

Breathing system pressure, often misquoted as airway pressure, is measured at the machine end of the inspiratory limb of the system. Typically, values for peak, mean, and PEEP are displayed. The relationship between proximal inspiratory limb pressure and true airway pressure (ideally alveolar pressure) is very complex and is influenced by several factors. Extended inspiratory times, such as those produced by an inverse ratio ventilation, encourage airway pressures to reach system pressures. The level of PEEP displayed (*extrinsic* PEEP) is again a breathing system pressure and, in sick lungs with short expiratory times, gas may be trapped at the end of expiration and significant *intrinsic* PEEP may be produced.

Lung mechanics have been of interest in ventilated ICU patients for many years[6] and are now often displayed by the more expensive ventilators. Lung compliance is the tidal volume divided by the distending pressure required to achieve that volume. True lung compliance needs a measurement of intrapleural pressure or an estimate from oesophageal pressure. In practice, the ventilator uses system pressure again and a crude estimate of total respiratory system compliance is produced. Resistance is pressure divided by flow and again strictly needs oesophageal pressure, although values calculated using system pressure do indicate significant changes. Volume–pressure and flow–pressure loops are displayed by the latest machines and, with skilled interpretation, may enable the ventilator settings to be adjusted to achieve adequate ventilation with less induced lung damage.

## pH and blood gas monitoring

Blood gas analysers measure pH, $P_{CO_2}$, and $P_{O_2}$; they also calculate a range of derived values.[7] Modern analysers may incorporate electrolyte, metabolite, and haemoglobin measurements into one device. The pH is measured using a miniaturised glass electrode, $P_{CO_2}$ with a membrane-covered pH electrode (Stow–Severinghaus), and $P_{O_2}$ with a miniature polarographic electrode (Leland–Clarke).

Samples for analysis should be collected anaerobically into syringes and mixed well with the anticoagulant. Analysis should be within 10 minutes and, if not possible, then the sample should be stored on ice. Home-made syringes with liquid heparin introduce significant errors and should be replaced with syringes using dry heparin pellets. Only certain blood gas syringes are suitable for ionised calcium measurements.

Cartridge-based near-patient analysers are commercially available and combine a reduced delay before sampling with a much higher analysis cost. Continuous intra-arterial blood gas analysis is also available using fibreoptic pH, $P_{CO_2}$, and $P_{O_2}$ electrodes. The sensor can be inserted through a 20-gauge arterial cannula and will give continuous readings for over 72 hours.

Interpretation of blood gas results needs a clear understanding of respiratory and cardiovascular physiology. Arterial $P_{O_2}$ should be interpreted only when the inspired oxygen concentration is known. An increase in our understanding of the damage that mechanical ventilation can do to lungs has led to a revision of target blood gas levels. It should also be appreciated that blood gases are only a very rough guide to the severity of pulmonary disease.

## CO oximetry and pulse oximetry

Oxyhaemoglobin and deoxyhaemoglobin absorb light differently in the red wavelengths but in a very similar fashion at the near-infrared wavelength of 805 nm, their isobestic point. This allows a spectrophotometer using two wavelengths theoretically to measure total and oxygenated haemoglobin and so calculate haemoglobin saturation. The addition of several other wavelengths allows measurements to be made of other haemoglobin species and is the principle of the CO-oximeter. Carboxyhaemoglobin is not distinguished from oxyhaemoglobin by the pulse oximeter, and CO-oximeter measurements must be made if carbon monoxide poisoning is suspected. Methaemoglobin measurements are made in patients receiving inhaled nitric oxide therapy. Spectrophotometry requires a known pathlength and a solution with minimal light scattering; blood in a sample CO-oximeter is lysed to reduce the scattering.

Transcutaneous measurements fulfil neither of these requirements and have made the development of non-invasive devices much more complex. In the pulse oximeter, red and near-infrared light are alternately passed through a digit and the ratio of absorption calculated. It is assumed that the pathlength is fixed for the brief periods of illumination ($< 1/400$ second) but is not stable enough for measurements of total haemoglobin to be made. Using complex digital signal processing, just the pulsatile component (about 2%) of the received signal is used and a built-in calibration table allows saturation to be displayed.

The pulse oximeter is a very useful and widely used monitoring device in ICU patients, but again caution is required in interpretation under certain circumstances. In very anaemic or poorly perfused patients, the pulsatile signal falls to very low levels and a marked deterioration in the precision of saturation measurement occurs.[8] The devices do not drift, however, and a maintained trend will be a true reflection of patient change. Saturation has a complex relationship with $Pao_2$ as described by the dissociation curve and is influenced by several factors including $Paco_2$ levels. In the patient with severe lung disease low $Pao_2$ and high $Paco_2$ levels often coexist, and blood gas measurements will be needed to distinguish the causes of a fall in saturation.

## Capnometry

End-tidal $CO_2$ tension ($Pe'co_2$) monitoring is widely used in anaesthetised patients both as an indicator of $Paco_2$ and as a ventilator disconnect alarm. The situation in ventilated ICU patients is more complex and lung damage affects the relationship between $Pe'co_2$ and $Paco_2$. Stable gradients between the two measurements have been described and allow $Paco_2$ to be estimated.[9] In many patients, however, the relationship is variable and a change in $Pe'co_2$ may reflect a change in pulmonary dead space and/or a change in pulmonary blood flow, rather than a change in $Paco_2$.

## Conclusions

Cardiovascular and respiratory monitoring are essential and important activities that occupy significant proportions of nursing and medical time in most ICU patients. Advances in physiological signal processing provide us

112

with both new monitoring tools and more reliable conventional monitors. Errors in monitoring usually arise from incorrect equipment use or from incorrect interpretation. True equipment faults are very rare today and unexpected results should always be checked when possible.

1 Gardner RM. Direct arterial pressure monitoring. *Curr Anaesth Crit Care* 1990;1:239–46.
2 Slogoff S, Keats AS, Arlund C. On the safety of radial artery cannulation. *Anesthesiology* 1983;**59**:42–7.
3 Clutton-Brock TH, Hutton P. Central venous and pulmonary artery catheterization. In: Hutton P, Prys-Roberts C, eds. *Monitoring in anaesthesia and intensive care.* London: WB Saunders, 1994: 145–55.
4 Roizen M, Berger D, Gabel R. Practical guidelines for pulmonary artery catheterization. *Anesthesiology* 1993;**78**:380–94.
5 Runciman WB, Ilsley AH, Roberts JG. An evaluation of thermodilution cardiac output measurement using the Swan-Ganz catheter. *Anaesth Intensive Care* 1981;**9**:208–20.
6 Tobin M. Respiratory monitoring. *JAMA* 1990;**264**:244–53.
7 Adams AP, Hahn CEW. *Principles and practice of blood gas analysis,* 2nd edn. Edinburgh: Churchill Livingstone, 1982.
8 Clayton D, Webb KK, Ralston AC, Duthie D, Runciman WB. A comparison of 20 pulse oximeters under conditions of poor perfusion. *Anaesthesia* 1991;**46**:3–10.
9 Fletcher R. Capnography. In: Hutton P, Prys-Roberts C, eds. *Monitoring in anaesthesia and intensive care.* London: WB Saunders, 1994: 214–31.

**Futher reading**

Hutton P, Prys-Roberts C, eds. *Monitoring in anaesthesia and intensive care.* London: WB Saunders, 1994.
Moyle JTB, Hahn CEW, Adams AP, eds. *Pulse oximetry.* London: BMJ Publishing Group, 1994.

# 12: Acute lung injury and respiratory support

S J BRETT and T W EVANS

For almost half a century it has been known that patients who initially survive an episode of acute illness or trauma are at risk of developing respiratory failure (Figure 12.1). The precipitating event need not involve the lungs, and the onset of such respiratory failure may herald a period of critical illness and often the demise of the patient. Respiratory failure in this context is often recognised as merely the pulmonary manifestation of a more global disease, in which vascular endothelial dysfunction is the pivotal pathological process.

In 1967, Ashbaugh and his colleagues described a heterogeneous group of 12 patients who developed acute respiratory failure in association with a variety of medical, surgical, and traumatic insults.[1] The authors characterised the key features of the syndrome, known variously as "shock lung", the "adult respiratory distress syndrome", or "acute respiratory distress syndrome" (ARDS). The important features noted were:

- dyspnoea
- tachypnoea
- cyanosis refractory to oxygen therapy
- loss of lung compliance
- diffuse alveolar infiltrates visible on the chest radiograph.

These features, with some refinements, remain the cornerstones of diagnosis today. The mortality rate of the original series was 58.3% with similar statistics being reported in many modern series.

## Spectrum of disease and definition

A variety of disease states is associated with the development of lung injury, the commonest of which are listed in Box 12.1. Estimates of the exact incidence of ARDS are problematic owing to differing definitions and study populations, but they vary between 1·5 and 75 cases per 100 000 population per year. Estimates of mortality rates are similarly difficult to interpret and range from 35 to 75%, related to the case-mix, as the risk of death is at least partially dependent upon the underlying disease. Thus, young patients with ARDS from trauma have a better outlook than elderly patients with faecal peritonitis. Furthermore, patients who die early *tend* to

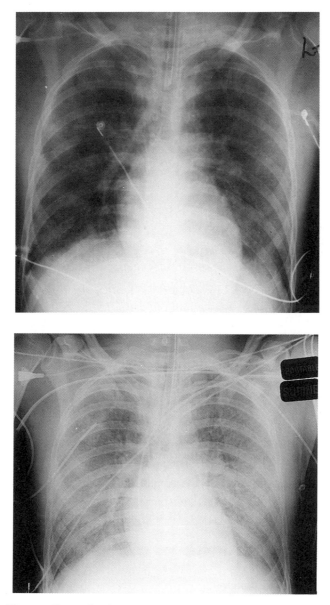

Fig 12.1   Chest radiograph of an 18 year-old man who had sustained a fractured femur in a road accident. (a) The radiograph was taken at the end of surgery to fix his femur internally. At this stage he had become hypoxaemic, and alveolar shadowing is evident. (b) Chest radiograph taken 24 hours later. Widespread, dense, alveolar shadowing is evident, as are central venous and pulmonary artery catheters and a chest drain.

---

**Box 12.1**   *Precipitating factors for ALI/ARDS*

**"Direct" injury to lung**

- Infection
- Aspiration
- Blunt trauma or blast injury
- Inhalation of toxic substances
- Near drowning

**"Indirect" injury to lung**

- Sepsis
- Polytrauma
- Fat embolism syndrome
- Cardiopulmonary bypass
- Prolonged hypotension
- Pancreatitis
- Massive blood transfusion
- Bone marrow transplant
- Certain drugs and toxins, *e.g.* paraquat

---

die from their underlying disease rather than from respiratory failure. By contrast, late deaths are attributable to sepsis and the failure of other organ systems. The combination of respiratory failure with either renal or hepatic failure carries a particularly poor prognosis.

The lack of unified diagnostic criteria has also created difficulties in interpreting the results of clinical trials. Consequently, an American–European Consensus Conference discussed the problem and published the results of their deliberations in 1994.[2] The key features of this unified diagnosis are outlined in Box 12.2. The definition has a number of merits: it is simple and does not rely on difficult or derived calculations;

---

**Box 12.2**   *Consensus definition of ALI/ARDS*[a]

- Appropriate precipitating condition, or one or more risk factors

- New bilateral fluffy infiltrates on chest radiograph[b]

- No clinical evidence of cardiac failure, fluid overload, or chronic lung disease (pulmonary artery occlusion pressure < 18 mm Hg)[c]

**PLUS**

Acute lung injury
- Oxygenation deficit as defined by:

$$Pao_2:Fio_2 \text{ ratio} < 40^d$$

**Acute respiratory distess**
- Oxygenation deficit as defined by:

$$Pao_2:Fio_2 \text{ ratio} < 20^d$$

[a] Adapted from Bernard *et al*,[2] with permission.
[b] Appearance on chest radiograph may lag behind clinical course.
[c] Patients with chronic lung disease may have abnormal radiological appearance or gas exchange prior to acute insult.
[d] Ventilatory maneuvres will alter this parameter and these must be carefully recorded.

---

complicated equipment is not required to produce the variables involved; and it is independent of the level of positive end-expiratory pressure (PEEP) applied during mechanical ventilation, making data from different groups more comparable, as PEEP strategies are notoriously variable. Other notable features include: the use of the term "acute" rather than "adult", in recognition that the syndrome can also afflict children, and the division of acute lung injury into two broad levels of severity – the term ARDS representing the severe and acute lung injury (ALI), the mild end of a spectrum of injury. These definitions are becoming widely employed in both clinical and scientific practice.

Because mortality is not related exclusively to the severity of lung injury, the development of severity of illness scoring systems specific to ALI/ARDS has been limited. Generalised systems are becoming highly developed and those said to be capable of producing an estimated predicted mortality for a given individual are currently undergoing clinical evaluation. The most applicable and widely quoted organ-specific score is the Lung Injury Score (LIS) of Murray and colleagues,[3] which involves calculating the aggregated score from four quantifiable variables:

- appearance on chest radiograph;
- the ratio of arterial oxygen tension to inspired fraction of oxygen ($Pao_2$/$Fio_2$ ratio);
- the level of PEEP applied;
- calculated respiratory system compliance (Box 12.3).

This system is simple, but insensitive in that a maximum possible score of 4 will have a limited capacity to define the severity of the whole spectrum of disease. Second, the increasing recognition of the systemic nature of ARDS makes such organ-specific scores redundant. Finally, the scoring of chest radiographs is subjective and in practice patients with anything other than limited disease invariably score 4, making this component a poor discriminator.

## Pathology

The lung has a limited repertoire of histological responses to injury, and morphological studies provide limited data concerning the underlying pathophysiology of ARDS. Interpretation of tissue specimens is rendered difficult by complications that occur commonly during the course of an episode of ARDS, such as nosocomial infection, iatrogenic lung damage caused by high pressure and volume ventilation, and the use of high concentrations of inspired oxygen. Furthermore, the disease is distributed in a non-homogeneous manner, with areas of spared, normal lung adjacent to diseased, consolidated tissue. Additionally, different parts of the lung may exhibit the features of different phases of the disease (see below).

Simultaneously, the procedure is accompanied by considerable risks, and therefore difficult to justify for an individual patient. Lung biopsy is therefore of limited value in clinical practice, and *antemortem* histological data are sparse.

The histopathological features result from disruption of the alveolar-capillary unit (termed "diffuse alveolar damage"), and may be divided into three phases which, although overlapping, correlate loosely with clinical progression.

### Exudative phase

The exudative phase occupies approximately the first week after the onset of respiratory failure. *Post mortem* the lungs are stiff, dull red in colour, and

---

**Box 12.3**   *Lung injury score*[a]

**1. Chest radiograph score**
- No alveolar consolidation                                    0
- Alveolar consolidation confined to 1 quadrant      1
- Alveolar consolidation confined to 2 quadrants    2
- Alveolar consolidation confined to 3 quadrants    3
- Alveolar consolidation in all 4 quadrants             4

**2. Hypoxaemia ($Pao_2/Fio_2$) score (calculated from $Pao_2$ in mm Hg)**
$\geq 300$      0
225–299    1
175–224    2
100–174    3
$< 100$       4

**3. PEEP score (when ventilated)**
$\geq 5$ cm $H_2O$       0
6–8 cm $H_2O$       1
9–11 cm $H_2O$     2
12–14 cm $H_2O$   3
$\geq 15$ cm $H_2O$     4

**4. Respiratory system compliance (when available)**
$\geq 80$ ml/cm $H_2O$      0
60–79 ml/cm $H_2O$      1
40–59 ml/cm $H_2O$      2
20–39 ml/cm $H_2O$      3
$\leq 19$ ml/cm $H_2O$      4

The final score is obtained by dividing the aggregate sum by the number of components that were used:

- No lung injury                              score = 0
- Mild to moderate lung injury      score = 0.1–2.5
- Severe lung injury                         score = > 2.5

[a] Adapted from Murray *et al*,[3] with permission.

---

greatly increased in weight (up to 1 kg each). The cut surface does not exude fluid, unlike cardiogenic oedema, because of the high protein content of alveolar fluid causing it to coagulate. Light microscopy reveals eosinophilic hyaline membranes, which are prominent in alveolar ducts and are characteristic of early ARDS. This material is composed of a mixture of plasma protein, which has leaked through the damaged endothelial–epithelial barrier, and cell debris. Focal aggregations of neutrophils are visible in capillaries. Alveolar septa demonstrate interstitial oedema, fibrin, and extravasated red cells. The alveolar epithelium displays necrosis of type-I cells. These slough from the basement membrane leaving a hyaline membrane and a population of type II cells, which are relatively resistant to damage and proliferate to replace the type I cells during repair. This process may start as early as day 3 after the initial insult.

## Proliferative phase

The proliferative phase is characterised by the organisation of intra-alveolar and interstitial exudates. Postmortem specimens obtained between the first and third week after injury exhibit the macroscopic appearance of solid lung, with a dull and slippery parenchymal texture attributable to the production of new connective tissue. Light microscopy demonstrates a new cuboidal epithelium covering the previously raw basement membrane. These cells stain immunohistochemically with features of type II cells. Fibroblasts and myofibroblasts proliferate in the alveolar wall and migrate into the exudate within the intra-alveolar space, producing granulation tissue that is ultimately converted into fibrous tissue. Collapsed and damaged alveolar walls may become sealed in apposition by overexuberant repair mechanisms. This process, termed "collapse induration", leads to fewer but larger alveoli and dilated alveolar ducts. The vascular lumina become compromised from the accumulation of cellular and protein debris, contributing to a loss of cross-sectional area of the pulmonary circulation.

## Fibrotic phase

The fibrotic phase may begin as early as day 10 after lung injury, and is associated with an increase in lung collagen. The lung surface is coarse and the cut parenchymal surface is spongy with microcystic air spaces and patchy scarring. Healed abscesses and chronic interstitial emphysema cause larger cysts in chronic ARDS. Extensive remodelling of the pulmonary vasculature occurs. Arteries become tortuous with mural fibrosis and narrowed lumina, and muscularisation of pre- and intra-acinar vessels is demonstrable. These processes undoubtedly contribute to the irreversible pulmonary hypertension which is a feature of pulmonary fibrosis secondary to ARDS.

Postmortem examination of lungs reveals thromboemboli in up to 95%

119

of cases. Postmortem angiograms demonstrate macrothrombi (in arteries >1 mm in diameter) in 86% of patients, but these are more common in specimens from patients succumbing early in the course of their disease. These thrombi may be embolic or produced *in situ*. ARDS patients are certainly predisposed to embolic events by their immobility, central cannulation, cardiac rhythm disturbances, and (often) underlying disease. Haemorrhagic infarcts and areas of necrosis are common, particularly in areas of peripheral lung adjacent to visceral pleura.

## Pathophysiology

It has become clear that many illnesses, under certain circumstances, elicit a host response that may be harmful. This takes the form of an uncontrolled or inappropriate activation of mechanisms normally involved in immune or inflammatory function, and pivotal to this is the cytokine series discussed in Chapter 7. These compounds, including tumour necrosis factor $\alpha$ (TNF$\alpha$), interleukins (IL)-1$\alpha$, -2, -6, and -8, platelet-activating factor (PAF), and a variety of others, are released from immune and/or endothelial cells. Once started, this process becomes amplified by positive feedback mechanisms. This activation has three important consequences:

- a number of these compounds are directly toxic to endothelium;
- upregulation and activation of neutrophils occurs;
- there is an increased expression of adhesion molecules on activated endothelial cell membranes.

The mean diameter of a pulmonary capillary is approximately 7·5 μm, and that of a neutrophil 6·8 μm. There is considerable overlap, and neutrophil traffic through the lung is therefore dependent on neutrophil deformability. Activated neutrophils are less deformable; moreover activation leads to an increased expression of surface adhesion molecules. These are ligands for endothelial adhesion molecules whose expression is upregulated by the presence of bacterial endotoxin, cytokines, and complement system products. IL-8 (released by endothelial cells) and certain products of complement activation create a chemotactic gradient increasing neutrophil recruitment to the lungs, and their adhesion to the vascular endothelium.[4,5] Subsequent events may include endothelial penetration and extravasation with the appearance of neutrophils in alveolar spaces (recoverable by bronchoalveolar lavage). Non-activated neutrophils do not exhibit these features, and there is experimental evidence that endothelial adhesion molecule blockers prevent the development of lung injury from endotoxin infusion.

Neutrophils injure the endothelium and alveolar epithelium by releasing proteolytic enzymes, reactive oxygen species, and inflammatory mediators.

The endothelium loses its integrity, and fluid and plasma protein leak into the interstitium and thence to the alveoli, producing the so-called "non-cardiogenic" pulmonary oedema.

The physical stability of the alveolus is dependent on the surface tension-reducing properties of a lung surface-active phospholipid (surfactant), produced by type II pneumocytes. The presence of plasma protein reduces the effectiveness of surfactant and the alveoli become pneumatically unstable and tend to collapse.[6] La Place's law relates the radius of a bubble, its internal pressure, and surface tension. If surface tension remains constant, pressure is inversely related to radius, that is, the smaller the bubble, the greater the pressure. Small alveoli would therefore empty into larger neighbours. The heavy, oedematous nature of the lung exacerbates this tendency, and these two physical factors probably account for the dependent distribution of atelectasis and oedema so characteristic of ARDS (Figure 12.2).

There is increasing evidence that inflammatory responses cause the expression of inducible forms of various enzymes such as nitric oxide synthase (iNOS)[7] and cyclo-oxygenase (COX II),[8] which are not under normal regulatory control and produce large quantities of vasoactive products. The nature of pulmonary vascular dysfunction in ALI is complex. Pulmonary hypertension is common and almost certainly due to a combination of mechanical blockage of the vasculature with fibrin and cellular debris, hypoxic pulmonary vasoconstriction (HPV), and impaired local vascular control. There are areas of the lung with profound

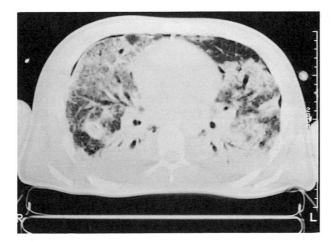

Fig 12.2 Typical CT scan of a patient with severe ARDS. Dense consolidation is visible, with a predominantly dependent distribution. Non-consolidated lung demonstrates typical "ground-glass" shadowing; there is almost no normal lung visible.

121

vasoconstriction, and yet simultaneously other areas exhibiting vasodilatation, contributing to a markedly increased shunt fraction. This may be reduced using almitrine dimesylate, a drug that improves the efficiency of HPV, although at the cost of worsening pulmonary hypertension. This failure of ventilation–perfusion matching has been shown to be responsible for the entire gas exchange deficit seen in ALI, without any increased barrier to diffusion.[9]

## Clinical presentation

Acute lung injury is normally apparent within 1–3 days of the start of a precipitating illness, although direct insults to the lung may present more acutely. Patients most commonly complain of dyspnoea, with increasing respiratory rate, hypoxaemia, and evidence of new infiltrates on the chest radiograph. Patients already mechanically ventilated tend to require increased inspired oxygen concentration ($F_{IO_2}$), in association with decreasing lung compliance. In the early stages of the disease, arterial blood gas analysis often shows normo- or hypocapnia.

The chest radiograph shows patchy alveolar shadowing (see Figure 12.1a). Hydrostatic and hypo-oncotic oedema are excluded by normal pulmonary artery occlusion pressure (PAOP) and serum albumin respectively. Frequently, respiratory failure becomes apparent after an episode of volume resuscitation for severe cardiovascular instability, in spite of careful efforts to avoid fluid overload.

The diffential diagnosis of acute respiratory failure includes pneumonia, and assessing the contribution of infection at presentation is important. Inappropriate use of antibiotics encourages colonisation with resistant nosocomial organisms. Pneumonia may itself precipitate an episode of ALI. Features associated with infection include a history of cough and/or the production of purulent sputum, fever (or hypopyrexia), and leukocytosis (or occasionally leukopenia). The chest radiograph may be initially unimpressive or show localised areas of increased shadowing; ALI may present with predominantly unilateral radiological changes, but this is unusual. Atypical pneumonias often present with gastrointestinal disturbance, confusion, and hyponatraemia.

## Assessment, investigation, and monitoring

As there is currently no specific therapy for lung injury, the diagnosis and treatment of the underlying disease, and in particular the eradication of sepsis, are of critical importance. All organ systems require a degree of monitoring to allow maximisation of support. The response of individual patients to particular therapeutic interventions is difficult to predict and constant re-evaluation is important.

## Cardiovascular system

Adequate tissue oxygen delivery ($Do_2$) is required, and therefore cardiac output must be maintained (Box 12.4). The dysfunctional nature of the pulmonary vascular endothelium means that adequate right ventricular output must be achieved with the lowest possible capillary pressures. This requires a careful titration of fluid balance and often inotropic support. Cardiac dysfunction is common in critical illness; moreover high intra-thoracic pressures may make the assessment of appropriate cardiac filling difficult. Assessment of pulmonary and systemic haemodynamics almost always requires the insertion of a pulmonary artery catheter. Estimates of

---

**Box 12.4** *Calculation of oxygen delivery and consumption*

**1. Oxygen delivery ($Do_2$)**

$$Do_2 = \text{cardiac output (l/min)} \times \text{arterial oxygen content } (Cao_2; \text{ml/l})$$

where

$$(Cao_2) = (1 \cdot 34 \times Hb[g/l] \times [Sao_2/100]).$$

$1 \cdot 34$ represents the binding capacity of haemoglobin for oxygen normally quoted as $1 \cdot 34$ ml $O_2$/g haemoglobin.

$Sao_2$ is the oxygen saturation of arterial blood, which should be the value measured with a co-oximeter, rather than the derived value from a blood gas analyser.

This equation ignores the minute amount of oxygen in physical solution in blood.

**2. Oxygen consumption ($\dot{V}o_2$)**

$$\dot{V}o_2 = \text{cardiac output} \times (Cao_2 - C\dot{v}o_2)$$

where

$C\dot{v}o_2$ is the mixed venous oxygen content. This is calculated by substituting mixed venous saturation instead of arterial saturation in arterial oxygen content equation.

This equation ignores the consumption of oxygen by the lungs.

Both $Do_2$ and $\dot{V}o_2$ are often indexed for body surface area ($Do_2I$ and $\dot{V}o_2I$ respectively), in which case the cardiac index is substituted for cardiac output in the appropriate equations.

---

cardiac output and preload allow a ventricular function curve to be produced, which allows the optimisation of volume status and output. A certain amount of volume loading may be required, even though the oedematous nature of the lungs prompts an attempt to achieve a negative fluid balance. A PAOP of 10–12 mm Hg would be a reasonable initial target, but patients with pre-existing cardiac disease or sepsis-induced cardiac dysfunction may require higher pressures.

## Respiratory system

The mainstays of respiratory system assessment are arterial blood gas analysis and the chest radiograph. The former permits the monitoring of both disease progression and the response to interventions, and the latter (normally performed on a daily basis) helps in assessing fluid balance, the search for infection, and the early detection of complications such as pneumothorax. The lateral "shoot through" film may be helpful in locating occult pneumothoraces.

In recent years computed tomography (CT) has played an increasing part in both research and clinical management of lung injury. An early CT scan may be helpful in assessing the amount and distribution of fluid overload and its degree of dependency. This aids in decisions concerning nursing the patient in the prone position or the use of high-frequency ventilation (see below). Later, CT scans can assist in defining the extent of lung fibrosis and are invaluable in the search for occult abscesses or loculated pneumothoraces and pneumatoceles, for which the plain radiograph is inadequate. In most hospitals, the CT scanner is physically separate from the intensive care unit, but on occasion the risks of moving the patient are easily outweighed by the clinical utility of the information provided.

Bronchoalveolar lavage (which should be performed by an experienced bronchoscopist) may provide useful specimens for microbiological investigation, and allow directed physiotherapy. Many patients pass through a phase during which their airways become inflamed and produce large quantities of mucus. At this time they are vulnerable to acute deteriorations caused by "plugging" of major airways, and careful and repeated bronchoscopy may be invaluable.

## Research techniques

A variety of devices and techniques has become available through research. These include:

124

- lung water computers;
- assessment of endothelial permeability to radiolabelled protein;
- measurement of damage to plasma constituents from reactive oxygen species;
- cytokine levels in plasma and lavage fluid;
- surfactant function;
- differential cell counts from bronchoalveolar lavage.

Although these techniques provide interesting data concerning pathological processes, they have yet to translate into useful clinical tools.


## Aspects of general patient care

Day-to-day management requires attention to detail. Scrupulous physical examination with a search for infection and evaluation of intravascular and other catheter sites is mandatory. Nutritional support is important and vigorous attempts should be made to provide nutrition via the enteral route. Only if this remains impossible is parenteral support acceptable. Mucosal protection using sucralfate or an $H_2$-receptor blocker is required, although the latter is associated with an increased incidence of nosocomial colonisation. Selective decontamination of the digestive tract is recommended by some authorities and reduces the incidence of nosocomial pneumonia, but mortality is uninfluenced, and the cost-effectiveness of the technique is open to question.

The diagnosis and management of nosocomial infection may be very difficult. Patients with active systemic inflammation frequently have fever, tachycardia, and a leukocytosis. Persistent attempts at culture may be negative and the picture can be complicated by previous antibiotic therapy. Clinical skill is important and changes in vital signs, haemodynamic stability, the quantity and quality of sputum, chest radiological appearences, and white cell count can provide the necessary evidence. If clinically warranted, blind antibiotic therapy should be initiated (after appropriate culture). Typically, therapy should cover Gram-negative and -positive organisms, each with two agents of differing pharmacological groups. This reduces the emergence of resistant strains. Such a regimen might consist of teicoplanin, piperacillin, and an aminoglycoside. Regimens should be adapted to local microbiological conditions and the advice of a microbiologist should be sought.

The isolation of fungal organisms from blood, or two or more extraoral sites, should prompt the consideration of systemic antifungal therapy. Fluconazole and amphotericin B are commonly used, and the newer colloidal or liposomal preparations of the latter are markedly less toxic.

125

# Ventilating the injured lung

## Continuous positive airway pressure

Patients with mild disease may occasionally be managed with simple respiratory support such as oxygen administered via a facemask with or without continuous positive airway pressure (CPAP). The latter is not easy to administer, but can reduce the increased work of breathing attributable to stiff, non-compliant lungs. In practice, most patients will require endotracheal intubation and mechanical ventilation.

## Indications for mechanical ventilation

There are a variety of blood gas criteria available as indications for ventilation (for example, a $Pao_2$ of 10 kPa with an $Fio_2$ of 0·5), but in practice most intensivists take a more holistic approach, regarding *changes* in variables (especially the $Pao_2/Fio_2$ ratio) as important. Additionally, an increasing respiratory rate, impending patient exhaustion, impaired conscious level, failure to cooperate with CPAP or physiotherapy, metabolic acidosis, and the requirement to eliminate the influence of large respiratory swings on haemodynamic measurements all contribute to the decision to ventilate. In patients with severe hypoxaemia, the requirement for reducing the oxygen consumption of overworked respiratory muscles is also important.

## Principles of mechanical ventilation

In recent years evidence from CT scanning has demonstrated the non-homogeneous nature of the condition with patchy collapse, consolidation, and areas of inflammation. Consolidated lung is not available for ventilation and vigorous attempts to expand these areas will lead to overdistension and damage (so-called volotrauma) to relatively disease-free lung. The lungs therefore behave as if they are functionally small. Collapsed but not consolidated lung may be amenable to what has become known as "alveolar recruitment" and this is discussed below.

## Targets for gas exchange

Until recently the conventional strategy for ventilating patients with ALI/ARDS employed normal blood gas tensions as therapeutic goals. This meant applying large tidal volumes (up to 15 ml/kg), and high levels of inspired oxygen and PEEP, often resulting in very high peak inspiratory pressures (> 45 cm $H_2O$), reducing venous return to the heart, causing direct cardiac compression which resulted in haemodynamic instability. Large inspiratory volumes and high levels of $Fio_2$ are almost certainly harmful and attempting to normalise blood gas tensions is not an appropriate therapeutic goal. A reasonable target for oxygenation is a $Pao_2$ of 7·5–8 kPa, while allowing the $Paco_2$ to rise to 10–14 kPa (known as "permissive hypercapnia"), provided that the acid–base status is acceptable and that there is no evidence of cerebral oedema. Damaged lungs may have a markedly increased physiological dead space and the achievement of normocapnia requires a large minute ventilation. In patients with ARDS (compared with severe asthma), however, the degree of permissive hypercapnia is sometimes limited by the associated rise in pulmonary artery pressures.

## Alveolar recruitment

### Definition

Pneumatic stability of the lung is impaired and, by opening collapsed alveoli and maintaining them in an inflated state throughout the respiratory cycle, the respiratory gas may be employed as a "pneumatic splint", preventing alveolar collapse on expiration and improving the mechanical characteristics of the stiff lung. This approach is termed "alveolar", or occasionally volume, recruitment.

### Positive end-expiratory pressure

Alveolar recruitment can be achieved in a number of ways, the most commonly used being the application of PEEP. At levels up to 14 cm $H_2O$ this prevents the end-expiratory collapse of alveoli opened by the previous inspiratory cycle. Experimental evidence shows that ventilation involving tidal alveolar collapse and re-recruitment is particularly harmful, and that this may be ameliorated by applying an adequate level of PEEP,[10] although improved oxygenation may often be seen only some 30–40 minutes later. Active recruitment using PEEP probably only occurs at levels > 12 cm $H_2O$, but this is often associated with haemodynamic disturbance.

As discussed earlier, PEEP may improve oxygenation at the expense of cardiac performance, and so a level of PEEP should be selected that maximises oxygen delivery, rather than $Pao_2$ itself. Increasing PEEP to high levels may also overdistend the lungs. Clearly, the level of PEEP applied must be continuously evaluated in order to avoid detrimental effects.

### Inverse ratio ventilation

Common ventilator modes are defined in Box 12.5. Ventilation may be either volume controlled, in whch the key parameter is a pre-set tidal volume delivered to the respiratory system regardless of pressure required, or pressure controlled, in which a fixed pressure is applied to the respiratory system creating a variable tidal volume dependent on the system mechanics (see below). The mean airway pressure throughout the respiratory cycle is an important determinant of alveolar recruitment and oxygenation. Provided that peak and plateau pressures can be kept low, a high mean pressure improves compliance and alveolar recruitment. A conventional inspiratory (I):expiratory (E) ratio is 1:3 and is standard for ventilating patients with normal lungs in the operating room (Figure 12.3). Prolonging the inspiratory time means that the respiratory system is under positive pressure for a greater proportion of the cycle and therefore the mean pressure is increased. The inspiratory time can be prolonged until the I:E ratio is reversed (that is, inverse ratio ventilation, IRV). A similar effect can be achieved by using high-frequency jet ventilation with frequencies around the resonant frequency of the lung (5 Hz). However, high mean airway

---

**Box 12.5**  *Common terms associated with ventilators*

- **Intermittent positive-pressure ventilation (IPPV)**
  Standard mode of ventilation in which all breaths are machine initiated and controlled. No provision is made for patient breaths. This is standard operating room type ventilation which requires deep sedation and often neuromuscular blockade. This is sometimes termed "controlled mechanical ventilation" or CMV.

- **Intermittent mandatory ventilation (IMV)**
  This mode allows the patient to breathe from the ventilator which has an additional circuit with a constant gas flow. This may be useful during weaning. Patient need not be deeply sedated, and the number of machine breaths may be progressively reduced. The main disadvantage is that the machine may provide an inspiratory volume as the patient is attempting to exhale.

- **Mandatory minute ventilation (MMV)**
  Modification of IMV that allows the patient to receive a pre-set minute volume despite variable spontaneous respiration, that is, the machine makes up for any shortfall. Not used frequently.

- **Synchronised intermittent mandatory ventilation (SIMV)**
  Modification of IMV that allows spontaneous breathing from an additional circuit which has a sensitive demand valve. A patient breath inhibits a machine breath and prevents machine-driven inspiration during patient exhalation. This is currently a very common form of support, especially during weaning.

- **Pressure support**
  The machine senses a spontaneous respiratory effort, by detecting either a pressure or flow change, and increases the pressure in the breathing circuit (to, for example, 20 cm $H_2O$). This reduces the work of breathing considerably, and is often used to support patient breaths during SIMV. It is also a very common weaning tool, during which the pressure support level is progresively reduced. Some ventilators have this feature labelled as "assisted spontaneous breathing" or ASB.

---

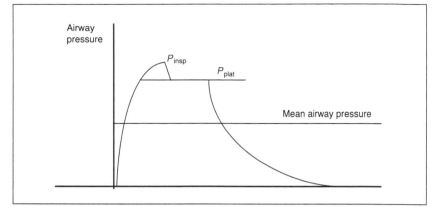

Fig 12.3  Detail of typical pressure–time profile for a volume-controlled ventilator inspiratory stroke, with a short inspiratory pause. $P_{insp}$ and $P_{plat}$ represent peak and plateau pressures, respectively. The pressure drop between these two values is due to redistribution of gas between lung units with different time constants.

pressures can also be transmitted to the pulmonary and systemic circulations and reduce cardiac preload. This again impairs cardiac performance and renders estimates of preload such as central venous and pulmonary artery occlusion pressures difficult to interpret.

Volume-controlled inverse ratio ventilation can result in high inflation pressures and progressive "stacking" of breaths, due to incomplete expiration before the next inspiratory volume is delivered. Pressure-controlled inverse ratio ventilation (PC-IRV) with the I:E ratio up to 2:1 is less likely to cause this. The lungs are inflated to a pre-set pressure, which is maintained until the machine cycles to expiration, resulting in a decelerating gas inflow pattern (Figure 12.4). This technique provides good gas exchange and haemodynamic stability, although gas trapping can occur. This is most likely when PC-IRV is combined with PEEP, or if the patient has pre-existing obstructive pulmonary disease. Gas trapping is manifest as thoracic overdistension, falling compliance, and worsening haemo-dynamics, signs that should be actively sought in all patients.

Tidal volume is controlled by the interrelationship of the preselected pressure level, typically between 30 and 40 cm $H_2O$, and the respiratory system mechanics. This often results in a tidal volume of 8–12 ml/kg, but this will change if compliance or airway resistance changes and careful monitoring is mandatory. Levels of peak pressure > 40 cm $H_2O$ are associated with lung damage such as pneumothorax and interstitial emphysema. One major disadvantage of IRV is that it is uncomfortable for the patient and largely not tolerated without profound sedation and often paralysis. Although this approach is theoretically attractive, and in Europe is

129

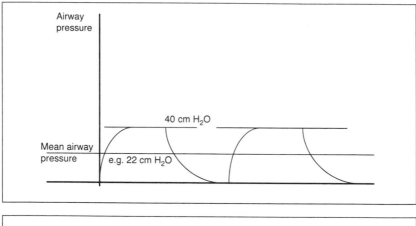

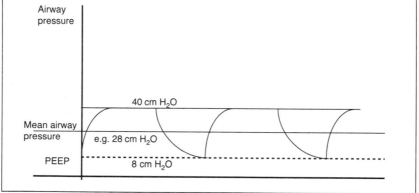

Fig 12.4(a)   Two pressure-controlled inspiratory strokes with an I:E ratio prolonged to approximately 1:1. $P_{insp}$ has been eliminated and $P_{plat}$ is controlled by the
ventilator setting. (b) Pressure-controlled ventilation with an I:E ratio of approximately 2:1; note that the application of PEEP prevents the system pressure ever
declining to zero. There is no $P_{insp}$ effect; mean airway pressure remains high but
acceptable.

becoming a standard strategy,[11-13] it has not been shown definitively to
improve outcome.

### High-frequency jet ventilation

High-frequency jet ventilation (HFJV), using frequencies of 4–8 Hz, is
currently undergoing evaluation as a means of minimising peak and plateau
pressures, while increasing mean airway pressure and therefore alveolar
recruitment, and controlling $Pa_{CO_2}$. The technique requires considerable
expertise and treatment is commonly associated with the development of
multiple pneumothoraces. Early problems encountered with monitoring

the patient–ventilator interaction and inadequate humidification have largely been overcome.

## Prone positioning

CT scans demonstrate the non-homogeneous distribution of lung lesions, with a predominantly dependent distribution (see Figure 12.2). Nursing the patient prone, for periods of 6–8 hours, can improve gas exchange and alveolar recruitment, both by improving $\dot{V}/\dot{Q}$ (ventilation–perfusion) matching and by altering the distribution of oedema.[14] The dangers and difficulties of turning critically ill patients are considerable.

## Recovery and weaning

After 7 days of mechanical ventilatory support, few patients wean quickly from the ventilator, and a tracheostomy is desirable to avoid the complications of long-term oral intubation, such as subglottic stenosis. Subsequent to this the sedation can often be lightened and frequently the patient will tolerate ventilatory support while awake.

A good index of recovery is the $F_{IO_2}$ required to produce adequate oxygenation ($P_{aO_2} > 8$ kPa), and when this has been diminished to 0·4–0·5 ventilatory support may be reduced. This involves normalising the I:E ratio and reducing PEEP, and at this point it is often possible to allow some spontaneous ventilation with the use of ventilator modes such as synchronised intermittent mandatory ventilation (SIMV) plus inspiratory pressure support. The support can be withdrawn over days or weeks as necessary, while the patient's respiratory muscles improve. A period of CPAP is often provided prior to decannulation.

# Non-ventilatory respiratory support

Attempts to provide extrapulmonary gas exchange to "rest" the lung, thereby facilitating repair and diminishing iatrogenic pulmonary damage, have met with only limited success and have yet to become standard therapy. Gas exchange may be achieved using an extracorporeal circuit incorporating a membrane oxygenator similar to that used during cardiac surgery (extracorporeal membrane oxygenation, ECMO). Initial studies employed total pulmonary bypass with arterial and venous cannulation and total circuit heparinisation; this resulted in significant coagulopathy and haemorrhage and so were not successful. Recently, advances in cannula design, the availability of heparin-bonded circuits, the development of vortex centrifugal pumps, and alterations in therapeutic strategy have lead to a resurgence of interest. Later studies have used venovenous cannulation (with reduced blood loss), with the aim of increasing mixed venous $O_2$ tension and reducing $CO_2$ tension. The extracorporeal circuit is used in

131

combination with low-frequency, low-volume mechanical ventilation to facilitate oxygenation.[15] This approach, termed extracorporeal $CO_2$ removal, has been associated with success in some centres, but the only controlled prospective trial has shown no advantage in outcome compared to conventional ventilation.

An alternative approach is to insert a gas-exchanging device intracorporeally. The intravenous oxygenator or IVOX (Cardiopulmonics Inc., Salt Lake City, USA) is a hollow fibre device which can be inserted percutaneously into the vena cava and right atrium. Oxygen is drawn through the device under negative pressure and gas exchange occurs at the fibre–blood interface.[16] Apart from isolated cases, the performance of the device was disappointing and it was withdrawn from use, although research is continuing.

Overall, the results of extrapulmonary gas exchange in adults have been mixed. A reasonable role is to employ such techniques only when all other (conventional) approaches have failed to achieve satisfactory gas exchange.

## Maintenance of tissue oxygen delivery

The prevention of dysfunction and failure in other organ systems is dependent upon the adequate provision of oxygen and nutrients via the blood stream. The delivery of oxygen to tissues ($Do_2$) may be estimated from the product of the cardiac output and the oxygen content of arterial blood (see Box 12.4). More acurately, this represents merely the dispatch of oxygen into the aorta; however, the concept does have some clinical value. Tissue oxygen consumption ($\dot{V}o_2$) can be estimated from the arteriovenous oxygen content difference and the cardiac output, or can be measured directly with a metabolic monitor. The maintenance of $Do_2$ therefore requires a balance between providing adequate cardiac performance and using judicious fluid and inotrope support, in combination with adequate oxygenation, achieved with minimal ventilator-induced cardiovascular depression. Trials investigating the effects of artificially elevating $Do_2$ and $\dot{V}o_2$ in patients with established multiple organ failure have produced conflicting results. However, many intensivists would consider actively increasing the $Do_2$ when faced with evidence of inadequate tissue oxygenation.

## Pharmacological approaches to lung injury

Drug therapy in ALI/ARDS has been developed in a number of key areas:

- to improve oxygenation and pulmonary haemodynamics;
- to modify the global inflammatory process;

- using agents aimed at inhibiting specific mediators of the disease process at a molecular level.

Recently, there have been attempts to improve alveolar stability using artificial surfactant.

## Pulmonary vascular manipulation

A number of vasodilators have been employed in attempts to reduce pulmonary hypertension and right ventricular dysfunction. Conventional vasodilator agents (such as sodium nitroprusside, glyceryl trinitrate, or calcium channel blockers) delivered to the pulmonary circulation produce systemic hypotension, in addition to any effect seen on the pulmonary vasculature. Furthermore, non-specific pulmonary vasodilatation produces a worsening in gas exchange owing to an increase in perfusion of non-ventilated alveolar units.

The delivery of agents with short duration of action via the ventilator has some theoretical advantages. Such inhaled drugs are only delivered to ventilated lung units, producing local vasodilatation and recruiting blood flow to aerated alveoli. This improves $\dot{V}/\dot{Q}$ matching (hence reducing shunt fraction), and reduces pulmonary vascular tone. Provided that the drug half-life is sufficiently short, there should be little systemic haemodynamic effect. Inhaled prostacyclin, administered via a nebuliser, has shown promising results both in improving oxygenation and in reducing pulmonary pressures.[17]

Nitric oxide (NO), an endogenous endothelially derived vasodilator, can also be administered via the ventilator. At concentrations of 0·1–50 parts per million, NO causes vasodilatation in ventilated areas improving $\dot{V}/\dot{Q}$ matching and oxygenation. Reductions in pulmonary artery pressures are also apparent.[18–21] Although this therapy shows promise, the technical aspects of administration are complex and no study has demonstrated a convincing improvement in survival. Moreover, concerns about direct NO-mediated toxicity have yet to be adequately addressed.[22] Such toxicity studies as have been performed have involved animals with healthy lungs, and there are theoretical reasons why NO may have enhanced toxicity in inflamed lungs.

## Anti-inflammatory therapy

Non-steroidal anti-inflammatory drugs, such as ibuprofen, inhibit the cyclo-oxygenase-mediated aspects of the inflammatory process. High-dose studies in animal models have shown some promise and the results of a clinical trial in human disease are awaited. The place of high-dose steroid therapy remains unclear, but some experts believe that they have a valuable role in patients without systemic infection who are progressing to the chronic phase of ALI.[23]

## Specific molecular therapy

A multiplicity of compounds that interfere with the inflammatory molecular cascade has been studied in animal models and some in clinical trials. Antibodies to endotoxin and TNF$\alpha$, the IL-1$\alpha$ receptor antagonist, and oxpentifylline (pentoxifylline) (a methylxanthine that prevents the expression of mRNA for TNF$\alpha$) are the best known. These compounds have not lived up to the promise of early laboratory experiments and most are being fundamentally re-evaluated. Problems of definition and mixed patient populations have hindered the conduction of effective clinical trials.

## Surfactant therapy

The pathological similarities of ALI/ARDS to infant respiratory distress syndrome and the demonstration of the importance of surfactant dysfunction in the latter has led to interest in supplementing natural surfactant with exogenous artificial surfactant materials. The ratio of surfactant to plasma protein in alveolar fluid is important for maintaining adequate surface-active properties. Initial success in small trials was followed by disappointment and early termination of a multicentre placebo-controlled study. There were difficulties in administering the original trial agents, and it may be appropriate to re-examine this avenue.

# Complications

Most patients surviving an episode of ARDS experience complications attributable to either the disease or its treatment. Nosocomial pneumonia is common and has been discussed elsewhere. Pneumothoraces and lung cysts are difficult to detect with a conventional radiograph and commonly require a CT scan for both diagnosis and management (Figures 12.5 and 12.6). The chest radiograph commonly exhibits widespread shadowing for a considerable time and may hide impressive lung abscesses (only apparent on CT) which will require therapy. Patients may require months of respiratory system support, and the attendant immobility and difficulties in maintaining nutritional status during the illness mean that recovery of both skeletal and respiratory musculature is prolonged.

# The long-term sequelae of ARDS

Data concerning the respiratory function of patients surviving severe ALI have only recently become available. Many are difficult to interpret and compare because of variations in patient demographics, the underlying diseases, severity of illness, and the treatment strategies applied.

In general survivors are surprisingly free of symptoms, but objective tests of lung function (for example, total lung diffusing capacity for carbon monoxide, $T\textsc{lco}$) and alveolar volume demonstrate persistent abnormalities. Most patients have reduced lung volumes after an episode of ALI, which tend to return to normal over 12–18 months. A permanent reduction

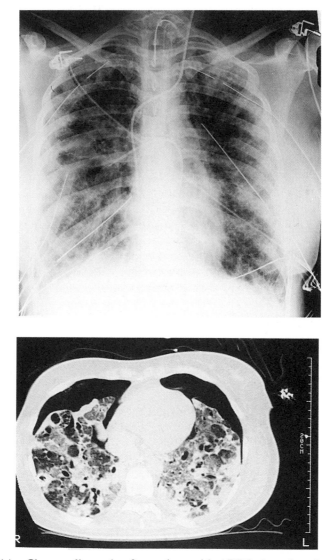

(a)

(b)

Fig 12.5(a)   Chest radiograph of a patient with ARDS 6 weeks after a smoke inhalation injury. A tracheostomy has been performed and a pulmonary artery catheter is still required. A number of chest drains are *in situ* to drain multiple loculated pneumothoraces. (b) CT scan performed on the same day. Substantial pneumothoraces remain undrained; these were not obvious from the conventional film. The lung fields remain very abnormal with areas of patchy consolidation, cystic change, and ground-glass shadowing.

135

in $T_{LCO}$ is a common finding in survivors, but this is mild and not clinically significant. Blood gas tensions tend to be normal at rest, but may become abnormal on exercise.[24] Thoracic CT scans performed during convalescence are often surprisingly normal when compared with the degree of destruction demonstrated by acute studies. The psychological sequelae of a

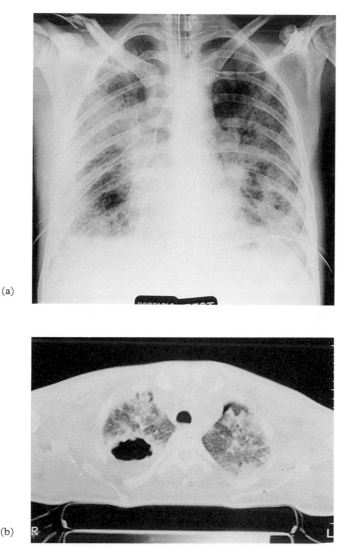

(a)

(b)

Fig 12.6(a)  Chest radiograph of a 21-year-old man with severe ARDS 6 weeks after multiple trauma. The lung fields remain extensively infiltrated. (b) A CT scan performed the following day; a substantial abscess is visible in the right lung, which was not obvious from the conventional radiograph.

period of long-term ventilatory support and intensive care have been inadequately investigated.

## The future

Recent research efforts into the pathophysiology of ARDS have yet to be translated into efficacious therapies. It seems unlikely that blocking individual components of the inflammatory cascade will be helpful. Therapy directed at either the final common pathway to lung injury or initiating processes may be more successful. However, treating all patients at risk for ALI/ARDS could hardly be justified on a cost–benefit basis. In the field of organ support, it remains to be demonstrated that any one mode of ventilation is convincingly better than any other. Extrapulmonary support remains controversial and confined to centres of enthusiasm.

1 Ashbaugh DG, Bigelow DB, Petty TL, Levine BE. Acute respiratory distress in adults. *Lancet* 1967;**ii**:319–23.
2 Bernard GR, Artigas A, Brigham KL, *et al.* The American–European Consensus Conference on ARDS. *Am J Respir Crit Care Med* 1994;**149**:818–24.
3 Murray JF, Mathay MA, Luce JM, Flick MR. An expanded definition of the adult respiratory distress syndrome. *Am Rev Respir Dis* 1988;**138**:720–3.
4 Streiter MR, Lukacs NW, Standiford TJ, Kunkel SL. Cytokines and lung inflammation: mechanisms of neutrophil recruitment to the lungs. *Thorax* 1993;**48**:765–9.
5 MacNee W, Selby C. Neutrophil traffic in the lungs: role of haemodynamics, cell adhesion and deformability. *Thorax* 1993;**48**:79–88.
6 Lewis JF, Jobe AH. Surfactant and the adult respiratory distress syndrome. *Am Rev Respir Dis* 1993;**147**:218–33.
7 Liu SF, Adcock IM, Old RW, Barnes PJ, Evans TW. Lipopolysaccharide treatment *in vivo* induces widespread tissue expression of inducible nitric oxide synthase mRNA. *Biochem Biophys Res Commun* 1993;**196**:1208–13.
8 Vane JR, Mitchell JA, Appleton I, *et al.* Inducible forms of isoforms of cyclooxygenase and nitric-oxide synthase. *Proc Natl Acad Sci USA* 1994;**91**:2046–50.
9 Dantzker DR, Brook CJ, Dehart P, Lynch JP, Weg JG. Ventilation-perfusion distributions in the adult respiratory distress syndrome. *Am Rev Respir Dis* 1979;**120**:1039–52.
10 Marini JJ. Ventilation of the acute respiratory distress syndrome – looking for Mr. Goodmode. *Anesthesiology* 1994;**80**:972–5.
11 Rappaport SH, Shpiner R, Yoshihara G, Wright J, Chang P, Abraham E. Randomised, prospective trial of pressure limited versus volume-controlled ventilation in severe respiratory failure. *Crit Care Med* 1994;**22**:22–32.
12 Hickling KG, Walsh J, Henderson S, Jackson R. Low mortality rate in adult respiratory distress syndrome using low-volume, pressure-limited ventilation with permissive hypercapnoea: a prospective study. *Crit Care Med* 1994;**22**:1568–78.
13 Lessard MR, Guérot E, Lorino H, Lemaire F, Brochard L. Effects of pressure-controlled with different I:E ratios versus volume-controlled ventilation on respiratory mechanics, gas exchange and hemodynamics in patients with adult respiratory distress syndrome. *Anesthesiology* 1994;**80**:983–91.
14 Pappert D, Rossaint R, Salma K, Gruning T, Falke KJ. Influence of positioning on ventilation-perfusion relationships in severe adult respiratory distress syndrome. *Chest* 1994;**106**:1511–16.
15 Brunet F, Belghith M, Mira JP, *et al.* Extracorporeal carbon dioxide removal and low-frequency positive pressure ventilation. Improvement in arterial oxygenation with reduction of risk of pulmonary barotrauma in patients with adult respiratory distress syndrome. *Chest* 1993;**104**:889–98.

16 High KM, Snider MT, Richard R, *et al.* Clinical trials of an intravenous oxygenator in patients with adult respiratory distress syndrome. *Anesthesiology* 1992;**77**:856–63.

17 Walmrath D, Scneider T, Pilch J, Gimminger F, Seeger W. Aerosolised prostacyclin in adult respiratory distress syndrome. *Lancet* 1993;**342**:961–2.

18 Frostell CG, Blomquist H, Hedenstierna G, Lundberg J, Zapol WM. Inhaled nitric oxide selectively reverses human hypoxic pulmonary vasoconstrction without causing systemic vasodilation. *Anesthesiology* 1993;**78**:427–35.

19 Gerlach H, Pappert D, Lewandowski K, Rossaint R, Falke KJ. Long term inhalation with evaluated low doses of nitric oxide for selective improvement of oxygenation in patients with adult respiratory distress syndrome. *Intensive Care Med* 1993;**19**:443–9.

20 Puybasset L, Rouby JJ, Mourgeon E, *et al.* Inhaled nitric oxide in acute respiratory failure; dose response curves. *Intensive Care Med* 1994;**20**:319–27.

21 Rossaint R, Falke KJ, Lopez F, Slama K, Pison U, Zapol WM. Inhaled nitric oxide for the adult respiratory distress syndrome. *N Engl J Med* 1993;**328**:399–405.

22 Brett SJ, Evans TW. Inhaled vasodilator therapy in acute lung injury – first do NO harm. *Thorax* 1995;**50**:821–3.

23 Meduri GU, Chinn AJ, Leeper KV, *et al.* Corticosteroid rescue treatment of progressive fibroproliferation in late ARDS. Patterns of response and predictors of outcome. *Chest* 1994;**105**:1516–27.

24 Hert R, Albert RK. Sequelae of the adult respiratory distress syndrome. *Thorax* 1994;**49**:8–13.

# 13: Ventilatory failure

C S GARRARD

Ventilatory failure (type II) occurs when carbon dioxide excretion by the lungs is less than the volume of carbon dioxide being produced by the body tissues. As a consequence, arterial and alveolar $P\text{CO}_2$ rise. This leads to a fall in alveolar $P\text{O}_2$ (alveolar gas equation) and the risk of hypoxaemia. In a patient with hypoventilatory respiratory failure and normal lungs the $(\text{A--a})D\text{O}_2$ (alveolar–arterial difference in oxygen diffusion) will remain normal (Figure 13.1).[1]

## Pathophysiology

Inadequate alveolar ventilation may be due to impaired central nervous respiratory drive, reduced respiratory neural transmission to the diaphragm, muscle weakness, or ventilation maldistribution as in chronic obstructive lung disease. Box 13.1 summarises the disorders that can result in hypoventilatory respiratory failure classified according to the site of the defect.

## Clinical features

In general, patients in the early stages of hypoventilatory failure may not complain of dyspnoea, and present with diminished chest wall movement and air entry. The underlying cause of hypoventilation may be clinically evident (Box 13.1), such as neuromuscular weakness in myasthenia gravis, or coma from a cerebrovascular accident or drug overdose. Tachypnoea may be present in conditions affecting the chest wall or bellows function of the lung, whilst slow respiration may reflect CNS depression, for example, by opioids. Cyanosis is usually a late sign. Hypercapnia contributes significantly to the clinical features that are commonly associated with acute respiratory failure, independent of hypoxaemia. Symptoms include headache, irritability, inability to concentrate, and drowsiness. Clinical examination demonstrates vasodilatation, bounding pulses, systemic arterial hypertension, engorged fundal veins, myoclonus, depressed spinal reflexes, stupor, and coma.

Hypoventilatory failure should be distinguished from acute hypoxaemic respiratory failure, or type I respiratory failure. Hypoxaemic respiratory failure is caused by diseases associated with lung damage producing

139

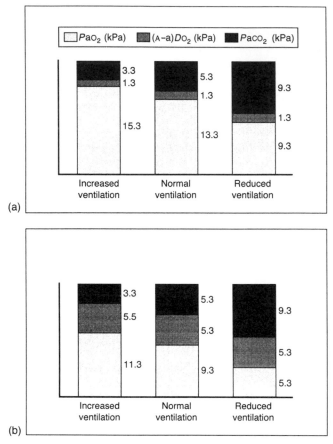

Fig 13.1 (a) Arterial blood gases and $(A-a)Do_2$ at three levels of ventilation in a patient with normal lungs. With a reduction in ventilation and rising $Paco_2$, $Pao_2$ falls as a consequence of the alveolar gas equation. (b) Arterial blood gases and $(A-a)Do_2$ at three levels of ventilation in a patient with abnormal lung pathophysiology and respiratory failure. With a reduction in ventilation and rising $Paco_2$, the degree of hypoxia is increased. (From Lane DJ, *Respiratory disease*, pp. 293, London: Heinemann, 1976.)

ventilation–perfusion maldistribution and impaired gas exchange (see Chapter 12). Some patients may exhibit both type I and type II respiratory failure. In diseases such as asthma, which usually cause hypoxaemic respiratory failure, the onset of fatigue and exhaustion leads to an increasing $Paco_2$ and mixed respiratory failure finally develops. Conversely, hypoventilation (e.g. poliomyelitis) may lead to basal lung collapse, microaspiration, lung damage, and hypoxaemic respiratory failure.[2]

Hypoventilatory failure is best demonstrated not by arterial blood gases but by simple tests of ventilatory capacity such as vital capacity, negative

**Box 13.1** *Some causes of hypoventilatory respiratory failure classified according to anatomical site of defect*

*Central nervous system*
- Brain-stem vascular lesions (haemorrhage, thrombosis, embolism)
- Primary central hypoventilation
- Pharmacological depressants (opioids, sedatives)
- Brain-stem herniation
- Traumatic injury

*Spinal cord*
- Traumatic cervical spine injury (above C3)
- Motor neuron disease
- Transverse myelitis
- Poliomyelitis
- Multiple sclerosis

*Peripheral nerve (phrenic nerves)*
- Peripheral neuropathy
  - vasculitides
  - Guillain–Barré disease
  - diabetes mellitus
  - heavy metal poisoning

*Motor nerve end-plate*
- Myasthenia gravis
- Neuromuscular blocking agents
  - depolarising
  - non-depolarising
- Organophosphate poisoning
- Eaton–Lambert syndrome
- Botulism

*Diaphragmatic muscle*
- Muscle dystrophies
- Myopathies
- Muscle spasm
  - Strychnine poisoning
  - Status epilepticus

*Chest wall and pleural cavities*
- Trauma and flail segment
- Kyphoscoliosis
- Ankylosing spondylitis
- Extreme obesity
- Bilateral pneumothoraces, pleural effusion, haemothoraces

*Lung and airways*
- Chronic pulmonary obstructive disease/emphysema
- Bronchial asthma
- Cystic fibrosis, bronchiectasis
- Extrathoracic airways
  - tracheal trauma
  - neck haemorrhage
  - airway tumours
  - obstructive sleep apnoea

inspiratory force (NIF), or maximum breathing capacity. In patients with normal lungs, $CO_2$ retention is a relatively late indicator, whilst a vital capacity $< 10$ ml/kg or an NIF $< -25$ mm Hg indicates severely impaired ventilatory effort. Arterial blood gases should be performed before anaesthesia or surgery to quantify the degree of $CO_2$ retention and metabolic compensation. If, as often happens, a pre-intervention blood gas sample is not available, the presence of a base excess on the first available sample may suggest chronic $CO_2$ retention.

## Management

Management is aimed at initial resuscitation followed by diagnosis and longer-term support. The resuscitation measures are summarised in Box 13.2.

### Establish an airway

Simple manoeuvres to re-establish a clear airway are essential. These include positioning and maintaining the head and neck in the "sniff position", inspection of the oropharynx, suctioning, and, if necessary, the insertion of an oral or pharyngeal airway. Ensure adequate ventilation using a self-inflating resuscitation bag and supplemental oxygen while clarifying the diagnosis and planning an interim management strategy, such as endotracheal intubation.[3]

### Endotracheal intubation

If simple measures do not restore the airway or respiratory function, endotracheal intubation must be performed. Orotracheal intubation is best for emergency intubation; nasotracheal intubation requires more time and skill, and must not be performed in the presence of coagulation defects as it may cause serious bleeding. Intubation should be performed by the most experienced clinician available, and neuromuscular relaxant drugs should be given only by medical staff trained in their use. The complications of endotracheal intubation are caused by occlusion or displacement of the tube, and airway trauma. The appropriate endotracheal tube size for most

---

**Box 13.2**  *Treatment of ventilatory failure*

- Establish and maintain an airway
- Maintain adequate ventilation
- Identify and treat the underlying cause
- Monitor $Sao_2$ (pulse oximetry), ECG, and vital signs
- Administer oxygen if hypoxia persists (if combined type I and II)

---

men is 8–9 mm internal diameter and for women 7–8 mm. For children, a rough calculation using

$$(\text{child's age in years}/4) + 4$$

will provide the tube internal diameter in millimetres. These smaller tubes are generally uncuffed.

The endotracheal tube must be securely anchored and the cuff inflation pressure < 30 cm $H_2O$.[4] Only high-volume, low-pressure cuffed tubes should be used, and cuff inflation pressures should be checked at least daily with an anaeroid manometer. Higher cuff pressures do not improve airway protection against aspiration, and will produce ischaemic damage to the tracheal mucosa with late subglottic stenosis.

Endotracheal intubation may be difficult in patients with a short "bull" neck or receding lower jaw, and those with restricted neck or jaw movements (rheumatoid arthritis or cervical spine injury) or abnormal oropharyngeal anatomy (tumour or trauma).[5] Management options in these circumstances include inhalational anaesthesia followed by muscle relaxants if the airway remains patent, awake intubation with topical anaesthesia, or the use of a fibreoptic bronchoscope or laryngoscope.[6] All these techniques require skill and training. In some instances difficulty with intubation may not be anticipated; a long curved-tip introducer should always be immediately available, and a management plan organised for failed intubation.

**Tracheostomy**

Tracheostomy should replace endotracheal intubation only for specific indications and not merely after the elapse of a predefined time interval. With modern endotracheal tubes and techniques, endotracheal intubation can be tolerated without permanent harm to the airway for months if necessary. Most mucosal damage occurs within the first week of intubation with little additional change thereafter. Common indications for tracheostomy include the need for long-term ventilation, to help weaning after previously failed attempts at extubation or to facilitate oral nutrition, or the presence of upper airway complications of endotracheal intubation. The same principles of cuff pressure management apply to tracheostomy tubes as to endotracheal tubes. Tracheostomy is associated with fewer but more serious complications than endotracheal intubation. These include tube displacement or obstruction, pneumothorax, haemorrhage, and wound infection.

Tracheostomy can be performed as an elective surgical procedure or percutaneously with a Seldinger wire technique.[7] This latter approach is a rapid, convenient, and safe procedure when undertaken by suitably trained intensive care clinicians within the ICU. Percutaneous tracheostomy has the added advantage of fewer infections, less bleeding, and a better cosmetic result. Complications from performing a "blind" procedure (misplacement, false tracts) may be minimised by adrenaline infiltration, a vertical skin incision, and blunt dissection down to the pretracheal fascia. Replacement of the tube is difficult should it become dislodged.

Cricothyroidotomy may be needed in life-threatening, upper airway obstructions where endotracheal intubation is not feasible and there is insufficient time to perform a tracheostomy. Performed under local anaesthesia, a full-sized tracheostomy tube can be inserted (6–8 mm internal diameter) to facilitate mechanical ventilation.

## Maintain adequate ventilation

In the emergency situation ventilation can be maintained successfully using a self-inflating resuscitation bag. The maximum $FIO_2$ achievable is about 0.6 unless a reservoir is added, in which case 100% oxygen can be delivered. Adequacy of ventilation should be monitored by inspection of chest movements, auscultation, pulse oximetry, and arterial blood gases. A heat and moisture exchanger (HME) must be interposed between the endotracheal tube and the bag.

## Define cause of hypoventilation

Defects in the central drive to respiration, neural transmission, the respiratory muscle response, or ventilation distribution within the lung can all result in diminished ventilatory response and hypoventilation.[8-13] These are summarised in Box 13.1. Specific therapies may be available and relieve hypoventilation.

## Oxygen therapy

In most cases of hypoventilatory failure correction of the ventilation defect results in adequate oxygenation. However, coexisting lung disease or associated pulmonary collapse may require supplemental oxygen therapy or the application of continuous positive airway pressure (CPAP). Oxygen can be delivered by a variety of means depending upon the concentration desired and the patient's minute ventilation.

Oxygen should be given in a concentration sufficient to prevent episodes of hypoxaemia. In patients with chronic obstructive lung disease the administered concentration must be controlled, and the response monitored to avoid suppression of ventilatory drive.[14,15] Monitoring should employ continuous pulse oximetry ($Sao_2$) and intermittent arterial blood gas sampling.[16] Failure to correct hypoxaemia should trigger referral to intensive care.

## Other systems

Patients with chronic hypoventilation may have co-morbid conditions such as myocardial or neuromuscular disease complicating or precipitating respiratory failure. Hypotension following intubation and ventilation is common, and is multifactorial (dehydration, loss of sympathetic drive with $CO_2$ clearance). In most cases it can be minimised by prior administration of intravenous colloids to expand circulating volume. Failure to respond should suggest impaired myocardial function and the need for right heart catheterisation.

## Chronic obstructive pulmonary disease (COPD)

This includes chronic bronchitis, emphysema, and chronic asthma, and may complicate bronchiectasis and cystic fibrosis. Pulmonary function tests demonstrate airway obstruction ($FEV_1$/FVC%; flow/volume loops; plethysmographic airway resistance) and hyperinflation (particularly with emphysema) with an increase in residual volume (RV), functional residual capacity (FRC), and total lung capacity (TLC). If there is more than 10–15% reversibility of the $FEV_1$, asthma is more likely. Resting arterial blood gases may be normal but usually reveal hypoxaemia and varying degrees of hypercapnia.[17]

The commonest precipitating events for acute respiratory failure in patients with COPD are lung infection, sputum retention, intercurrent illness, heart failure, general anaesthesia, and surgical stress (Box 13.3). Inadvertent oversedation, particularly with opioids, or the administration of too high an $FIO_2$ may further exacerbate $CO_2$ retention in these patients.[18-20]

### Assessment

Patients usually have increased cough and sputum production, increasing dyspnoea, increased lethargy and, in severe cases, confusion and obtundation. Physical examination generally reveals a breathless patient with wheezy or faint breath sounds. Cyanosis may be present and the patient may be unresponsive to verbal commands. Differential or concurrent diagnoses include left ventricular failure, obstructive sleep apnoea, upper airway obstruction, pulmonary embolism, and pneumothorax.

Arterial blood gases should be measured and arterial oxygen saturation monitored by pulse oximetry. Uncompensated respiratory acidosis (low pH, elevated $Paco_2$) is consistent with acute respiratory decompensation. For each 1·33 kPa (10 mm Hg) rise in $Pco_2$ above 5·33 kPa (40 mm Hg), the pH will fall approximately 0·1 unit. In severely ill patients a metabolic acidosis may occur from tissue hypoxia and hypoperfusion. In long-standing or chronic hypercapnia the serum bicarbonate is elevated (> 30 mmol/l) and the base excess will be > 4 mmol/l indicating that renal compensation has occurred.

The 12-lead ECG may be unremarkable or may show signs of RA or RV hypertrophy and RV strain. Continuous ECG monitoring is recommended to detect dysrhythmias. A chest radiograph is needed to identify precipitating causes such as pneumonia or heart failure, and to exclude pneumothorax, lung collapse, or concurrent bronchogenic malignancy. Sputum Gram stain and culture should be performed to identify lower respiratory tract pathogens. Initial antibiotic treatment can be much influenced by the Gram stain which might reveal *Staphylococcus* spp., *Streptococcus pneumoniae*, or *Haemophilus* spp. Culture of expectorated sputum contributes little to management. On full blood count a poly-

---

**Box 13.3**   *Precipitants of acute respiratory failure in COPD patients*

*Acute infection*
• Acute bronchitis
  – influenza viruses
  – respiratory syncitial virus
  – *Haemophilus influenza*
  – *Branhamella catarrhalis*
  – Viridans streptococci
• Pneumonia
  – *Streptococcus pneumoniae*
  – *Haemophilus influenzae*
  – *Mycoplasma pneumoniae*
  – *Legionella pneumophila*
  – *Staphylococcus aureus*
  – Influenza A virus

*Sputum retention*
• Intercurrent illness
• General anaesthesia
• Major surgery
• Severe polytrauma (e.g. fractured ribs)
• Mental obtundation.

*Bronchospasm/hyperreactivity*
• Common allergens
• Chemical irritants
• Infection

*Heart failure*
• RV failure with pulmonary hypertension
• LV failure from ischaemic heart disease

*Uncontrolled oxygen administration*
• High $F_{IO_2}$ given by low-flow systems

*Other causes*
• Oversedation
• Pneumothorax
• Pulmonary embolism

---

cythaemia suggests chronicity and hypoxia. A leukocytosis and left shift indicate infection.

Spirometry at the time of admission to the ICU may not be possible given severe respiratory distress. Review of earlier measurements will provide a useful guide to the severity of pre-existing lung dysfunction and prognosis. Typically the $FEV_1/FVC$ ratio is < 50% or the $FEV_1$ < 1·0 litre.

## Management: conservative measures

If the patient is stable then conservative management can be followed. These measures are aimed at relieving hypoxia, stimulating respiratory efforts and coughing, reversing some of the airway obstruction, and correcting any precipitating cause. Survival rates (>90%) and avoidance of mechanical ventilation (<3% of cases)[21] have changed little since the 1960s.

### Oxygen therapy

Hypoxaemia should be reversed using oxygen delivery systems that are controllable, such as the Venturi mask at 24 or 28%. Nasal cannulae or low-flow oxygen facemasks might inadvertently deliver a higher than intended $F_{IO_2}$ and therefore suppress central hypoxic drive. This complication can be avoided by proper monitoring of the dose–response; if hypoxaemia does not correct it, expert help should be obtained. The aim of treatment is to achieve modest improvement in oxygenation ($Sao_2$ to the 90–93% range) without causing a progressive rise in $Paco_2$. A clinical improvement in mental or cardiovascular status is often more important than the actual $Sao_2$ or $Paco_2$. It is essential that, once oxygen therapy is begun, it is not stopped precipitously. Complete removal of supplemental oxygen from a patient whose $Paco_2$ is rising may result in profound hypoxia, and precipitate emergency intubation.[22,23]

### Drug therapy

Start nebulised $\beta_2$-specific sympathomimetics (e.g. salbutamol 2·5–5·0 mg 4–6 hourly) immediately. It is important that the same $F_{IO_2}$ (24–28%) be administered during aerosol therapy. Inhaled ipratropium bromide may have an additional bronchodilator effect. Aminophylline is an alternative in a loading dose 5 mg/kg i.v. over 30 min, followed by continuous infusion at 0·5–0·9 mg/kg per h; although it has the theoretical benefit of improving respiratory muscle contractility and delaying diaphragmatic fatigue, its advantage over inhaled bronchodilators is largely unproven.

Corticosteroids contribute little bronchodilatation in these patients (<10%) compared with those with asthma, and should be avoided if bacterial infection is present. Hydrocortisone 3 mg/kg or methylpredniso-lone 0·5 mg/kg 6 hourly can be given for two to three days before reducing this to a maintenance dose. Maximum effect may not appear for up to 10 days.[24,25]

Antibiotics are probably overprescribed. They should be given when bacterial infection is likely and after an organism has been identified on Gram stain. A combination of cefuroxime and erythromycin will cover bacterial pathogens such as *Streptococcus pneumoniae*, *Staphylococcus aureus*, *Haemophilus influenzae*, and atypical organisms.

*Other measures*

Chest physiotherapy will encourage coughing, sputum clearance, and deep breathing. The external oscillator/ventilator (Hayek oscillator) may also be of value to assist expectoration and improve ventilation. Mucolytic agents, such as acetylcysteine in cystic fibrosis, are of no proven benefit in COPD. Pleuritic chest pain or rib fractures may contribute to respiratory insufficiency; this pain may be difficult to manage. Non-steroidal anti-inflammatory drugs in an hypoxaemic patient with impaired myocardial function may precipitate renal injury.

Malnutrition is associated with reduced respiratory muscle mass, reduced contractility, and earlier onset of respiratory muscle fatigue. Enteral feeding should be started as soon as possible to prevent further muscle wasting. Specialised feeds are available (Pulmocare) that reduce excessive $CO_2$ production from carbohydrate,[26] but alternatively one should simply avoid overfeeding with standard feeds. Co-morbid conditions must be actively identified and treated, particularly heart failure, atrial fibrillation, and electrolyte disturbances such as hypokalaemia, hypo-phosphataemia, and hypomagnesaemia. Immobile, polycythaemic patients must receive prophylaxis for deep vein thrombosis.

Respiratory stimulants have been used in the management of hypoventi-latory respiratory failure,[27] and may help to avoid mechanical ventilation in some patients. Doxapram and almitrine are probably the most effective.[28,29] Doxapram acts on peripheral carotid chemoreceptors and the respiratory centre. Almitrine sensitises peripheral chemoreceptors to both hypoxia and hypercapnia. The need for respiratory stimulants should trigger ICU referral.

## Mechanical ventilation

In a minority of patients conservative measures will fail. ICU staff should be contacted well before the patient is *in extremis*, to allow early assessment and informed discussions about the appropriateness and extent of treatment with the patient and family. The treatment priority is to restore adequate tissue oxygenation. This involves removing respiratory work by providing mechanical support, using a sufficient $FIO_2$ to achieve an $SaO_2$ of up to 93%, and taking measures to maximise cardiac output. Hypotension occurring shortly after establishing adequate ventilation should be prevented by giving adequate intravenous colloids, as discussed above.

*Ventilator settings*

The aim is to maintain adequate oxygenation and prevent further rise in $Pa\text{CO}_2$ (or worsening of respiratory acidosis) with the use of the lowest tolerable minute ventilation. Tidal volumes and I:E (inspiratory:expiratory) ratios are adjusted to minimise "auto-PEEP" (dynamic pulmonary hyperinflation)[30,31] in these patients who already have severe airway obstruction. The I:E ratio should be 1:2 or more; if the respiratory rate is < 12 breaths/min, and the tidal volume 6–8 ml/kg (compared to the standard setting of 10–12 ml/kg), expiratory times approaching four seconds may be possible. If the ventilator rates are increased in an attempt to increase minute ventilation, the $Pa\text{CO}_2$ may paradoxically rise as hyperinflation and the $V\text{D}/V\text{T}$ ratio (proportion of tidal volume ventilating the dead space) increase and alveolar ventilation falls. The $Pa\text{CO}_2$ should be reduced very slowly *towards* but not *to* normal levels over 6–8 hours. The $F\text{IO}_2$ should be adjusted initially to achieve an $Sa\text{O}_2$ of up to 93%. Positive end-expiratory pressure (PEEP) should be minimised.

Synchronised intermittent mandatory ventilation (SIMV) or pressure support alone has been used successfully in COPD patients,[32,33] but no particular mode of ventilation appears advantageous. It is often necessary initially to sedate the patient heavily and suppress spontaneous respiration with opioids if mechanical support and intubation are not tolerated. The choice of a sedative regimen depends upon the weaning plan; alfentanil with propofol may be easier to control if the period of support is likely to be less than three days. Otherwise, morphine and intermittent or continuous benzodiazepines are more economical. The use of muscle relaxants should be minimised. Weaning is discussed below.

# Bronchial asthma

The prevalence of and mortality from asthma are increasing in many countries. Possible reasons include atmospheric pollution and $\beta$-receptor down-regulation from exposure to adrenergic agents. Most deaths occur outside hospital but an increasing number of patients are admitted to hospital with an acute exacerbation, of whom around 1% will need mechanical ventilatory support.

## Management

*Early and continuous monitoring*

Failure to recognise the asthmatic patient who is at risk may result in an avoidable death. Life-threatening attacks of asthma tend to occur in steroid-dependent patients who have previously required ICU admission or mechanical ventilation (Box 13.4). High-risk patients should be admitted to an ICU or high dependency unit (HDU)[34] for continuous monitoring of ECG, pulse oximetry, and arterial catheterisation for serial arterial blood gas (ABG) analysis and continuous blood pressure monitoring. The patient's clinical condition should be continually reassessed. Specific indications for ICU admission have been defined by the British Thoracic Society (Box 13.5). Given proper management in an ICU, death is rare.

*Drug treatment*

Oxygen must be given in the highest concentration available, together with inhaled and intravenous bronchodilators and high-dose systemic

---

**Box 13.4**   *Severe asthma attack*[35]

**Characteristics**
*Potentially life-threatening features*
• Unable to complete sentences in one breath
• Respiratory rate >25 breaths/min
• Heart rate >110 beats/min
• PEFR (peak expiratory flow rate) <40% of predicted normal or of best normal if known
• PEFR <200 l/min if best normal not known
• Arterial paradox >10 mm Hg

*Immediately life-threatening features*
• Silent chest on auscultation
• Cyanosis
• Bradycardia
• Exhaustion, confusion, unconsciousness

**Action**
*Observation and monitoring*
• Vital signs every 15 min
• Continuous ECG
• Oxygenation: pulse oximetry
• Intermittent $P$a$co_2$
• Intravascular volume status
• Electrolytes, $K^+$
• Pulmonary function testing ($FEV_1$)

*Therapy*
• Bronchodilators
• Corticosteroids
• Oxygen
• Mechanical ventilation
• Rehydration
• Potassium

---

---

**Box 13.5**  *Indications for admission to intensive care*[35]

- $Pao_2$ <8 kPa despite $Fio_2$ >0·6
- $Paco_2$ >6 kPa
- Exhaustion
- Depressed level of consciousness
- Respiratory arrest

---

steroids (Box 13.6).[35] The most important and frequently neglected aspect of care is maintaining adequate oxygenation, even with referrals to a specialised centre.[36] Pulse oximetry is mandatory and the $Sao_2$ must be maintained at >95%. Nebulised $\beta_2$-specific adrenergic agonists given 2–4 hourly form the mainstay of bronchodilator therapy. If this is ineffective, continuous nebulisation of 5 mg doses of salbutamol (each dose lasting 5–10 minutes) for 45–60 minutes can be given up to a total dose of 30–40 mg, provided the heart rate is closely monitored.[37]

## Mechanical ventilation

### Indications

Mechanical ventilation is not a treatment for asthma, but buys time for specific bronchodilator and anti-inflammatory therapy to take effect. The benefits of ventilation must be balanced against the risks of hypotension, barotrauma, and lung infection.[38] Delaying intubation to the point of exhaustion and cardiorespiratory arrest may prove fatal since a number of these patients suffer significant cerebral anoxic injury at the time of arrest. If maximal medical therapy fails to produce improvement, mechanical ventilation is indicated (Box 13.7).

A normal or increased $Paco_2$ indicates ventilatory failure, but trends in $Paco_2$ are more important than single values. If the patient is not deteriorating clinically and is not hypoxaemic, medical measures should be continued despite hypercapnia. Other indicators of severity include heart rate, respiratory rate, peak expiratory flow rate (PEFR), degree of arterial paradox (the fall in systolic blood pressure on inspiration), and ability to

---

**Box 13.6**  *Medical therapy for life-threatening acute asthma*[35]

- *High-dose inhaled $\beta_2$ agonists* (e.g. salbutamol 2·5–5·0 mg or terbutaline 5–10 mg repeated 2–4 hourly; monitor heart rate)
- *High-dose systemic steroids* (e.g. prednisolone 30–60 mg/day orally or hydrocortisone 200 mg i.v., or both)
- *Intravenous bronchodilators* (aminophylline 250 mg i.v. in 30 min, or salbutamol 200 g i.v. in 10 min; maintenance doses: aminophylline 0·5–0·9 mg/kg per h i.v. or salbutamol 3–20 g/min i.v.)

---

---

**Box 13.7** *Indications for mechanical ventilation in patients receiving maximal medical bronchodilator therapy*

*Warning signs*
- Increasing distress
- Increasing $Paco_2$
- Increasing arterial paradox
- Increasing heart rate
- Increasing respiratory rate
- Decreasing PEFR or $FEV_1$
- Decreasing ability to converse

*Impending collapse*
- Worsening hypoxaemia
- Decreasing level of consciousness
- Exhaustion

---

speak. The importance of correcting hypoxaemia with high concentrations of inspired oxygen cannot be overemphasised.

*Endotracheal intubation*

Endotracheal intubation of a patient with acute asthma is associated with a definite morbidity and risk of death, and must be performed only by a skilled individual.[39] At least one large-bore (minimum size 16 gauge) intravenous catheter should be in place and fluid ready for rapid infusion. A full range of resuscitation drugs should be available as induction of anaesthesia and initiation of positive pressure ventilation can produce profound hypotension. Rapid fluid resuscitation will restore blood pressure in most cases. Preoxygenation with 100% oxygen, an intravenous induction, and cricoid pressure by a competent assistant to prevent aspiration should be employed in all cases. Fentanyl (3–5 $\mu$g/kg) combined with midazolam (0·05–0·15 mg/kg) for anaesthesia and suxamethonium (1–1·5 mg/kg) for muscle relaxation comprise one of several suitable induction regimens.

*Complications*

Deaths in ventilated asthmatics may follow anoxia from cardiorespiratory arrest before mechanical ventilation, arrhythmias, sepsis, and barotrauma. Attempts to achieve normocapnia may require airway pressures of more than 60 cm $H_2O$ and result in barotrauma presenting as a simple or a tension pneumothorax, pneumomediastinum, pneumopericardium, or pneumoperitoneum. Tension pneumothorax is a medical emergency and is rapidly fatal if not treated. An asthmatic presenting in cardiac arrest (especially with electromechanical dissociation), or who suffers sudden cardiovascular deterioration during mechanical ventilation, should be assumed to have a tension pneumothorax. There is rarely time to obtain a chest radiograph, and emergency decompression should be performed by insertion of a large-bore (14 gauge) intravenous cannula, into the side of the clinically suspected pneumothorax, followed immediately by formal chest drain insertion (using blunt dissection and without using the trochar that is often supplied).

*Aims and mode of ventilation*

Correction of hypoxaemia is essential, but normalisation of $P\text{a}CO_2$ must take second place to minimisation of the risk of barotrauma from high pressures and volumes. Low-volume, pressure-limited ventilation with permissive hypercapnia[40,41] is often required in the acute phase. A prolonged expiratory time (I:E $> 1{:}2$) is needed to reduce air trapping, but this will shorten inspiratory time and increase flow rate and peak inspiratory pressure (PIP). PEEP is not recommended. Box 13.8 summarises initial ventilator settings. The ventilated asthmatic must be continuously reassessed both clinically and by measurement of airway pressures and ABGs. The risks of air trapping and volume and pressure damage must be recognised by all staff. Most asthmatic deaths are related to cardiorespiratory arrest *before* intensive care admission, indicating the need for early detection and referral to intensive care.

*Sedation and muscle relaxation*

Asthmatic patients are often exhausted and many tolerate ventilation well, but hypnotic agents are always needed for patient comfort, and are essential if neuromuscular blocking drugs are used to increase total lung compliance when airway pressures remain high, or to facilitate permissive hypercapnia. The volatile anaesthetic halothane is a potent bronchodilator at low concentrations and may also reduce pulmonary artery and right ventricular end-diastolic pressures; scavenging systems are required if it is used. The intravenous dissociative anaesthetic ketamine also has bronchodilator properties and has been shown to be effective in children (10–40 micrograms/kg per min by infusion); it is a good choice for inducing anaesthesia at intubation of these patients because it has central

---

**Box 13.8** *Recommended initial ventilator settings in acute asthma*

1. $FiO_2$ unrestricted (start at 1·0)
2. Low tidal volume (5–8 ml/kg)
3. Slow rate (8–12 breaths/min)
4. I:E $\geq$ 1:2
5. Low PIP pressure limit $< 40$ cm $H_2O$
6. Zero CPAP/PEEP

---

sympathetic stimulant properties which prevent hypotension. Other agents may be used for sedation according to local policy, and there is little evidence favouring any particular regimen.

Muscle relaxants may be necessary short term. Their use is associated with a severe, usually reversible myopathy causing prolonged ventilator dependence. This may be more common with the potent steroidal relaxants in conjunction with systemic corticosteroids. They should therefore be used for the shortest period possible, and preferably < 24 h.[50,51]

*Other treatments*

Magnesium sulphate (i.v.) has been reported to reverse bronchospasm in anecdotal reports. However, randomised, controlled studies have failed to demonstrate a significant bronchodilator effect or suppression of hyper-reactivity. Heliox, a mixture of 30–50% oxygen in helium, increases peak expiratory flow and reduces dyspnoea during acute asthma. The benefits are marginal although this modality may reduce the need for mechanical ventilation.[52] Extracorporeal membrane oxygenation (ECMO) has been employed,[53] but its place in managing these patients is uncertain.

*Weaning from mechanical ventilation*

The majority of patients require ventilation for < 24 h and can be weaned rapidly. If bronchospasm recurs during this process, extubation can be performed under sedation with an inhalational agent or propofol. Weaning will not be successful until full pharmacological control of bronchospasm is achieved. Weaning from longer-term ventilation is discussed below.

# Non-invasive ventilatory support

## Mask CPAP

Continuous positive airway pressure is applied using close-fitting masks and a pressurised circuit with a reservoir to allow for peak inspiratory flow. Patients should be carefully selected and managed in an ICU, HDU, or respiratory unit. The patient must be fully alert, cooperative, and unlikely to vomit. Mask CPAP is particularly suited to hypoxaemic patients with basal collapse following surgery, or those with cardiogenic pulmonary oedema or interstitial pneumonia (e.g. *Pneumocystis carinii* pneumonia). CPAP levels > 10–15 cm $H_2O$ should not be employed. Continuous assessment is essential, and air swallowing may result in gastric distension.

## Positive pressure non-invasive ventilation (PPNIV)

Non-invasive assisted ventilation provides an alternative to endotracheal intubation in some patients with COPD and acute respiratory failure. Positive pressure techniques support the respiratory muscles and avoid upper airway obstruction. PPNIV for acute exacerbation of COPD is provided using volume-cycled ventilation, bilevel positive airway pressure (BiPAP), or pressure support via closely fitting face or nasal masks.[54,55] Success rates of 40–76% have been reported.[56] However, it has not yet been shown that non-invasive ventilation improves survival compared with intubation and mechanical ventilation, and it is difficult for patients to tolerate it for more than a few days.

The following requirements must be satisfied before attempting PPNIV, otherwise intubation and positive pressure ventilation is the preferred option:[57]

• staff familiarity with the technique;
• close monitoring in an ICU or HDU;
• cooperative patient protecting own airway and clearing sputum;
• physiologically stable with no other acute organ-system failure.

## Negative pressure ventilation

Negative pressure ventilation (NPV) is achieved by applying subatmospheric pressures to the surface of the thorax during inspiration.[4] The pressure gradient between the mouth and the alveoli produces inspiratory flow. Expiration occurs passively by the elastic recoil pressure of the lungs and chest wall, although there are systems that actively aid expiration. Negative pressures can be applied to the whole body ("iron lung"), to the chest wall, or to the chest and abdomen (cuirasse).[58] Some devices maintain a negative pressure at end-expiration to improve alveolar recruitment (NEEP). NPV with NEEP has been used in patients with acute respiratory distress syndrome.[59] The haemodynamic effects of NPV are variable and depend on whether negative pressure is applied to the whole body or only to the thorax.[60]

Negative pressure ventilation using "iron lungs" has been used mostly in patients with neuromuscular disorders, such as poliomyelitis,[57] or diseases of the chest wall[61] and for postoperative weaning of muscular dystrophy patients.[62] It has also been used to rest the ventilatory muscles of COPD patients and for acute exacerbations of COPD.[63]

The negative intratracheal pressures generated during NPV may adduct the vocal cords producing laryngeal obstruction. As a result, NPV is not ideal for diseases that may be complicated by upper airway obstruction, such as Guillain–Barré syndrome and myasthenia gravis.[64] For similar reasons, NPV may be ineffective in patients with sleep apnoea. In contrast, the application of nasal CPAP (positive pressure) to such patients is recognised as reliably preventing upper airway obstruction.

### Hayek oscillator

The Hayek oscillator is an enhanced NPV device that applies high-frequency external oscillation with variable I:E ratio to the chest wall and upper abdomen. The pressure profile is both positive and negative and can produce large tidal volume excursions. This approach may offer an advantage in terms of gas exchange or even the removal of lung secretions. The Hayek oscillator has been used in the management of a patient with predicted difficult tracheal intubation after failed awake fibreoptic intubation and in patients undergoing microlaryngeal surgery.[65,66] It has also been effectively used in severe COPD and respiratory failure to assist ventilation and relieve muscle fatigue.[67] The Hayek oscillator has been shown to support blood perfusion and lung ventilation as effectively as standard cardiopulmonary resuscitation for humans in cardiac arrest.[68]

## Discontinuation of mechanical ventilation (weaning)

Weaning from mechanical ventilation should be attempted as soon as clinical conditions allow. In most cases extubation can follow weaning provided the patient is cooperative, and able to protect the airway and clear secretions. In general terms, clinical assessment is more important than arterial blood gas analyses at determining suitability for weaning and extubation.[69] Weaning methods vary. Many patients receiving respiratory support postoperatively can be weaned rapidly by clinical evaluation of their spontaneous ventilation on a "T-piece" or similar circuit. Those who have received respiratory support for longer periods require a progressive reduction in ventilatory support, with objective measurement of spontaneous tidal volumes, respiratory rate, and effort (Box 13.9).[70] If these criteria can be met, ventilatory support can be reduced rapidly. Prolonged use of a T-piece may be associated with progressive basal collapse, as this method prevents the patient from generating positive airway pressure.

---

**Box 13.9** *Patient variables when considering withdrawal of mechanical ventilation*

1. Adequate oxygenation ($Pa_{O_2}$ > 10 kPa or 80 mm Hg on an $FI_{O_2}$ < 0·4)
2. Adequate ventilatory effort to prevent atelectasis (vital capacity > 10 ml/kg or negative inspiratory force (NIF) > 20–25 cm $H_2O$)
3. Acceptable ventilatory demand (minute ventilation to maintain normal $Pa_{CO_2}$ ideally < 12 l/min)
4. Ability to meet this demand (patient's spontaneous minute ventilation equals minute ventilation on ventilator)
5. Acceptable breathing pattern (frequency tidal volume index [f/VT] < 100 breaths/min per l)
6. Alert and responsive – able to protect own airway
7. Any other procedures planned in the near future requiring intubation and mechanical ventilation (e.g. re-laparotomy, head CT scan)

---

# Weaning from prolonged acute respiratory failure

Patients who have undergone prolonged mechanical ventilation may take several weeks to gain respiratory independence.[71] Modes of ventilation such as SIMV or pressure support (PS) are well suited to this process. A clear weaning plan understood by all members of staff should be established for each patient, and reviewed frequently. Causes of failure to wean are summarised in Box 13.1. Particular attention should be paid to correcting metabolic and electrolyte disturbances,[72,73] drug effects, excessive $CO_2$ production,[6] and mechanical problems such as the size of the endotracheal tube, abdominal distension, phrenic nerve injury, or pain. Patients requiring levels of end-expiratory pressure $>5$ cm $H_2O$, with high oxygen requirement, or with a persisting tachypnoea, will probably require the intermediary step of a tracheostomy.

Weaning of COPD patients requires expertise, experience, and patience. Principles include maximising respiratory drive, minimising respiratory work, and optimising the efficiency of mechanical support. Target arterial blood gases should reflect ambulatory status before acute deterioration (i.e.

---

**Box 13.10**   *Causes of failure to wean from mechanical ventilation*

*Ventilatory muscle function impaired*
• Hypokalaemia
• Hypomagnesaemia
• Muscle relaxants, aminoglycosides
• Hypophosphataemia
• Severe malnutrition and cachexia
• Neuromuscular disease (e.g. myasthenia gravis, Guillain–Barré syndrome)

*Reduced central ventilatory drive*
• Sedatives, hypnotics, opioids
• Metabolic alkalosis
• Hypothyroidism (and impaired muscle function)

*Increased ventilatory demand*
• Metabolic acidosis
• Bicarbonate loading
• Excessive calorie intake

*Failure of other organ systems*
• Neurological (coma, confusion, impaired airway protection)
• Cardiac (increased preload + myocardial work during spontaneous ventilation in patients with impaired myocardial function)
• Renal (fluid overload, metabolic acidosis)
• Hepatic (encephalopathy)

if $P$ao$_2$ is normally 7 kPa on air at home, do not aim for values significantly higher). The $F$io$_2$ should be adjusted to the minimum level consistent with target $P$ao$_2$. In practice try to get $F$io$_2$ < 0·3. The $P$aco$_2$ may have to rise to high levels (e.g. 8–10 kPa). Optimise bronchodilator therapy with $\beta$-adrenergic agonists, anticholinergics, and steroids if necessary. Avoid excess $CO_2$ production by providing no more than adequate calorie intake and lipid/carbohydrate balance.[74] Gradually reduce ventilatory support (either SIMV rate or level of PS) every 2–4 hours allowing pH to correct after each rise in $P$aco$_2$ (metabolic compensation). Finally, discontinue all sedation and opioid analgesia.

## Extubation

Once weaning from intermittent positive pressure ventilation has been achieved, extubation should be considered. The patient must be able to maintain a patent airway and clear secretions. Adverse factors include mental obtundation, oropharyngeal neuromuscular weakness, and oedema or stenosis of any part of the upper airway.[75] The presence of a strong cough on endotracheal suctioning and vigorous gag reflex suggests that extubation can be safely undertaken.

The patient should be awake and responsive, and given an explanation and reassurance. Extubation should be preceded by oropharyngeal and tracheal suctioning to remove secretions. This will not reach secretions trapped in the subglottic space, which are removed by performing extubation with a positive pressure inflation of the lungs with 100% oxygen as the endotracheal tube cuff is deflated; the secretions will be blown forward into the mouth, and should be cleared with a Yankauer sucker. The presence of a large leak around the endotracheal tube at this point largely excludes significant airway oedema and the potential for postextubation stridor or obstruction. Experienced staff and equipment should always be available to deal with the rare occasions when extubation is followed by stridor or ventilatory failure.

## Conclusions

### Ventilatory failure

- The causes of ventilatory failure include central brain-stem pathology, neural transmission defects to the respiratory muscles, chest wall, pulmonary, and extrapulmonary disease.
- Ventilatory failure is usually associated with a normal $(\text{A–a})D\text{o}_2$.
- Vital capacity and NIF are good indicators of ventilatory reserve.

- Management is aimed at:
  - resuscitation (ABC)
  - establishing and maintaining airway
  - maintaining alveolar ventilation
  - identifying underlying cause
  - giving supplemental oxygen if needed.
- Apply specific therapies for underlying cause if available.

## Chronic obstructive pulmonary disease

- Precipitating events for acute-on-chronic respiratory failure include:
  - lung infection
  - sputum retention
  - intercurrent illness
  - heart failure
  - general anaesthesia
  - surgical stress
  - inadvertent oversedation
  - too high an $F_{IO_2}$ exacerbating $CO_2$ retention.
- Treatment initially aimed at:
  - relieving hypoxia
  - stimulating respiratory efforts and coughing
  - reversing some of the airway obstruction
  - correcting any precipitating cause.
- Survival rates without mechanical ventilation exceed 90%.
- Mechanical ventilation is required by a minority of patients.
- Mechanical ventilation provides time to reverse precipitating cause.
- Weaning from mechanical ventilation can be protracted.

## Bronchial asthma

- Most deaths from asthma occur outside hospital.
- Most hospital deaths indicate either inadequate observation or under-treatment.
- Severe acute asthma should be managed in an ICU or HDU.
- Hypoxaemia must be reversed.
- Hypovolaemia and hypokalaemia are important complications.
- Maximal bronchodilator therapy must be applied before implementing mechanical ventilation.
- Intubation should be undertaken by an experienced anaesthetist or intensivist.
- Ventilator settings are aimed at reducing lung pressure/volume injury.
- Anticipate tension pneumothoraces in ventilated asthmatics.
- Practise permissive hypercapnia.
- Halogenated inhalational anaesthetics are powerful bronchodilators.

• The patient with asthma requiring mechanical ventilation is at high risk of death from future asthma attacks.

## Non-invasive ventilatory support

• Non-invasive assisted ventilation:
  - may offer an alternative to endotracheal intubation;
  - may employ positive (PPNIV) or negative (NPV) pressure techniques;
  - requires HDU/ICU monitoring and staff experienced in airway management;
  - cannot be used in uncooperative, confused, physiologically unstable patients;
  - does not provide airway protection from aspiration;
  - may cause upper airway obstruction in some patients.

## Weaning and extubation

• Most patients are successfully weaned from ventilation with the use of clinical criteria.
• Formal measurement of vital capacity and NIF may be useful in patients who have undergone prolonged respiratory support.
• SIMV and PS are the most useful weaning modes.
• A weaning plan and regular clinical assessment are required.
• Before extubating a patient, ensure that all facilities for reintubation are immediately available.

1 Mellemgaard K. Alveolar–arterial oxygen difference: size and components in normal man. *Acta Physiol Scand* 1966;**67**:10–17.
2 Lane DJ, Hazleman B, Nichols PJR. Late onset respiratory failure in patients with previous poliomyelitis. *Q J Med* 1974;**43**:551.
3 Schwartz DE, Matthay MA, Cohen NH. Death and other complications of emergency airway management in critically ill adults. A prospective investigation of 297 tracheal intubations. *Anesthesiology* 1995;**82**:367–76.
4 Seegobin RD, van-Hasselt GL. Endotracheal cuff pressure and tracheal mucosal blood flow: endoscopic study of effects of four large volume cuffs. *BMJ Clin Res Ed* 1984;**288**:965–8.
5 Frerk CM. Predicting difficult intubation. *Anaesthesia* 1991;**46**:1005–8.
6 Dellinger RP. Fiberoptic bronchoscopy in adult airway management. *Crit Care Med* 1990;**18**:882–7.
7 Leinhardt DJ, Mughal M, Bowles B. Appraisal of percutaneous tracheostomy. *Br J Surg* 1992;**79**:255–8.
8 Bergofsky EH, Turino GM, Fishman AP. Cardiorespiratory failure in kyphoscoliosis. *Medicine (Baltimore)* 1959;**38**:263–8.
9 Kilburn KH, Eagan JT, Sieker HO, Heyman A. Cardiopulmonary insufficiency in myotonic and progressive muscular dystrophy. *N Engl J Med* 1959;**261**:108–9.
10 Mellins RB, Balfour HH, Turino GM, Winters, RW. Failure of automatic control of ventilation (Ondine's curse). *Medicine (Baltimore)* 1970;**49**:487–94.
11 Zwillich CW, Pierson DJ, Hofeldt FD, Lufkin EG, Weil, JV. Ventilatory control in myxoedema and hypothyroidism. *N Engl J Med* 1975;**292**:662–7.
12 Hughes RAC. *Guillain–Barré syndrome*. London: Springer Verlag, 1990.

13  Leventhal R, Orkin FK, Hirsch RA. Prediction of the need for postoperative mechanical ventilation in myasthenia gravis. *Anesthesiology* 1980;**53**:26–30.

14  Flenley DC, Franklin DH, Millar JS. Hypoxic drive to breathing in chronic bronchitis and emphysema. *Clin Sci* 1970;**38**:503–7.

15  Warrell DA, Edwards RHT, Godfrey S, Jones NL. Effect of controlled oxygen therapy on arterial blood gases in acute respiratory failure. *BMJ* 1970;**1**:452–5.

16  Hutton P, Clutton-Brock T. The benefits and pitfalls of pulse oximetry. *BMJ* 1993;**307**:457–8.

17  Gilbert R, Keighley, J, Auchincloss, JH. Mechanisms of chronic carbon dioxide retention in patients with obstructive pulmonary disease. *Am J Med* 1965;**38**:217–21.

18  Mithoefer JC, Keighley JF, Karetzky MS. Response of the arterial $Po_2$ to oxygen administration in chronic pulmonary disease: interpretation of findings in a study of 46 patients and 14 normal subjects. *Ann Intern Med* 1971;**74**:328–35.

19  Fahey PJ, Hyde RW. "Won't breathe" versus "can't breathe". Detection of depressed ventilatory drive in patients with obstructive pulmonary disease. *Chest* 1983;**84**:19–25.

20  Lane DJ, Howell JBL, Giblin B. The relation between airways obstruction and $CO_2$ tension in chronic obstructive airways disease. *BMJ* 1968;**3**:707–12.

21  Campbell EJM. The mangement of acute respiratory failure in chronic bronchitis and emphysema. *Am Rev Respir Dis* 1967;**96**:626–31.

22  Warrell DA, Edwards RHT, Godfrey S, Jones NL. Effect of controlled oxygen therapy on arterial blood gases in acute respiratory failure. *BMJ* 1970;**2**:452–7.

23  Asmundsson T, Kilburn KH. Survival of acute respiratory failure: a study of 239 episodes. *Ann Intern Med* 1969;**70**:471–5.

24  Sahn SA. Critical review. Corticosteroids in chronic bronchitis and pulmonary emphysema. *Chest* 1978;**73**:389–95.

25  Albert RK, Martin TR, Lewis SW. Controlled clinical trial of methylprednisolone in patients with chronic bronchitis and acute respiratory insufficiency. *Ann Intern Med* 1980;**92**:753–8.

26  Wilson DO, Rogers RM, Hoffman RM. Nutrition and chronic lung disease. *Am Rev Respir Dis* 1985;**132**:1347–65.

27  Galko BM, Rebuck AS. Therapeutic use of respiratory stimulants. An overview of newer developments. *Drugs* 1985;**30**:475–81.

28  Moser KM, Luchsinger PC, Adamson JS, *et al.* Respiratory stimulation with intravenous doxapram in respiratory failure: a double blind cooperative study, *N Engl J Med* 1973;**288**:427–32.

29  Powles ACP, Tuxen DV, Mahood B, Pugsley SO, Campbell EJM. The effect of intravenously administered almitrine, a peripheral chemoreceptor agonist, on patients with chronic air-flow obstruction. *Am Rev Respir Dis* 1983;**127**:284–9.

30  Benson MS, Pierson DJ. Auto-PEEP during mechanical ventilation of adults. *Respir Care* 1988;**33**:557–68.

31  Brown DG, Pierson DJ. Auto-PEEP is common in mechanically ventilated patients: a study of incidence, severity, and detection. *Respir Care* 1986;**31**:1069–74.

32  Slutsky AS. Mechanical ventilation: American College of Chest Physicians' Consensus Conference. *Chest* 1993;**104**:1833–59.

33  Tuxen DV, Lane S. The effects of ventilatory pattern on hyperventilation, airway pressures, and circulation in mechanical ventilation of patients with severe air-flow obstruction. *Am Rev Respir Dis* 1987;**136**:872–9.

34  Cockcroft DW. Management of acute severe asthma. *Ann Allergy Asthma Immunol* 1995;**75**:83–9.

35  Statement by the British Thoracic Society, Research Unit of the Royal College of Physicians of London, King's Fund Centre and Campaign. Guidelines for management of asthma in adults II. *BMJ* 1990;**301**:797–800.

36  Lipworth BJ, Jackson CM, Ziyaie D, Winter JH, Dhillon PD, Clark RA. An audit of acute asthma admissions to a respiratory unit. *Health Bull Edinb* 1992;**50**:389–98.

37  Buck ML. Administration of albuterol by continuous nebulization. *AACN Clin Issues* 1995;**6**:279–86.

38  Branthwaite MA. An update on mechanical ventilation for severe acute asthma. *Clin Intensive Care* 1990;**1**:4–6.

161

39 Rosengarten PL, Tuxen DV, Dzuikas L, Scheinkestel C, Merrett K, Bowes G. Circulatory arrest induced by intermittent positive pressure ventilation in a patient with severe asthma. *Anaesthes Intensive Care* 1991;**19**:118–21.

40 Darioli R, Perret C. Mechanical controlled hypoventilation in status asthmaticus. *Am Rev Respir Dis* 1984;**129**:385–7.

41 Hickling KG, Henderson SJ, Jackson R. Low mortality associated with low volume pressure limited ventilation with permissive hypercapnia in severe adult respiratory distress syndrome. *Intensive Care Med* 1990;**16**:372–7.

42 Quist J, Andersen JB, Pemberton M, Bennike KA. High level PEEP in severe asthma. *N Engl J Med* 1982;**307**:1347–8.

43 Tuxen DV. Detrimental effects of positive end-expiratory pressure during controlled mechanical ventilation of patients with severe airflow obstruction. *Am Rev Respir Dis* 1989;**140**:5–9.

44 Marini JJ. Should PEEP be used in airflow obstruction? *Am Rev Respir Dis* 1989;**140**:1–3.

45 Tuxen DV, Williams TJ, Scheinkestel CD, Czarny D, Bowes G. Use of a measurement of pulmonary hyperinflation to control the level of mechanical ventilation in patients with acute severe asthma. *Am Rev Respir Dis* 1992;**146**:1136–42.

46 Robertson CE, Steedman D, Sinclair CJ, Brown D, Malcolm SN. Use of ether in life-threatening acute severe asthma. *Lancet* 1985;**i**:187–8.

47 Rock MJ, De la Rocha SR, L'Hommedieu CS, Treumper E. Use of ketamine in asthmatic children to treat respiratory failure refractory to conventional therapy. *Crit Care Med* 1986;**14**:514–16.

48 Echeverria M, Gelb AW, Wexler HR, Ahmad D, Kenefick P. Enflurane and halothane in status asthmaticus. *Chest* 1986;**89**:152–4.

49 Strube PJ, Hallam PL. Ketamine by continuous infusion in status asthmaticus. *Anaesthesia* 1986;**41**:1017–19.

50 Griffin D, Fairman N, Coursin D, Rawsthorne L, Grossman JE. Acute myopathy during treatment of status asthmaticus with corticosteroids and steroidal muscle relaxants. *Chest* 1992;**102(2)**:510–14.

51 Margolis BD, Khachikian D, Friedman Y, Garrard C. Prolonged reversible quadriparesis in mechanically ventilated patients who received long–term infusions of vecuronium. *Chest* 1991;**100**:877–8.

52 Kass JE, Castriotta RJ. Heliox therapy in acute asthma. *Chest* 1995;**107**:757–60.

53 Tajimi K, Kasai T, Nakatani T, Kobayashi K. Extracorporeal lung assist for patient with hypercapnia due to status asthmaticus. *Intensive Care Med* 1988;**14**:588–9.

54 Brochard L, Isabey D, Piquet J, *et al*. Reversal of acute exacerbations of chronic obstructive lung disease by inspiratory assistance with a face mask. *N Engl J Med* 1990;**323**:1523–30.

55 Bott J, Carroll MP, Conway JH, *et al*. Randomised controlled trial of nasal ventilation in acute ventilatory failure due to chronic obstructive airways disease. *Lancet* 1993;**341**:1555–7.

56 Hill NS. Noninvasive ventilation: does it work, for whom, and how? *Am Rev Respir Dis* 1993;**147**:1050–5

57 Hill NS. Clinical applications of body ventilators. *Chest* 1986;**90**:897–905.

58 Cropp A, DiMarco AF. Effects of intermittent negative pressure ventilation on respiratory muscle function in patients with severe chronic obstructive pulmonary disease. *Am Rev Respir Dis* 1987;**135**:1056–61.

59 Sanyal S, Bernal R, Hughes WT. Continuous negative chest–wall pressure: Successful use for severe respiratory distress in an adult. *JAMA* 1976;**236**:1727–8.

60 Kinnear W, Petch M, Taylor G. Assisted ventilation using cuirass respirators. *Eur Respir J* 1988;**1**:198–203.

61 Wiers PWJ, LeCoultre R, Dallinga OT. Cuirass respiratory treatment of chronic respiratory failure in scoliotic patients. *Thorax* 1977;**32**:221–8.

62 Alderson SH, Warren RH. Ventilatory management of muscular dystrophy patients following spinal fushion. *Respir Care* 1984;**29**:829–32.

63 Celli B, Lee H, Criner G. Controlled trial of external negative pressure ventilation in patients with severe chronic airflow obstruction. *Am Rev Respir Dis* 1989;**140**:1251–6.

64 Rodrigues JF, York EL, Nair CPV. Upper airway obstruction in Guillain–Barré syndrome. *Chest* 1984;**86**:147–8.

65 Broomhead CJ, Dilkes MG, Monks PS. Use of the Hayek oscillator in a case of failed fibreoptic intubation. *Br J Anaesth* 1995;**74**:720–1.

66 Dilkes MG, McNeill JM, Hill AC, Monks PS, McKelvie P, Hollamby RG. The Hayek oscillator:a new method of ventilation in microlaryngeal surgery. *Ann Otol Rhinol Laryngol* 1993;**102**:455–8

67 Spitzer SA, Fink G, Mittelman M. External high-frequency ventilation in severe chronic obstructive pulmonary disease. *Chest* 1993;**104**:1698–701.

68 Smithline HA, Rivers EP, Rady MY, Blake HC, Nowak RM. Biphasic extrathoracic pressure CPR. A human pilot study. *Chest* 1994;**105**:842–6.

69 Sahn SA, Lakshminarayan S. Bedside criteria for discontinuation of mechanical ventilation. *Chest* 1973;**63**:1002–5.

70 Yang KL, Tobin MJ. A prospective study of indexes predicting the outcome of trials of weaning from mechanical ventilation. *N Engl J Med* 1991;**324**:1445–50.

71 Pierson DJ. Weaning from mechanical ventilation in acute respiratory failure: Concepts, indications, and techniques. *Respir Care* 1983;**28**:646–62.

72 Dhingra S, Solven F, Wilson A, McCarthy DS. Hypomagnesemia and respiratory muscle power. *Am Rev Respir Dis* 1984;**129**:497–8.

73 Aubier M, Murciano D, Lecocguic. Effect of hypophosphatemia on diaphragmatic contractility in patients with acute respiratory failure. *N Engl J Med* 1985;**313**:420–4.

74 Dark DS, Pingletons K, Kerby GR. Hypercapnia during weaning: complication of nutritional support. *Chest* 1985;**88**:141–3.

75 Colice GL, Stukel TA, Dain B. Laryngeal complications of prolonged intubation. *Chest* 1989;**96**:877–84.

# 14: Cardiovascular failure and support

J-L VINCENT

## Pathophysiology

Circulatory failure is a clinical syndrome characterised by abnormal oxygen utilisation by the tissues, in which oxygen availability is insufficient to maintain normal aerobic metabolism. In low-flow states, the pathophysiology is quite straightforward, related to reduced oxygen delivery to the cells. In septic shock things are more complex but, as in other forms of acute circulatory failure, it should be seen as an imbalance between oxygen demand and oxygen supply. In sepsis, oxygen demand is typically increased by the inflammatory response, while at the same time there is a reduction in peripheral oxygen extraction capability with consequent cellular hypoxia. Myocardial depression in sepsis may also contribute to tissue hypoxia because, even though oxygen supply is normal or high, it may be insufficient to satisfy the elevated oxygen demand of the tissues.[1]

Cardiovascular failure may be due to one, or any combination, of four major pathophysiological mechanisms: hypovolaemia, heart failure, obstruction, or maldistribution of blood flow. In the first three types of circulatory failure, the primary problem is reduction in blood flow. The systemic vascular resistance (SVR), calculated as the ratio of pressure over blood flow, is typically increased. An accurate clinical history is the most important element in determining the cause or causes of cardiovascular failure.

- *Hypovolaemic shock* is the most common form of circulatory failure. The fall in cardiac output is due to a fall in venous return. Common causes include haemorrhage (including trauma) and increased fluid losses in the absence of an adequate fluid intake (profuse diarrhoea, extensive burns, postoperative patients). The cardiac filling pressures are usually low.
- *Cardiogenic shock:* the fall in cardiac output is due to a marked reduction in pump function of the heart. Myocardial infarction is a common cause. Cardiogenic shock is likely if more than 40% of the myocardial mass is involved in the necrotic process. Cardiac filling pressures are typically elevated in these conditions.

164

- *Obstructive shock:* the primary problem here is an obstruction, usually of the pulmonary circulation as in pulmonary embolism, or of cardiac contraction as in tamponade. In the former case, the pulmonary artery pressures and the right atrial pressure are particularly elevated. In the latter case, the left- and right-sided filling pressures are equally elevated.
- *Maldistributive shock:* in this fourth case, the release of a number of inflammatory mediators, including tumour necrosis factor α (TNFα), interleukin-1, oxygen free radicals, and nitric oxide, is implicated in a fall of vascular tone, associated with a relatively low oxygen extraction. Hence, the cardiac output is usually normal or high (especially after initial fluid resuscitation), the SVR low, and the mixed venous oxygen saturation relatively high. Interestingly, the same mediators are incriminated in the development of myocardial depression, so that myocardial contractility can be depressed even though cardiac output is normal or high. Septic shock is the most common form of maldistributive shock. In these conditions, the degree of mediator release is directly related to the prognosis. Hence the severity of peripheral vasodilatation and myocardial depression have both been related to the likelihood of death.[2] Low SVR states may be difficult to diagnose on clinical features alone (Table 14.1) and require invasive monitoring for accurate measurement and management.

Very often, shock results from a combination of these mechanisms. The reason is that any form of circulatory failure is associated with some degree of activation of the immune system, with a resulting release of cytokines. Tissue hypoxia, either generalised or localised to certain regions of the body

Table 14.1 Principal characteristics of the four forms of acute circulatory failure

| Characteristics | Type of shock | |
| --- | --- | --- |
| | Hypovolaemic, cardiogenic, or obstructive | Maldistributive |
| Arterial hypotension | Present | Present |
| Cardiac output | Decreased | Normal or increased (seldom reduced) |
| Systemic vascular resistance | Increased | Decreased |
| Cutaneous vasoconstriction (poor capillary return, cyanosis, sweating) | Present | Often absent |
| Urine output | Low | Generally low |
| Mental status | Altered | Altered |
| Intestinal peristalsis | Often absent | Often absent |
| Coagulation abnormalities | Sometimes present | Often present |
| Hyperlactataemia or base deficit | Present | Present |

165

such as the gut, is an important trigger of this cytokine release. Conversely, the release of mediators can cause a reduction in global blood flow associated with hypovolaemia, from alterations in permeability or sequestration of blood, or a predominant myocardial depression. In addition, several events may take place simultaneously. A good example is *anaphylactic shock* in which reduced venous return, myocardial depression, and a fall in vascular tone occur concurrently.

## Clinical signs

Principal signs of circulatory failure are presented in Table 14.1. Hypotension is the most important but its absence does not of course imply circulatory sufficiency. It is usually defined as a systolic blood pressure of < 90 mm Hg despite fluid administration. However, to diagnose circulatory failure one also requires the presence of some sign of tissue hypoperfusion, such as reduced urine output, altered consciousness, or altered skin perfusion.

There is a great need for selective markers of tissue hypoxia. The best biological indicator of shock remains an increase in blood lactate level. The normal lactate level is around 1 $\mu$mol/l and a level higher than 2 $\mu$mol/l is compatible with the diagnosis of shock. However, hyperlactataemia is not pathgnomonic of hypoxia. For instance, seizures or intense shivering with hyperventilation can also result in high lactate levels, as can high doeses of $\beta_2$-agonist catecholamines. Although patients with liver failure usually have a normal lactate level, these patients have reduced lactate clearance by the liver, so that, if elevated their lactate levels may remain high for longer than in a patient with no liver failure. Some investigators have argued that the hyperlactaemia in sepsis may not be due to tissue hypoxia but rather to an inactivation of pyruvate dehydrogenase.[3] This is certainly true when a bolus of endotoxin is administered in animals, but the observation of a normal lactate level in septic patients without shock argues against such a phenomenon being an important one. In any case, there is agreement on the fact that hyperlactataemia in sepsis is associated with a worse prognosis especially when it persists, so that its presence requires aggressive treatment.

Measurement of gastric intramucosal $CO_2$ and the derivation of intramucosal pH (pH$_i$) has created both interest and controversy.[4] This measurement is based on the fact that the gut may be compromised in acute circulatory failure and that the gut mucosa is easily accessible via a nasogastric tube. The technique is described in Chapter 11. Measurement of pH$_i$ or regional $P$co$_2$ ($P$rco$_2$) is more complicated than the use of blood lactate levels. Nevertheless, the combination of lactate with pH$_i$ ($P$rco$_2$) could be valuable in assessing the degree of tissue hypoperfusion.[5] Technology in this field is still evolving. Instead of calculating pH$_i$

intermittently from $P\text{rco}_2$ and arterial bicarbonate concentration, continuous measurement of $P\text{rco}_2$ may represent an almost continuous assessment of splanchnic perfusion, and might provide an early marker of inadequate tissue oxygenation.

## Treatment

The treatment of any severe situation should follow the VIP rule proposed by Weil many years ago. The rule employs the three essentials of ventilate, infuse, and pump.

### Ventilate

The management of cardiovascular failure is unlikely to be effective if respiratory management is inadequate (compare the ABC rule of cardio-pulmonary resuscitation). Hypoxaemia must be avoided, as it compromises both the arterial content of the blood and the myocardial oxygen supply. Oxygen administration must be prompt and generous.

The use of mechanical ventilation should be actively considered in all cases of cardiovascular failure, not only to improve gas exchange, but also to reduce the oxygen demand of the respiratory muscles. Some experimental studies have indicated that the early use of mechanical ventilation can improve the outcome from shock. Severe metabolic acidaemia can reduce myocardial contractility and the use of mechanical ventilation will help to correct this by lowering $P\text{aco}_2$. This option is preferable to the administration of sodium bicarbonate, which should be reserved for exceptional circumstances, as it produces only a temporary correction of the laboratory results and not of the patient's pathophysiology.

### Infuse

Fluid therapy must always be considered before any form of vasoactive support. Even in cardiogenic shock, where pulmonary oedema may be present, the prudent administration of fluids (together with inotropic agents) may sometimes improve cardiac output by the Starling mechanism. In fact, those patients who survive an episode of cardiogenic shock are often those who favourably respond to fluid administration.

Many clinicians are too afraid of the possible development of pulmonary oedema. Even though an excessive increase in cardiac filling pressures may increase the risk of pulmonary oedema development, the maintenance of hypovolaemia will result in underresuscitation with persistent tissue hypoxia, which could lead to failure of the lungs and other organs. Some clinicians prefer the use of vasopressors to further fluid administration, but this will increase cardiac filling pressures and produce a false impression of fluid repletion while disguising a fluid deficit. Fluid administration requires close monitoring to avoid the development of iatrogenic pulmonary oedema. The use of a fluid challenge technique is necessary in these conditions,[6] and cannot satisfactorily be performed without central venous pressure measurement as a minimum. The most appropriate fluids for this purpose are probably colloids rather than crystalloids as the dose–response relationship is more readily observed.

## Pump

Once oxygenation is restored and fluid therapy optimised, the use of vasoactive agents should be considered. In the presence of cardiovascular failure, adrenergic agents are the agents of choice. Their use should be based first on the restoration of perfusion pressure, and second on the optimisation of cardiac output.

### Blood pressure

The first question to ask is whether blood pressure is sufficiently maintained. No patient should be left hypotensive. An obvious question is how to define hypotension. As a simple rule, the mean arterial pressure should always be kept >60 mm Hg, and this usually corresponds to a systolic blood pressure of around 90 mm Hg. However, some patients, especially the elderly, or those with pre-existing hypotension, may require higher pressures. The definition of an adequate blood pressure must be guided by clinical evaluation of the patient. The kidney is one of the first organs to demonstrate an inadequate perfusion pressure, so that the minimal pressure required can sometimes be guided by urine output monitoring. A minimal pressure would be one sufficient to maintain urine flow.

In low SVR states, vasopressers administered via a central venous cannula are commonly required in the initial stages of resuscitation to restore a minimal tissue perfusion pressure. By combining $\alpha$- and $\beta$-adrenergic properties, dopamine is widely used for this purpose. The vasoconstrictive effects of dopamine become increasingly potent as the doses are increased. However, if despite adequate fluid resuscitation the patient remains hypotensive with 20–25 µg/kg per min of dopamine, the administration of noradrenaline is usually recommended. Noradrenaline has potent $\alpha$-stimulating effects and is usually more effective at restoring vascular tone in severe sepsis with fewer tachyarrhythmias than caused by dopamine. However, it is not clear in high-output states to what extent vasoconstriction is beneficial, once minimal tissue perfusion pressures have been restored. Vasoconstriction may mask hypovolaemia, limit peripheral oxygen availability, and increase organ damage; vasoconstrictors should not be used in the absence of regular assessment of the adequacy of circulating volume, which may require repeated fluid challenges with measurement of cardiac filling pressures and cardiac output.

*Cardiac output*

The second aim is to maintain sufficient blood flow to the organs and to prevent adverse vasoconstriction. The synthetic inotropic agent dobutamine has become the agent of reference, and in states of low cardiac output a dose of 5–10 $\mu$g/kg/ per min is usually sufficient to increase cardiac output significantly, although higher doses (up to 20 $\mu$g/kg per min) are sometimes required in severe heart failure. Higher doses may induce severe tachycardia and hypotension from vasodilatation. The persistence of a low cardiac output despite dobutamine at 20 $\mu$g/kg per min should prompt a revision of the diagnosis, the substitution of adrenaline, and perhaps the use of aortic balloon counterpulsation. Dobutamine has also been used to obtain further increases in cardiac output in septic patients even when cardiac output is high, in order to increase oxygen delivery ($D_{O_2}$) to the tissues and to counteract the sepsis-related myocardial depression, which is associated with increased mortality rates.[2] Noradrenaline may be required to counteract the combined vasodilatory effects of sepsis and dobutamine. If a reduction in arterial pressure occurs during dobutamine administration, this should also raise the possibility of unrecognised hypovolaemia. Alternatively some centres use adrenaline alone to support flow and pressure.

It is difficult to define an optimal level of cardiac output and $D_{O_2}$ that one should try to achieve with inotropic support. Although higher $D_{O_2}$ and oxygen consumption ($V_{O_2}$) values have sometimes been proposed as target values, most investigators would consider such levels arbitrary and even potentially harmful. This is primarily because oxygen demand can vary markedly in septic patients, according to the type and severity of disease and many other associated factors including therapy, environmental conditions, etc. It is preferable to tailor therapy according to careful clinical evaluation, accompanied by repeated monitoring of blood lactate levels and perhaps $pH_i$.

*Should SVR guide therapy?*

Titration of therapy according to SVR alone is potentially dangerous. Since SVR is calculated as the ratio of pressure to flow, increasing it would correspond to either a further increase in blood pressure, which may not be useful once a minimal perfusion pressure has been restored, or a reduction in blood flow, which is likely to be detrimental. Moreover, myocardial depression is a feature of both hyperkinetic and hypokinetic states, and can be present even when cardiac output is normal or high, as indicated by the analysis of ventricular function curves (relating ventricular strike work to the corresponding cardiac filling pressure or volume) or the determination of ventricular ejection fraction. The primary goals of therapy must therefore be to restore both flow and pressure, not an arbitrary vascular resistance.

## Distribution of blood flow

The concept of maximising blood flow to specific key organs is attractive. The infusion of dopamine at 2–3 μg/kg per min is often proposed to preserve renal perfusion, and this does indeed produce a perferential increase in renal blood flow in animals and humans. However, these effects are less evident in the presence of sepsis, and protective effects of dopamine on renal function have never been well demonstrated. In consequence the use of dopamine for potential protective renal effects is now being questioned. Dopexamine is a newly developed synthetic catecholamine with β- (primarily $\beta_2$) and dopaminergic properties. The haemodynamic effects of dopexamine, combining vasodilating and inotropic effects, may be useful in patients with congestive heart failure, although at higher doses it produces mild hypotension and tachycardia. Dopexamine is probably best used to increase blood flow to the renal and especially the splanchnic circulations, and the dose should not exceed 4–5 μg/kg per min. However, the precise indications and benefits for this form of intervention are not yet well defined.

## The place of non-adrenergic agents

In view of its weak inotropic effects, digoxin has a very limited place in the management of septic shock, except in the presence of atrial tachyarrhythmias. Substances selectively inhibiting the phosphodiesterase (PDE) III of the myocardium have been used successfully in the management of patients with severe heart failure. By inhibiting the degradation of cyclic adenosine monophosphate (cAMP), these substances have positive inotropic and vasodilating effects. As a result, they can increase cardiac output without major risk of myocardial ischaemia in patients with coronary heart disease.

The particular interest of PDE inhibitors lies in their combination with adrenergic agents, which also increase intramycardial cAMP content by stimulating adenylate cyclase.

Unfortunately, all PDE inhibitors have a relatively long half-life, which has limited their widespread administration in the acutely ill, and especially in hypotensive patients. Even newer products with a shorter half-life, such as piroximone, cannot be easily titrated. For this reason, we prefer to administer PDE inhibitors as repeated short-term infusions or even as repeated slow boluses rather than by constant infusion.[7] With all these agents, a sustained reduction in arterial pressure may occur which may be difficult to reverse even with noradrenaline. As with other vasodilators, PDE inhibitors can also reduce venous return, but this should be relatively well tolerated when fluid administration is simultaneously titrated to maintain cardiac filling pressures.

170

The place of PDE inhibitors in septic shock is unsettled. Although the combination of PDE inhibitors with catecholamines has been proposed in animal studies, the clinical application of these observations is still uncertain because of the limited possibilities for administering vasodilators when vascular tone is already decreased in these inflammatory states.

**Vasodilators**

Although the use of vasodilators is contraindicated in the acute phase of cardiovascular collapse, prudent administration of nitrates should be considered in the treatment of heart failure. Sodium nitroprusside is a potent vasodilator that influences both the arterial and the venous sides of the vasculature. Dosage is between 40 and 250 µg/min. Prolonged administration of high doses can lead to cyanide toxicity, especially in the presence of renal failure, and in these conditions thiocyanate levels should be monitored. If cyanide poisoning occurs, it should be treated by the intravenous administration of sodium thiosulphate.

Nitroglycerin is sometimes preferred for its predominant effects on the venous side of the vasculature, particularly desirable in the management of pulmonary oedema, or when there is a risk of hypotension. Nitroglycerin may also have better effects on the coronary distribution of blood flow. The doses are approximately equivalent to those of nitroprusside.

Hydralazine is a vasodilating agent, acting more on the arteriolar side of the vasculature; it also has some adrenergic-mediated positive inotropic effects. As a result, it increases heart rate, a property that may be useful in patients with relative bradycardia. Hydralazine is also of therapeutic use as an oral substitute for dobutamine when patients are being weaned from intravenous therapy.

Angiotension-converting enzyme (ACE) inhibitors improve the perform-ance of the failing heart, particularly in patients with an elevated SVR during weaning from prolonged mechanical ventilation. They may, how-ever, produce marked hypotension and renal failure, and should only be introduced, in low dose, in patients who are adequately monitored.

**The particular problem of right ventricular failure**

The combination of pulmonary hypertension and arterial hypotension can compromise right ventricular function by decreasing the coronary perfusion to the right ventricle. In these particular, but very unusual, circumstances, a vasopressor agent such as dopamine and even noradrena-line may represent the only therapeutic option to restore right ventricular perfusion, but at the expense of an increase in pulmonary vascular resistance. In the absence of a profound systemic hypotension, dobutamine is the best agent for the management of right ventricular dysfunction secondary to pulmonary hypertension.

Prostaglandin $E_1$ combined with vasopressors such as noradrenaline can represent a valuable option. More recently, inhaled nitric oxide has been used selectively to decrease pulmonary vascular tone, and has largely replaced the use of pulmonary vasodilators with systemic effects.

### Should hypocalcaemia or hypophosphataemia be corrected?

Calcium is essential to myocardial contraction as well as to the maintenance of vascular tone. Hypocalcaemia may contribute to the development of hypotension. Some direct association has been made in aseptic animals between the mortality rate and the blood calcium level. Experimental studies have also indicated that calcium entry blockers could exert protective effects in septic shock. Hence, routine correction of hypocalcaemia in septic patients may not be indicated. However, in the presence of persisting cardiovascular collapse, slow calcium administration may alleviate or reduce the need for vasoactive support.[8] Recent studies have emphasised the contribution of hypophosphataemia to inadequate cardiac function in septic patients. Hypophosphataemia should be routinely corrected.

# Conclusion

The goal of resuscitation is to normalise cellular oxygen metabolism, and the management of cardiovascular failure should be based on a VIP approach. After optimisation of respiratory support and oxygenation, fluid administration should be considered as a priority. Hypotension is often a late sign of circulatory inadequacy. Vasopressors may be necessary to restore perfusion pressure, although the risk of arteriolar vasoconstriction must not be neglected. The maintenance of blood flow to the organs remains a fundamental goal, and the use of limited doses of dobutamine may be helpful for this purpose. With profound vasodilatation as in sepsis, the need for vasoconstriction should not obscure the accompanying myocardial depression which may further limit oxygen availability to the cells.

Manipulation of the distribution of blood flow with adrenergic agents is still open to question. Resuscitation should be guided by a careful clinical evaluation, accompanied by repeated assessment of the adequacy of oxygen supply such as urine output and blood lactate levels.

1 Vincent JL. Diagnostic and medical management/supportive care of patients with gram-negative bacteremia and septic shock. *Infect Dis Clin North Am* 1991;5:807–16.
2 Vincent JL, Gris P, Ceffernils M, *et al.* Myocardial depression characterizes the fatal course of septic shock. *Surgery* 1992;111:660–7.
3 Gutierrez G, Wulf ME. Lactic acidosis in sepsis: A commentary. *Intensive Care Med* 1996;22:6–16.

4 Groeneveld AB, Kolkman JJ. Splanchnic tonometry: a review of physiology, methodology, and clinical applications. *J Crit Care* 1994;**9**:198–210.
5 Friedman G, Berlot G, Kahn RJ, Vincent JL. Combined measurements of blood lactate levels and gastric intramucosal pH in patients with severe sepsis. *Crit Care Med* 1995;**23**:1184–93.
6 Vincent JL. Fluids for resuscitation. *Br J Anaesth* 1991;**67**:185–93.
7 Vincent JL, Roman A, Kahn RJ. Dobutamine administration in septic shock: Addition to a standard protocol. *Crit Care Med* 1990;**18**:689–93.
8 Jankowski S, Vincent JL. Calcium administration in the critically ill. When is it indicated? *J Intensive Care Med* 1995;**10**:91–100.

# 15: Intensive care of the cardiothoracic surgical patient

J F BION and B E KEOGH

The majority of patients undergoing cardiothoracic surgical procedures have an uncomplicated postoperative course and require only a few hours of stabilisation in the intensive care unit before transfer to high dependency and then ward care. Overall mortality rates of 2–4% are the norm, but within this total population are subsets with higher mortality risk, such as patients requiring valve replacements in combination with coronary grafts or those with poor left ventricular function or pulmonary hypertension; in patients undergoing non-cardiac thoracic surgery there may be co-morbid illnesses such as chronic renal impairment or ischaemic heart disease. Technical advances mean that an increasing proportion of these higher-risk patients is being offered surgery, and will require specialist intensive care management.

## Preoperative assessment

Postoperative intensive care should start preoperatively. Psychological preparation of the patient and family by medical and nursing staff is essential, as understanding improves cooperation and minimises anxiety. Most cardiothoracic surgical patients will have undergone a routine "work-up" including standardised clinical examination and investigations (for example, cardiac catheter/spirometry, chest radiograph, blood count, biochemistry, arterial blood gases) as determined by their clinical state, and planned surgery. The purpose of these investigations is to quantify the severity of the primary diagnosis, and to detect significant co-morbid disease which may adversely affect outcome (Box 15.1). Some clues may be easily missed, for example, a history suggestive of transient ischaemic attacks from carotid atheroma, or a marginally elevated serum creatinine concentration indicating limited renal reserve. Patients receiving long-term oral anticoagulants (warfarin, aspirin), or heparin infusions for unstable angina may be at increased risk of operative and postoperative bleeding.

Patients scheduled for non-cardiac major surgery who have impaired myocardial function (which may be occult or relatively asymptomatic) are

---

**Box 15.1** *Risk factors for patients undergoing cardiothoracic surgery*

*Cardiorespiratory*
- Emergency status
- Recent myocardial infarction
- Re-do surgery
- Valve + ischaemic heart disease
- Poor left ventricular function
- Pulmonary hypertension
- $FEV_1$ < 1 litre
- Hypoxaemia

*Other co-morbid disease*
- Renal impairment
- Diabetes
- Peripheral vascular disease
- Malnutrition
- Age > 70 years

---

at particular risk of cardiac events and sudden death. Static measures (history, ECG) do not provide as accurate a guide to the adequacy of cardiac reserve as dynamic measures, such as exercise testing and measurement of the anaerobic threshold, but these are more difficult to obtain. These patients require skilled perioperative management, including optimisation of circulating volume and cardiac output, before they are subjected to the metabolic stress of surgery.

## Perioperative management

### Optimisation of the high-risk surgical patient

Patients undergoing major surgery, particularly those with cardiac disease, have an increased mortality risk which can be minimised by the simple process of optimisation of circulating volume and cardiac output around the time of induction of anaesthesia. This can be achieved by incremental boluses of intravenous colloids until there is no further increase in stroke volume. The response to volume loading can be measured either by pulmonary arterial catheter or by oesophageal Doppler, although the latter technique can be employed only once the patient is anaesthetised and intubated. Patients who respond to fluids with or without inotropic agents by increasing their cardiac index to around 4·5 l/min per $m^2$ have a lower perioperative mortality than those who are managed without fluid loading. Preoperative optimisation is likely to be beneficial for two reasons: it increases systemic tissue oxygen supply at a time when the metabolic stress of surgery may double oxygen requirements; and it also identifies the "responders" who have a greater cardiac reserve and therefore better outcomes. Although a cardiac index of 4·5 l/min per $m^2$ is often quoted as an important goal, it is probably the process of fluid optimisation that is important, rather than achievement of an absolute value with large doses of inotropic drugs. This is particularly true in patients with valvular heart disease where the mechanical limitation to forward blood flow may prevent a significant increase in cardiac output.

### The cardiac surgical patient

Cardiac surgical patients differ from general surgical high-risk patients in that they are undergoing a corrective procedure to restore cardiac function. They are also intensively monitored, and the majority receive volume expansion (500–1000 ml colloid) at the time of induction of anaesthesia which helps to maintain cardiovascular stability in the period before cardiopulmonary bypass. Bypass is associated with varying degrees of metabolic acidosis and a systemic inflammatory response. These features may represent a combination of impaired tissue perfusion, neutrophil activation by the extracorporeal circuit, endotoxin release, and endothelial dysfunction. Although clinically unimportant in the majority of patients, these phenomena can contribute to postoperative instability. Adequate rewarming and volume expansion are essential at the end of bypass to avoid late hypothermia from reperfusion of cold tissues (the "heat sink"), resulting in vasoconstriction, an inadequate cardiac output, and impaired coagulation postoperatively. Maintaining an adequate body temperature can be difficult in patients undergoing thoracic non-cardiac surgery.

## Postoperative care

In the majority of cases, postoperative intensive care management is standardised, uncomplicated, and brief. The main aims should be the interrelated goals of adequate analgesia, restoration and maintenance of normal core temperature, oxygenation, circulating volume, and respiratory effort. Essential prerequisites are a cooperative physiologically stable patient, and accurate transfer of information between anaesthetic, surgical, and intensive care staff. An overall strategy should be established for patient management based on the initial assessment at handover (Box 15.2). It should be possible at this stage to categorise patients as:

- uncomplicated and suitable for weaning from respiratory support;
- requiring a period of stabilisation;
- unstable or high risk requiring complex organ system support.

In the absence of contraindications, patients should be allowed to wake and wean from mechanical ventilation without delay. Drug treatment should be based on protocols for uncomplicated patients; a basic regimen for coronary bypass patients includes 24 hours of prophylactic antibiotics and an $H_2$-receptor antagonist, and long-term low-dose aspirin.

---

**Box 15.2** *Initial assessment: the three Ps*

*Past history*
- Co-morbid disease and prior health status
- Presurgical cardiorespiratory state
- Intraoperative events

*Present state:*
- Current therapeutic support
- Review organ system function

*Plan for the next few hours:*
- *Determine clinical and physiological goals*
- *Minimal pain, cooperating with care*
- *Breathing and oxygenation satisfactory*
- *Base deficit diminishing towards normal*
- *Cardiovascular variables (BP, CVP) stable*
- *Core temperature >36°C*
- *Drain blood loss <100 ml/h and falling*
- *Haemoglobin concentration >7·5 g/l*
- *Inotrope requirements (if any) diminishing*
- *Urine output ≥ 1 ml/kg per h*
- *Serum creatinine not rising*
- *Serum K⁺ 4·5–5·5 mmol/l*

---

## Cardiovascular and fluid management and monitoring

*Fluid management*

In general, the aim should be to provide an "optimal" circulating volume and cardiac index using intravenous colloid and minimal inotropic agents. In stable patients who meet the criteria in Box 15.2, this can be achieved with colloid boluses to maintain a given central venous pressure (CVP), together with 0·5–1·0 ml/kg per h of dextrose saline to replace water losses and provide a vehicle for potassium supplements. The CVP, however, is not a reliable guide to circulating volume, and requires intelligent clinical interpretation, particularly in patients who emerge from the operating room hypothermic and hypovolaemic, in which case active volume resuscitation will be required with regular review of the patient every few minutes. The majority of cardiac patients benefit from a nitrate infusion for both coronary and systemic vasodilatation, which will facilitate volume expansion.

Fluid overload may contribute to pulmonary oedema in patients who have undergone lung surgery (particularly transplantations) and worsen cardiac performance in patients with impaired ventricular function. Depending on the cause, heart failure may present as either increased compliance with progressive myocardial distension in response to fluids, or reduced compliance with failure of relaxation (diastolic dysfunction). In these patients fluid management can be difficult without measurement of filling pressures and flow. A pulmonary artery catheter or oesophageal Doppler should be used if there is evidence of impaired end-organ perfusion and cardiovascular instability, and assessment made of physiological responses to fluid challenges or inotropic agents is appropriate. Too often these measurements are made at a late stage when clinical guesswork is proving ineffective and the patient's condition has deteriorated significantly. In general terms, if urine flow is >1 ml/kg per h, and the base deficit and serum lactate are correcting, it is likely that cardiac output and circulating volume are adequate.

Blood transfusion should be avoided in the absence of a good reason for providing what is in effect a tissue transplant. Transfusion should not be needed in cardiac patients who are physiologically stable, not bleeding, and who have a haemoglobin >7·5 g/l, because much of the "anaemia" is bypass haemodilution and will disappear with a diuresis. Drain losses > 100 ml/h may be a consequence of preoperative anticoagulation (aspirin, warfarin, heparin), insufficient protamine following bypass, or inadequate surgical haemostasis; inform the surgeon if losses are increasing or the patient is unstable. Aprotinin is often used to reduce thrombolysis and clotting cascade activation in complex or re-do procedures, and is best employed prophylactically; rare adverse effects include anaphylaxis (particularly following prior exposure) and the potential for a hypercoagulable state. Following oesophagectomy, colloid requirements in the first 24 hours may be substantially greater than anticipated from drain losses if surgical dissection was extensive.

*Blood pressure control*

Although it is the adequacy of cardiac output and oxygen delivery that are the important variables, bedside therapy is usually driven by interpretation of blood pressure. The patient's preoperative blood pressure should be documented and taken into account in interpreting postoperative values. The commonest causes of hypertension are pain or the stimulus of the endotracheal tube, and should be treated with adequate analgesia or extubation as appropriate. Intravenous nitrates or sublingual nifedipine are suitable for short-term control of hypertension. An exaggerated reduction in pressure in response to hypotensive agents may indicate relative hypovolaemia.

*Hypotension*

Hypotension is a common phenomenon in the first few hours following cardiac surgery (Box 15.3) while the patient is still receiving mechanical ventilation. It is usually a consequence of rewarming and relative hypovolaemia in patients with temporarily limited capacity to increase cardiac output. Elevation of the legs to increase venous return will often clarify the diagnosis. Other common causes include sedation with propofol,

---

**Box 15.3** *Common causes of hypotension after cardiac surgery*

- Hypovolaemia
- Impaired myocardial contractility
- Vasodilatation
- Valsalva effect (shivering)
- Tamponade
- Dysrhythmias
- Sedative agents
- Hypokalaemia, hypocalcaemia

---

atrial fibrillation or an atrioventricular nodal rhythm, or persistent effect of preoperative ACE inhibitor-induced vasodilatation. An adequate arterial diastolic pressure is important for coronary perfusion in patients with pre-existing left ventricular hypertrophy if hypotension is associated with ECG evidence of ischaemia.

A common source of anxiety is those patients who develop a rising CVP in association with hypotension and tachycardia, and whose peripheral perfusion appears to be poor. The picture may be complicated by changes in thoracic drain volumes. Although cardiac tamponade or tension pneumothorax must be thought of first, the cause is usually a Valsalva-type phenomenon produced by increasing muscle tone in a cold patient starting to emerge from anaesthesia. The two can be distinguished by giving an intravenous bolus of an opioid, or in the unconscious patient a small dose of a muscle relaxant which will abolish muscle tone and allow restoration of venous return and arterial pressure in the absence of tamponade. Inform the surgical staff immediately if hypotension persists or is severe: true tamponade is a surgical emergency.

Many cardiac surgical patients develop a "subclinical" systemic inflammatory response during and after bypass, which may be marked by an associated pyrexia lasting up to 24 hours, and an increase in inflammatory markers including serum amylase. In severe instances a true pancreatitis may develop. The accompanying vasodilatation may be sufficiently marked to cause hypotension, particularly in those patients who cannot increase cardiac output to compensate, or those receiving ACE inhibitors preoperatively. In these patients, vasoconstrictors may be needed in addition to colloid loading. Vasoconstriction with a useful degree of inotropy can often be achieved with relatively low-dose dopamine infusions, but some patients require noradrenaline for effective constriction. Vasoconstrictors should not be used in the absence of measurement of cardiac index (CI) and systemic vascular resistance (SVR) if there is doubt about the physiology, if the patient is unstable, or if there is clinical evidence of inadequate perfusion. The commonest cause of hypotension is an inadequate circulating volume, and vasoconstrictors will disguise this. The absence of a base deficit does not guarantee an adequate systemic oxygen supply.

*Inotropic drugs*

The two main "triggers" for prescribing inotropic drugs are hypotension or clinical evidence of an inadequate cardiac output, and it is important to exclude causes other than impaired myocardial contractility first (for example, hypovolaemia, vasodilatation, sedative drugs, or tamponade). If inotropic drugs are needed, adrenaline is effective and cheap; dobutamine can produce excessive vasodilatation, but its chronotropic effect may be useful, as many patients have a fixed stroke volume, and cardiac output is therefore rate dependent. High doses of $\beta_2$ agonists are associated with a lactic acidosis, which may be misinterpreted as evidence of an inadequate cardiac index requiring an even higher infusion rate. A perceived need for inotropes in a patient with previously normal ventricular function should suggest either the wrong diagnosis or a surgical complication.

*Dysrhythmias*

Disorders of heart rhythm are more likely to occur following complex surgery (for example, valve replacement where sutures pass close to the conduction tissue) or recent infarcts. Atrial fibrillation is relatively common after cardiac surgery (25–30%), pneumonectomy, and oesophageal surgery, and usually resolves rapidly on treatment with antidysrhythmic agents. Exclude or correct hypokalaemia (serum $K^+$ should be >4·5 mmol/l), hypomagnesaemia, hypovolaemia, and hypoxaemia. Left lower lobe collapse and sepsis are common precipitants. Adenosine may help to clarify the underlying rhythm if this is not clear. Amiodarone (300–450 mg i.v. over 30 minutes, 1200 mg i.v. over the next 24 hours, followed by 600 mg/day i.v. or 1200 mg orally) will facilitate spontaneous resolution. However, if cardiac output is compromised, cardioversion should be considered since the atria contribute around 20% to cardiac output, and sinus rhythm should be restored whenever possible. Digoxin 1·0–1·5 mg i.v. may be a better choice if ventricular function is impaired, but the maintenance dose should be reduced in the presence of renal impairment. Bradycardias may need treatment if cardiac output is low or escape rhythms develop: options include atropine, isoprenaline, or pacing, and the choice will depend on the nature of the underlying problem.

*Intra-aortic balloon pump*

The intra-aortic counterpulsation balloon pump simultaneously improves coronary perfusion while reducing left ventricular impedance and work. It does this by inflating during diastole, which increases diastolic pressure in the aortic root and arch, and collapsing in systole, which facilitates left ventricular ejection. It is particularly effective for short-term

(<5 days) support of patients with ischaemic left ventricular failure in whom the diastolic arterial pressure needs to be high for coronary perfusion but low for ventricular ejection. It is usually inserted percutaneously via the femoral artery, with the balloon tip positioned just distal to the origin of the left subclavian artery. Leg pulses must be checked and the results documented immediately after insertion, and every hour thereafter, to detect any signs of distal arterial occlusion and ischaemia. The patient should be heparinised to prevent clot formation on the catheter.

## Respiratory management

Most cardiothoracic surgical patients require only a brief period of respiratory support and will be extubated within a few hours of the end of surgery. This period permits physiological stabilisation, adjustment of analgesia, and exclusion of short-term complications such as bleeding. Initial "default" ventilator settings for the cardiac surgical patient may include an $F_{IO_2}$ of 0·5 synchronised intermittent mandatory ventilation (SIMV) proceeding rapidly to pressure support, and positive end-expiratory pressure (PEEP) of 5 cm $H_2O$. Pre-existing respiratory disease should be noted, and taken into account when a weaning plan is being made: the clinical appearance of the patient may be a better guide to "extubatability" than arterial blood gases in patients with chronic lung disease. Cardiac surgery involving a left internal mammary artery graft and opening of the pleura is usually associated with basal collapse of the left lung and a small pleural effusion visible on the radiograph. This is usually of limited clinical significance, but patients with poor reserve may require interventions to achieve basal expansion or fluid drainage. Patients who have undergone lung resection should be managed with minimal PEEP and the lowest airway pressures compatible with adequate ventilation in order to avoid barotrauma and air leaks.

Increased lung permeability following cardiopulmonary bypass is an expression of endothelial dysfunction. Usually the process remains sub-clinical, but a few patients develop acute lung injury following prolonged bypass with complications. Excess lung water will increase respiratory work and delay weaning from ventilation; lung function may be improved by promoting a diuresis and maintaining circulating volume with narrow band starch solutions or albumin rather than crystalloid or gelatin solutions.

## Analgesia

Adequate postoperative analgesia is essential not only for humanitarian reasons but also to facilitate sputum clearance and basal expansion of the lungs. The majority of cardiac patients will have received high doses of opioids during surgery, and adequate analgesia can be maintained with a morphine infusion or intermittent tramadol. Alfentanil is appropriate for patients with impaired renal function. Thoracic surgery patients may have an epidural catheter *in situ*; epidural opioids may be associated with respiratory depression and pruritis. Some patients experience severe pain or nausea which is difficult to control with standard drugs, but this is rare. Non-steroidal anti-inflammatory drugs should be avoided, or used only with extreme caution, during the first 48 hours following cardiac surgery, as these agents can cause significant renal dysfunction.

## Neurological complications

Clinically evident neurological complications following cardiopulmonary bypass are uncommon, though subclinical changes can be detected more frequently using psychometric testing. Causes include atheromatous or air emboli, cerebral atheroma, and transient cerebral oedema as part of systemic endothelial dysfunction. Risk factors are cerebrovascular disease (known and undetected), age, diabetes, and prolonged bypass. Confusion during the first few hours in the intensive care unit is relatively common, particularly in emergency cases as patients emerge from the combined effects of anaesthesia, surgery, and bypass. Overt neurological injury affects around 1% of routine cases, and often carries a much better prognosis than an equivalent "stroke" in medical patients. It may take up to two weeks before a clear prognosis can be given. Contrast-enhanced CT scanning may be helpful to clarify the diagnosis but rarely alters management or relates to clinical perceptions of severity.

## Miscellaneous conditions

### Pulmonary hypertension

Pulmonary hypertension is defined as a mean pulmonary arterial pressure (PAP) of >25 mm Hg. It may be acute (as in pulmonary embolism), subacute (complicating acute lung injury and sepsis), or chronic (primary pulmonary hypertension, or secondary to cardiac or hypoxaemic pulmonary disease). Patients with severe pulmonary hypertension (mean PAP >40 mm Hg) are at risk of right heart failure and sudden death. Particular care is required with intravenous fluids and vasoactive drugs. Pulmonary artery catheterisation may allow right and left heart function to be studied separately, but it can be difficult to "wedge" the catheter in these patients and there is additional risk from pulmonary arteriolar rupture. Reversibility can be assessed using a variety of pulmonary arterial vasodilators including intravenous $\beta_2$ agonists and nitrates, or inhaled volatile anaesthetic agents, nitric oxide, and nebulised prostacyclin.

### Pulmonary embolism

Pulmonary embolism may occur from air (intravenous pressure infusors, CVP catheter track), amniotic fluid during delivery, or fat from long bone fractures (both of which are often accompanied by features of disseminated intravascular coagulation), or most commonly from venous thrombus in predisposed patients. The surgical management of thromboembolism is confined to those cases in which the embolus is large but has not completely occluded the pulmonary circulation, and in which thrombolysis carries greater risks than the heparin anticoagulation required for bypass. Massive pulmonary embolism may present with variable combinations of acute hypotension or shock, oppressive chest pain, dyspnoea and hypoxaemia, ECG changes (often non-specific ST/T wave changes, uncommonly S1Q3T3), and chest radiograph evidence of air space shadowing or pleural fluid from lung infarction. Signs of peripheral venous thrombosis are often absent. Risk factors for deep venous thrombosis include recent immobility, dehydration, surgery, low cardiac output states, and failure to apply subcutaneous heparin prophylaxis. Pulmonary embolism occurring *de novo* is uncommon in intensive care patients, presumably because impaired coagulation and low blood viscosity from relative anaemia counterbalance the immobility of critical illness.

*Transplant recipients*

Solid organ transplantation is increasing as are survival times, so there is a greater chance that intensive care units may admit transplant recipients with an intercurrent infection, or following surgery for a non-transplant condition. The transplant centre responsible for their care must be contacted as soon as possible. Meticulous care must be taken to avoid cross-infection (catheters, handwashing, etc.) as for any immunosuppressed population. The diagnosis of primary infections is a priority, and requires a team approach with close liaison with microbiology. The transplanted heart is denervated; it will therefore not respond to vagolytic agents (atropine, digoxin), does not adjust contractility or rate promptly in response to shifts in circulating volume, and may be particularly sensitive to exogenous catecholamines. If possible, central cannulation should avoid the right internal jugular vein because this route needs to be preserved for regular biopsy monitoring of rejection.

# Further reading

Alfieri A, Kotler MN. Noncardiac complications of open-heart surgery. *Am Heart J* 1990;**119**:149–58.
Foex P, Leone BJ. Pressure-volume loops: a dynamic approach to the assessment of ventricular function. *J Cardiothorac Vasc Anaesth* 1994;**8**:84–96.
Hollenberg M, Mangano DT, Browner WS, *et al*. Predictors of postoperative myocardial ischaemia in patients undergoing noncardiac surgery. *JAMA* 1992;**268**:205–9.
Morgans DT, Browner WS, Hollenberg M, *et al*. Association of perioperative myocardial ischaemia with cardiac morbidity and mortality in men undergoing non-cardiac surgery. *N Engl J Med* 1990;**323**:1781–8.

Older P, Smith R, Courtney P, Hone R. Preoperative evaluation of cardiac failure and ischemia in elderly patients by cardiopulmonary exercise testing. *Chest* 1993,**104**:701–4.

Thromboembolic Risk Factors (THRIFT) Consensus Group. Risk of and prophylaxis for venous thromboembolism in hospital patients. *BMJ* 1992;**305**:567–74 (letters 1156).

Williams BT, Jindane A. New trends in the postoperative management of cardiac surgical patients: a review. *J Cardiovasc Surg* 1994;**35**:161–3.

# 16: Acute renal failure and renal replacement

## L HARPER and N T RICHARDS

## Definition

Few of the existing definitions of acute renal failure are of any clinical use. For epidemiological purposes, that used by the British Renal Association is probably the simplest and most useful: "A sudden and potentially reversible reduction in renal function, from which, if renal replacement is not provided, the patient will die."

## Epidemiology and pathophysiology

### Incidence

It is estimated that 50 per million population per year will develop acute renal failure requiring dialysis. However, the point prevalence at any hospital will vary depending on the age distribution of the local population and the type of hospital. Specialist hospitals, with renal units, undertaking major cardiac, hepatobiliary, and urological surgery will see a greater number of cases with a different spectrum of aetiology to that seen in a district general hospital.

The true incidence of acute renal failure is probably greatly underestimated. Feest et al, in a study set in two health districts, where acute renal failure was defined as a creatinine of >500 mmol/l for the first time in 2 years, estimated an incidence of 140·5 cases per million population.[1] The incidence increased rapidly with age (Table 16.1). This study suggested that acute renal failure is at least twice as common as previously reported from renal unit-based studies. The availability of renal services was also found to influence referral patterns, particularly in the elderly population. This is despite the conclusion of many studies that age does not influence outcome of acute renal failure.

### Aetiology

The many possible causes of acute renal failure may be categorised broadly as prerenal (hypovolaemia, cardiogenic, or septic shock), intrinsic (renal disease/damage), and postrenal (obstructive). In the ICU prerenal causes will predominate.

Table 16.1 Age-related incidence of acute renal failure

| Age (years) | Incidence (per $10^6$/population) |
| --- | --- |
| 16–49 | 17·1 |
| 50–59 | 82·7 |
| 60–69 | 185·9 |
| 70–79 | 660·3 |
| 80–89 | 949·0 |

## Pathophysiology

The histological end-point of acute renal failure, in the majority of cases, is acute tubular necrosis. The kidney has a number of protective compensatory mechanisms designed to maintain glomerular filtration rate and it is only when these have been overwhelmed that acute tubular necrosis develops.

### Susceptibility of the medulla to necrosis

The kidneys receive over 20% of the cardiac output. More than 90% of the blood that enters the kidney supplies the renal cortex, which is perfused at a rate of 500 ml/min per 100 g tissue. The renal cortex receives far more oxygen than its metabolic functions require. This is in order to maintain glomerular filtration. As a consequence of the anatomy of the renal microcirculation, oxygen delivery is not uniform, with the medullary blood supply being no more than adequate. Blood is delivered to the medulla via the vasa recta, capillaries derived from efferent arterioles originating in the cortex. The inner medulla receives a blood supply of only 20 ml/min per 100 g tissue. The vasa recta follow the loops of Henle in a similar hairpin arrangement. This arrangement allows the capillaries to function as countercurrent exchangers, in the same way as the loops of Henle. However, this arrangement is very inefficient at delivering oxygen. In a similar way to how countercurrent mechanism increases the sodium concentration of the tubular fluid, $Po_2$ is reduced (Figure 16.1).

Sodium reabsorption is the primary function of tubular cells and is a highly energy-dependent process accounting for >50% of renal oxygen consumption. The region of the kidney with the highest metabolic demand is the very region that is most susceptible to hypoxia (Figure 16.1).

The fraction of cardiac output perfusing the kidneys is dependent on the ratio of renal vascular resistance to systemic vascular resistance. The kidney has a number of mechanisms of modulating vascular resistance in order to maintain filtration in the face of falling pressure.

### Autoregulation

Tubuloglomerular feedback is designed to maintain salt and water homeostasis. During periods of actual or perceived hypoperfusion there

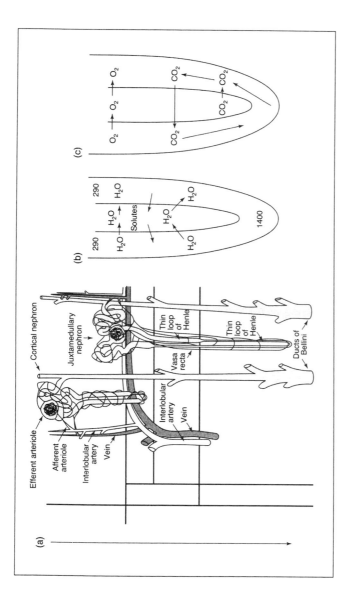

Fig 16.1 (a) Cortical (short-looped) and juxtamedullary (long-looped) nephrons, showing the differences in the blood supply to the two nephron types. Countercurrent exchange in the vasa recta. (b) As the descending vasa recta enter the increasingly hypertonic medullary interstitium, water is osmotically abstracted from the blood vessel so that osmolality of the blood and its viscosity are increased. In the ascending limb, water re-enters the blood vessel. The system ensures a low-flow rate through the deep parts of the vasa recta, and minimises washout of medullary solutes. (c) $O_2$ also undergoes countercurrent exchange in the vasa recta, so that the vasa recta are rather inefficient suppliers of $O_2$ and removers of $CO_2$ for cells deep in the medulla. (Reproduced with permission from Lote C. *Principles of renal physiology*, 3rd edn London: Chapman & Hall, 1994.)

is a decrease in solute delivery to the macula densa cells of the juxtaglomerular apparatus. This results in vasodilatation of the adjacent afferent glomerular arteriole, reducing renal vascular resistance and improving glomerular perfusion and filtration. This response predominantly involves the afferent arteriole and is limited such that renal blood flow remains constant until systolic pressure falls below 80 mm Hg when renal blood flow falls precipitously. However, in patients with pre-existing renal disease or renal artery narrowing, this adaptive mechanism is impaired, resulting in precipitous falls in renal blood flow with only minor degrees of hypotension. In these patients the maintenance of cardiac output and blood pressure is of considerable importance.

### Locally produced vasoactive substances

Prostaglandins are synthesised in the cortex and the medullary interstitium, and by collecting duct epithelial cells. The main ones are $PGE_2$, $PGI_2$ (prostacyclin), $PGF_{2\alpha}$, $PGD_2$, and thromboxane $A_2$, and are synthesised from arachidonic acid via the cyclo-oxygenase pathway. Both $PGE_2$ and $PGI_2$ are vasodilators and are produced in increasing amounts when renal blood flow falls, thus minimising renal cortical vasoconstriction. $PGI_2$, the main prostaglandin of the cortex, is also a mediator of renin release. The medullary prostaglandins (mainly $PGE_2$) act predominantly on collecting tubules, producing a natriuresis and diuresis, and impair the action of the antidiuretic hormone. These properties may limit the extent to which sodium reabsorption can be stimulated in the medulla, and hence are protective during hypovolaemia.

Thromboxane $A_2$ is a vasoconstrictor. Unlike other prostanoids, it has no role in the maintenance of renal function under physiological conditions. During episodes of hypovolaemia its synthesis is stimulated by angiotensin II and vasopressin. Renal blood flow and glomerular filtration rate are reduced by preferential constriction of the efferent arteriole and glomerular mesangial cells (reducing the glomerular surface area available for filtration).

Nitric oxide is a potent vasodilator derived from the $N$-terminal guanidino group of L-arginine by the action of the enzyme nitric oxide synthase within endothelial cells.[2] It promotes the conversion of guanosine triphosphate to cyclic GMP, resulting in a decrease in intracellular calcium and relaxation of smooth muscle. Nitric oxide also acts on mesangial and juxtaglomerular cells, influencing glomerular function. Within the kidney, there is basal secretion of nitric oxide through constitutive nitric oxide synthase. Nitric oxide may also be produced in much larger quantities (10-fold) by an inducible nitric oxide synthase.

Endothelins are a family of peptides of 21 amino acids produced by endothelial cells.[3] Endothelin-1(ET-1) is the predominant isoform found within the kidney and is the most potent vasoconstrictor described to date. The precise physiological role of ET-1 is yet to be defined but it is involved in regulation of vascular smooth muscle and mesangial cell tone, sodium and water excretion, and renal cell mitogenesis. The renal vasculature is extremely sensitive to the vasoconstrictor effects of ET-1 which acts on both afferent and efferent arterioles. Mesangial cells are stimulated to produce platelet-aggregating factor which may in part mediate its contractile effects. ET-1 induces the release of prostaglandins and nitric oxide from endothelial cells. ET-1 acts directly on the collecting duct to inhibit sodium and water transport, and reduces vasopressin-stimulated water reabsorption.

During hypovolaemia systemic blood pressure is maintained by a combination of increased sympathetic tone and systemic vasoconstrictors such as angiotensin II and vasopressin. Secondary generation of intrarenal vasodilators, such as prostaglandins and nitric oxide, ameliorate the effects of these constrictors on the renal vasculature, preventing a rise in renal vascular resistance and hence a fall in renal blood flow.

Septic shock is characterised by uncontrolled vasodilatation and marked cytokine production. Cytokines such as tumour necrosis factor $\alpha$ (TNF$\alpha$) may act directly on glomerular endothelial and mesangial cells, producing a marked increase in ET-1 release. Excessive production of ET-1 has been implicated in the intense vasoconstriction seen in established acute renal failure.[4,5]

Decompensation of the mechanisms used to maintain renal blood flow and hence glomerular filtration rate may be precipitated by injudicious therapeutic interventions such as non-steroidal anti-inflammatory agents (NSAIDs).

## Control of filtration fraction

The kidney has an unique anatomical arrangement in the form of the efferent arteriole which allows it to control renal blood flow and glomerular filtration. Selective vasoconstriction of the efferent arteriole produces a fall in glomerular plasma flow. Glomerular filtration rate does not fall because glomerular capillary pressure upstream of the constriction tends to rise, thereby augmenting glomerular filtration. Angiotensin II acts preferentially on the efferent arteriole to produce this effect, as do low concentrations of noradrenaline. The adrenergic nervous system may also be important in maintaining glomerular filtration in times of circulatory embarrassment. By this mechanism renal blood flow may be reduced at the expense of maintaining systemic blood flow without a reduction in glomerular filtration rate. However, at high concentrations, angiotensin II and noradrenaline constrict the afferent in addition to the efferent arteriole, reducing renal blood flow and glomerular filtration rate. This is a property shared by other circulating vasoconstrictors.

## Inflammatory mediators

Sepsis is a common cause of acute renal failure and septicaemia is a common event in a patient with acute renal failure, particularly in the setting of the intensive care unit. Infective agents may exert their effects by both direct and indirect mechanisms. Many of the indirect effects of bacteria may be mediated by endotoxin. Endotoxin may act directly on tubular cells but also stimulates cytokine production, particularly TNF$\alpha$, interleukin-1, and platelet-aggregating factor. These cytokines directly interact with renal cells, leading to the upregulation of intercellular adhesion molecules and indirectly cause damage through the accumulation of activated leukocytes. Leukocytes appear to accumulate within glomeruli and release proteases and oxygen-derived free radicals, resulting in cell damage. Cytokines activate the complement system, releasing vasoactive and chemotactic factors, and the coagulation and fibrinolytic cascades.

A number of cytokines can induce the release of ET-1 and induce expression of inducible nitric oxide synthase. Nitric oxide is then produced in large quantities in an uncontrolled manner. This results in prolonged vasoconstrictor-resistant vasodilatation. In these circumstances nitric oxide may act as a potent oxygen-derived free radical. There is alteration in the balance of arachidonic acid metabolites with a relative increase in the production of vasoconstricting thromboxane $A_2$ and leukotriene $D_4$.

Some infective agents have direct renal toxic effects and are associated with specific types of renal disease (Table 16.2).

Table 16.2 Infective agents and renal disease

| Infective agent | Renal disease |
| --- | --- |
| *Mycoplasma pneumoniae* *Leptospira icterohaemorrhagiae* *Yersinia enterolytica* *Legionella pneumophila* | Interstitial nephritis |
| Hepatitis B and C | Glomerulonephritis |
| Coxsackie A3, B9 | Rhabdomyolysis |
| Verotoxin-producing *E. coli* | Haemolytic uraemic syndrome |
| Gram-negative bacteria | Disseminated intravascular coagulation |

# Prevention of acute renal failure

Prevention of acute renal failure (ARF) is always a better option than treatment. Patients at risk can be identified, and certain simple measures can prevent its development. ARF is often multifactorial. The risk factors are listed in Box 16.1.

The risk of ARF is increased if several factors operate in conjunction. The

**Box 16.1**  *Risk factors for ARF*

- Pre-existing renal impairment
- Diabetes mellitus
- Hypertension and/or vascular disease
- Drugs, including NSAIDs, angiotensin-converting enzyme inhibitors
- Jaundice
- Multiple myeloma and other hyperviscosity states
- Sepsis and the systemic inflammatory response
- Dehydration and contrast media
- Age

elderly patient receiving an NSAID and an ACE inhibitor, who is admitted with a respiratory infection, dehydration, hypotension, and hypoxaemia, is certain to develop ARF in the absence of prompt resuscitation. In addition to the basic ABC of resuscitation, the preventive measures discussed below are of particular importance.

**Adequate hydration**

Hypovolaemia must be prevented in "at risk" individuals by maximising circulating volume; this may necessitate the use of central venous pressure monitoring. Vigorous hydration with physiological saline is mandatory in those at risk of acute renal failure, particularly before major surgery, in the jaundiced patient, and in those undergoing aortic surgery.[2] Studies performed in the 1980s by Eisenberg *et al* found no cases of ARF in high-risk patients undergoing major angiography who received 250 ml of saline by rapid infusion and a further 550 ml of saline infused throughout the procedure.[6] Recently, in a prospective study, patients with renal impairment who underwent coronary angiography were hydrated with 0·45% saline pre- and post angiography. Saline alone, compared with mannitol or the combination of saline and frusemide, significantly reduced the risk of renal failure.[7]

**Renal perfusion**

Both cardiac output and systemic arterial blood pressure are important determinants of renal blood flow, particularly in patients with pre-existing renal impairment. A blood pressure of 110/80 mm Hg may represent significant hypotension in a normally hypertensive individual, and may contribute to further renal ischaemic injury.

**Nephrotoxic agents**

All potentially nephrotoxic agents should be discontinued especially NSAIDs, the adverse effects of which are increased when prescribed in conjunction with ACE inhibitors.

## Renoprotective agents

### Dopamine

The role of dopamine as a renoprotective agent is controversial. Dopamine is used widely in the dose range 2–5 mg/kg per min and is said to act as a renal vasodilator. The evidence supporting this is largely anecdotal. There is significant overlap in the stimulation of $\beta$-adrenergic and $\alpha$-adrenergic receptors even at these low doses. The increase in renal blood flow seen is probably due to its inotropic effects and can be reproduced by other non-dopaminergic inotropes. The ability of dopamine and dobutamine, a non-dopaminergic inotrope, to improve renal function has been compared in a randomised, double-blind trial. Dopamine induced a diuresis but did not increase creatinine clearance whilst dobutamine increased creatinine clearance without a change in urine output.[8] The diuresis seen following dopamine administration is probably a direct tubular effect. Dopamine impairs the important tubuloglomerular feedback mechanism and may adversely affect the ratio between oxygen supply and demand, promoting the development of acute tubular necrosis.[9] It has recently been suggested that dopamine may prolong the duration of ARF, particularly in oliguric patients.[10]

Well-designed studies have shown no benefit from dopamine in the prevention of renal dysfunction in well-hydrated patients undergoing elective abdominal surgery[11] or in patients undergoing coronary artery bypass surgery.[12] There is one study in which dopamine appeared to protect against radiocontrast-induced renal failure in patients with pre-existing renal impairment.[13] It is important to note that the tubular and possibly other dopamine-1 receptor effects are inhibited by commonly used dopamine antagonists such as metoclopramide. There is little evidence that dopamine is a renoprotective agent and its routine use should be questioned.

### Mannitol

Mannitol is an osmotic diuretic which, if administered prophylactically to jaundiced patients undergoing surgery or invasive abdominal procedures, reduces the incidence of ARF.[14] However, in jaundiced patients mannitol has been shown to be no better than saline.[15] The beneficial effects of mannitol are thought to be due to decreased intratubular obstruction and improved renal haemodynamics from an increase in medullary blood flow. Whether its oxygen free radical-scavenging properties are of value in humans undergoing predictable renal ischaemia–reperfusion (such as aortic aneurysm surgery) is unknown, but its use should be considered for this purpose.

*Frusemide*

Loop diuretics inhibit $Na^+/K^+$ ATPase, and reduce renal tubular oxygen consumption. In circumstances where renal blood flow is likely to be impaired, the use of low-dose frusemide infusions (about 10 mg/h) may possibly be beneficial, provided that an excessive diuresis is not allowed to produce volume depletion.

## Management of acute renal failure

Patients with ARF are likely to have a condition requiring urgent specific therapy. They should be managed jointly by a nephrologist and an intensivist. The principles of management are:

- to diagnose and treat the cause of the renal failure;
- to support the patient by means of dialysis until renal function returns.

### Diagnosis and treatment

Diagnosis and treatment should proceed together. It is essential at the outset to treat prerenal causes and to exclude the possibility of renal tract obstruction, with the use of renal and bladder ultrasound. In the presence of oligo-anuria even mild degrees of pelvicalyceal dilatation should be considered significant and an anterograde urogram performed. Ultrasound will also confirm the number of kidneys, estimate the size and texture (small, bright kidneys indicating chronic disease), and confirm the presence of arterial and venous blood flow using Doppler.

In most cases the cause of ARF is readily apparent with obvious precipitating factors (surgery, trauma, sepsis). Unexplained ARF occurring in the ICU should prompt a search for a septic focus or ischaemic tissue. If the cause is either in doubt or not apparent, a renal biopsy should be performed as a matter of urgency. Previous studies have demonstrated that management can be altered in over 70% of cases of ARF in which a renal biopsy has been performed. Additional investigations under these circumstances should include, as a minimum, a full biochemical profile including creatine phosphokinase, urate and glucose, measurement of antinuclear antibodies, antineutrophil cytoplasmic antibodies, antiglomerular basement membrane antibodies, C3 and C4 components of complement, and a protein electrophoresis.

Urinalysis may be useful. In prerenal failure there is little in the way of cells, casts, or protein. In established acute tubular necrosis, there is an abundance of tubular cell debris and mild proteinuria. The presence of haematuria may be an indicator of glomerular disease. Urinary electrolytes and osmolality are influenced by previous renal disease, state of hydration, catabolic state, and previous diuretic administration, and in practice they are rarely used. In established acute tubular necrosis, the urine is dilute and tends to be iso-osmotic (osmolality 280–320 mosmol/kg); urinary sodium is generally >40 mmol/l. In prerenal failure, the urine should be concentrated and the sodium content is usually <10 mmol/l.

Nephrotoxic agents (for example, NSAIDs, ACE inhibitors, and aminoglycosides) should be discontinued if possible or appropriate dose alterations made. Assessment of intravascular volume status and cardiac output must be made. These should be corrected as necessary with the appropriate plasma volume expander or inotropes. Detailed and accurate management cannot be conducted without measures of circulating volume and cardiac output with the use of either thermodilution pulmonary artery catheterisaton or the oesophageal Doppler in skilled hands. Repeated fluid challenges in the presence of oliguria and the absence of monitoring are to be deplored, as they may precipitate left ventricular volume overload, pulmonary oedema, and the need for dialysis.

When obstruction has been excluded and intravascular volume and cardiac output optimised, a diuretic challenge with increasing doses of frusemide up to 2 mg/min for 3–4 hours or mannitol 20–30 g may be attempted. This can produce a diuresis and abort the establishment of acute tubular necrosis. More commonly, either there is no effect or the oliguric state is converted to a non-oliguric state, which simplifies management and may carry a better prognosis. The mechanisms of the effects of diuretics are complex and not fully understood. Diuretics inhibit sodium reabsorption and hence reduce tubular oxygen requirements. The diuresis may remove sloughed tubular cells, relieving tubular obstruction and reducing filtrate back-leak across tubular epithelial cells. There is also evidence that frusemide improves renal blood flow to the mid-cortical zone and, in some animal models, may reduce the duration of renal failure.

At present there are no acknowledged treatment strategies that reduce duration or mortality of ARF. However, recent animal studies have indicated that atrial natriuretic peptide (ANP) attenuates the severity and/or accelerates the recovery in experimental models of ARF. ANP increases glomerular filtration rate in pathological states by increasing glomerular capillary perfusion pressure, and has a direct diuretic and natriuretic effect on the distal tubule. In a randomised blinded study of 53 patients, ANP or placebo was given to patients with established ARF. ANP was infused intrarenally for 8 hours or intravenously for 24 hours. Independent of the route of administration, creatinine clearance increased significantly at 8 and 24 hours after discontinuing the infusion. ANP appeared to reduce the need for dialysis and increase creatinine clearance when given to patients with established ARF.[16] However, in a further placebo-controlled study of intravenous ANP in 504 patients with ARF, there was no difference in outcome, and specifically no reduction in dialysis requirements.[17] Subgroup analysis suggested less dialysis dependence and a trend towards improved survival in patients with oliguric renal failure.[18] Further studies are required.

## Electrolyte abnormalities

Hyperkalaemia and hyponatraemia are the commonest electrolyte abnormalities seen in ARF. Hyponatraemia is commonly dilutional, but may also be related to salt depletion. Hyperkalaemia is the most important electrolyte abnormality. The clinical consequences depend on the rate of rise and the degree of hyperkalaemia. Hyperkalaemia results in alterations in membrane excitability leading to cardiac dysrhythmias, an effect potentiated by hypocalcaemia.

The ECG signs of hyperkalaemia are :

I     Tall peaked T waves
II    Widening of the QRS complex
III   Lengthening of the PR interval
IV    Bradycardia
V     Asystolic cardiac arrest.

Treatment is urgent if ECG changes are present or if the potassium is > 6.5 mmol/l. Serum potassium may be reduced rapidly by facilitating intracellular uptake with the use of 50 ml of 50% dextrose and 8–10 units of soluble insulin intravenously. Insulin stimulates cell membrane $Na^+/K^+$ ATPase, leading to potassium influx and sodium efflux. This is an emergency measure until dialysis is established. Intravenous calcium salts (usually 10 ml of 10% calcium gluconate) may be given to reduce cardiac toxicity. The majority of hyperkalaemic patients with ARF also have a metabolic acidosis. If this is corrected with the use of intravenous sodium bicarbonate (usually in 100 mmol aliquots over 15–30 minutes), the serum potassium will fall. In general this is more effective than the use of insulin and dextrose. Care must be taken to avoid excessive sodium load.

Hypocalcaemia is relatively rare and may indicate a degree of chronicity, although this is not reliable. ARF due to rhabdomyolysis is associated with severe hypocalcaemia, hyperphosphataemia, and hyperkalaemia in the oliguric phase. The hypocalcaemia is caused by calcium deposition in injured muscle. Hypocalcaemia in this situation should not be treated unless the patient is symptomatic, as this may exacerbate ectopic calcification.

## Nutrition

Adequate nutrition is necessary to minimise protein breakdown and prevent malnutrition. Uncomplicated ARF has little effect on energy expenditure but, as part of the systemic inflammatory response syndrome, oxygen consumption increases by about 30%. This uncontrolled catabolism cannot be completely reversed by feeding. The aetiology of the protein breakdown is multifactorial, the most important elements being insulin resistance, the release of catabolic hormones, the presence of a metabolic acidosis, and activation of inflammatory mediators.

The nutritional requirements of each patient should be assessed. An excessive calorie load may result in fatty degeneration of the liver, increased release of stress hormones, and respiratory insufficiency. The predominant energy source should be carbohydrate. Insulin may be required because of impaired glucose utilisation and insulin resistance. Lipid given at the rate of 1 g/kg per day provides 20–25% of energy requirements while avoiding hypertriglyceridaemia. Intake of protein should be around 1.5 g/kg per day; greater amounts increase generation of urea and other nitrogenous waste products. Both essential and non-essential amino acids should be included.

It may be possible in the future to reverse or even prevent the development of the hypercatabolic state by various endocrine/metabolic interventions such as the administration of thyroxine, growth hormone, and insulin-like growth factor I. These are being evaluated at present. Insulin-like growth factor I has been shown to improve nitrogen balance and may accelerate renal recovery.[19]

## Infection

Infection is extremely common in patients with ARF, from a combination of the immunosuppressant effects of uraemia and the nature of the underlying problem. Lymphopenia is common in both acute and chronic renal failure, and is probably a consequence of an impaired blastogenic response of uraemic lymphocytes. The use of prophylactic antibiotics is of no benefit. Chest physiotherapy and scrupulous care of implanted foreign bodies such as dialysis access devices are important. Urinary catheters should be removed as soon as possible especially in patients who are oliguric, where they play no role. Many patients are infected at presentation. There should be a clear policy for the investigation and management of pyrexia.

## Gastrointestinal haemorrhage

Uraemic patients bleed spontaneously and have a prolonged bleeding time because of inhibition of the interaction between platelet glycoprotein IIb–IIIa and von Willebrand's factor, preventing platelet spread. The coagulation cascade is otherwise usually normal. Gastrointestinal blood loss is common, though $H_2$-receptor antagonists have reduced the mortality from this complication. $H_2$ Receptor antagonists or sucralfate should be prescribed for all patients with ARF.

## Uraemic encephalopathy

Various disturbances of consciousness may affect the uraemic patient. Lethargy, drowsiness, and eventually coma are part of the progression of uraemic encephalopathy. With advanced uraemia a number of abnormal movements including tremor, cramps, metabolic flap, myoclonic jerks, and seizures may occur. The presence of a significant uraemic encephalopathy is a sign of severe uraemia and should be treated by dialysis. Phenytoin should be prescribed to reduce the risk of fitting from acute reductions in urea during dialysis.

# Dialysis therapies

The standard technique of daily intermittent haemodialysis for ARF is now being replaced by continuous renal replacement techniques. There are a number of indications for dialysis (Box 16.2). Although there are no absolute levels of urea or creatinine at which dialysis should be started, it would usually be considered at a serum urea of 20–30 mmol/l and a serum creatinine of 500–700 mmol/l. Early dialysis has been shown to improve survival.

## Choice of therapy

There are a number of different dialysis modalities. These can be broadly divided into continuous therapies (peritoneal dialysis, haemofiltration, haemodiafiltration, ultrafiltration) and intermittent therapies (haemodialysis, peritoneal dialysis). The choice of therapy depends upon the therapeutic goal, the clinical condition of the patient, and, unfortunately, the equipment available. Initially either solute or fluid removal will be the goal. Haemodialysis is more efficient at removing solute, and haemofiltration has a greater capacity for fluid removal. When assessing a patient for dialysis, haemodynamic stability, abdominal status, respiratory status, degree of catabolism, and the state of anticoagulation are all important factors. Catabolic, haemodynamically unstable patients with multiple organ failure are better managed with continuous haemodiafiltration. For a

---

**Box 16.2** *Indications for dialysis*

- Hyperkalaemia
- Uraemic pericarditis
- Uncontrolled acidosis
- Pulmonary oedema
- Uraemic bleeding
- Uraemic encephalopathy

---

Table 16.3 Dialysis efficiencies

| Modality | Rate | Urea clearance | Inulin clearance |
|----------|------|----------------|------------------|
| CAVH | UFR 8 ml/min | 12 | 10 |
| CAVH | UFR 14 ml/min | 20 | 16 |
| CVVH | UFR 17 ml/min | 24 | 20 |
| CAVHD | $Q_d$ 1 l/h + UFR 3 ml/min | 28 | 3·5 |
| CVVHD | $Q_d$ 1 l/h + UFR 17 ml/min | 28 | 14 |
| HD | 4 hours | 38 | 2 |
| CPD | 20 l/day + 3 l UF | 23 | 7·5 |

CAVH, continuous arteriovenous haemofiltration; CAVHD, continuous arteriovenous haemodiafiltration; CVVH, continuous venovenous haemofiltration; CVVHD, continous venovenous haemodiafiltration; HD, haemodiafiltration; CPD, continuous peritoneal dialysis; $Q_d$, dialysis rate; UFR, ultrafiltration rate; UF, ultrafiltrate.

comparison of the efficiencies of the various therapies see Table 16.3. The normal glomerular filtration rate is approximately 120 ml/min, and at least 10% of this should be provided by any chosen therapy to ensure adequate solute and fluid removal.

## Peritoneal dialysis

Peritoneal dialysis uses the peritoneum as a semipermeable membrane. The dialysate is an electrolyte solution containing glucose, in varying concentrations, as the oncotic agent, and lactate as the buffer. Dialysate is infused into the peritoneal cavity via a semirigid Teflon catheter. The fluid is left for a time to equilibrate and then drained out. Usually hourly exchanges of 1–1·5 litres allow adequate removal of fluid and solute in a non-catabolic patient. Peritoneal dialysis cannot be used in patients following abdominal surgery or in those who have abdominal hernias. Complications of peritoneal dialysis are common, and include gut perforation both at the time of insertion and from later migration, haemorrhage, and peritonitis. Peritonitis is by far the commonest complication and is heralded by abdominal pain and cloudy dialysate fluid with a raised neutrophil count. This should be treated with intraperitoneal and systemic antibiotics, and catheter removal.

## Haemofiltration

Haemofiltration simulates the non-specific filtration that occurs in glomeruli, so that water and solutes are forced through a semipermeable membrane from the plasma by hydrostatic pressure (forced convection). There are no osmolar changes in the cells or extracelluar fluid, and this allows rapid replacement of the removed fluid and solute without hypotension. High ultrafiltration rates are achieved by the use of membranes with high hydraulic permeability. The solute concentration present in the filtrate equates to that in plasma, up to the molecular weight dictated by the membrane permeability. Larger molecules (mol. wt > 1000–10 000 daltons) are better removed by this method than by haemodialysis. Large volumes of filtrate are removed (up to 100 ml/min), replaced as necessary by administering balanced electrolyte solutions.

Continuous arteriovenous haemofiltration (CAVH) uses low transmembrane pressure gradients and achieves haemofiltration rates up to 20 ml/min. Vascular access is achieved usually via short, large-bore femoral arterial and venous catheters, or a Scribner shunt. CAVH has advantages in that arteriovenous pressure difference alone can achieve blood flow rates of up to 120 ml/min. There is no risk of air embolism and ultrafiltration is self-limiting .

Continuous venovenous haemofiltration (CVVH) has the addition of a blood pump in the system. Vascular access is achieved via a double-lumen central venous catheter. Arterial cannulation is avoided although there are other risks. Sophisticated monitoring equipment is required for the extracorporeal blood circuit to prevent air embolism and exsanguination. This type of pumped system is very efficient and is not dependent upon arterial blood pressure, so it is applicable to patients with cardiovascular compromise. Vacuum suction applied to the filtrate component enhances the ultrafiltration rate, but the resulting rise in blood viscosity can lead to earlier clotting of the haemofilter.

Substitution fluids can be varied according to the patient's clinical and metabolic requirements, and are infused at a rate that achieves the desired fluid balance. Lactate is usually used as the buffer in replacement solutions although systems exist that use bicarbonate. Exchange volumes in excess of 25 litres/day can be achieved.


### Haemodiafiltration

Haemodiafiltration is a modification of haemofiltration which provides enhanced solute clearance by adding the diffusion of dialysis to convective ultrafiltration. It is achieved by infusing dialysate through the filtrate compartment of the haemofilter, countercurrent to blood flow at a rate of 0·5–2·0 litres/hour. Solute clearances are superior to those achieved with haemofiltration alone.

Both continuous haemofiltration and haemodiafiltration are extremely well tolerated even in patients who are inotrope dependent. Both techniques produce good biochemical control, even in highly catabolic patients, and in addition allow complete control of fluid balance. Nutrition should be optimal as the volume of feed need not be constrained. Amino acid loss through, and drug clearance by, the filter depends on molecular size and charge, protein binding, and bulk convection.

## Complications of continuous haemofiltration

Exsanguination and air embolism should not occur if there are adequate numbers of skilled staff and sophisticated monitoring. Bleeding from over-anticoagulation with heparin will be avoided if the APTT (activated partial thromboplastin time) is measured frequently, and maintained at 2–2·5 times control values. Prolonged use of heparin may result in thrombocytopenia and other anticoagulants such as prostacyclin or low-molecular-weight heparin may be required (Table 16.4). In at-risk patients, heparin can be reversed by continuous infusion of protamine into the return circuit.

Table 16.4 Continuous therapies – advantages and disadvantages

| Advantages | Disadvantages |
| --- | --- |
| Continuous | Constant anticoagulation |
| Virtually unlimited fluid removal | Slow removal of toxins |
| Biocompatible membranes | Lactate-buffered dialysis |

## Haemodialysis

Daily haemodialysis is the most efficient technique for fluid and solute removal. Standard dialysis membranes remove solute by passive diffusion. The rate of diffusion depends largely on solute size and the concentration gradient of solute between plasma and dialysate. Small molecules (up to 200 daltons) are cleared in direct proportion to dialysing membrane permeability, duration of dialysis, and blood and dialysate flow rates. Clearance of medium-sized molecules (500–3000 daltons) is related to membrane porosity and dialysis duration. Ultrafiltration is dependent on the transmembrane hydro-oncotic pressure. Bicarbonate is the buffer of choice and there is good evidence that its use is associated with greater cardiovascular stability in patients with acute renal failure. Access to the circulation is achieved with double-lumen venous catheters into central veins. Blood flow rates are usually maintained at 150–250 ml/min depending on patient tolerance. Dialysate flow rate is in the region of 500 ml/min. Heparin is usually required to prevent clotting of the dialyser.

Hypotension is a common complication of haemodialysis, and this may preclude its use in critically ill patients. In contrast to haemofiltration, solute is removed preferentially from the intravascular space and extra-cellular fluid, resulting in a fall in extracellular osmolality. Relative intracellular hypertonicity causes fluid to move from the extracellular to the intracellular compartment, further depleting intravascular volume and possibly leading to cerebral oedema. Sequential dialysis with ultrafiltration may improve this problem. Approximately 10–15% of patients with multiple organ failure cannot tolerate haemodialysis and continuous therapies should be employed. Haemodialysis is generally performed intermittently (although slow continuous haemodialysis has been employed) and it does not have the capacity of continuous therapies to remove large quantities of fluid. Thus haemodialysis does not provide the same fine control of fluid balance as continuous therapies.

Non-cellulose biocompatible membranes should be used because cellophane-based membranes activate complement, leading to sequestration of activated polymorphs in the lungs and a worsening of hypoxaemia. Biocompatible membranes may reduce the duration of the dialysis-dependent phase of ARF.

## Outcome

There is a suggestion that the use of continuous therapies is associated with improved survival, although there a few hard data to support this. In a retrospective study performed by Kierdorf et al in 1989, patients treated by continuous renal replacement did significantly better than historical controls treated by intermittent haemodialysis. Of the 73 patients treated by CVVH, 22% survived compared with 7% of the historical controls.[20] McDonald and Metha in a further retrospective analysis showed a trend towards improved survival in those patients treated with CAVH or those who were changed from intermittent haemodialysis to CAVH.[21] When patients with similar disease severity were compared, there was a significant improvement in mortality in those managed with a continuous technique. In a study of patients with fulminant liver failure and ARF, randomised to receive either haemodialysis or continuous haemofiltration, the continuous technique was associated with better control of cardiovascular function and intracranial pressure, but this was not translated into improved survival. Intermittent haemodialysis was associated with significantly worse tissue oxygen extraction.[22] In high-risk patients haemofiltration or haemodiafiltration is the treatment of choice.

## Conclusions

In many cases, simple measures such as the prevention of intravascular volume depletion, the restoration of cardiac output and perfusion pressure, and the discontinuation of nephrotoxic agents may prevent the development of ARF. Patients at risk should be identified early. Prompt diagnosis and management are essential to maximise the chances of renal recovery. In established ARF, renal replacement therapy and adequate nutrition must be started early. In the ICU continuous therapies are the method of choice.

1 Feest TG, Round A, Hamad S. Incidence of severe acute renal failure in adults: results of a community based study. *BMJ* 1993;**306**:481–3.
2 Glauser MP, Zanetti G, Baumgartner JD, Cohen J. Septic shock: pathogenesis. *Lancet* 1991;**338**:732–5.
3 Takabatake T, Takuyki I, Ohta K, Kobayashi Y. Endothelin effects on renal function and tubuloglomerular feedback. *Kidney Int* 1991;**39**:S122–4.
4 Wardle EN. Acute renal failure and muti-organ failure. *Nephrol Dial Transplant* 1994;**66**:380–5.
5 Kohan DE. Role of endothelin and tumour necrosis factor in the renal response to sepsis. *Nephrol Dial Transplant* 1994;**9**(suppl 4):73–7.
6 Eisenberg RL, Bank WD, Hedglock MW. Renal failure after major angiography. *Am J Med* 1980;**68**:43–6.
7 Solomom R, Werner C, Mann D, D'Elia J, Silva P. Effects of saline, mannitol, and frusemide on acute decreases in renal function by radiocontrast agents. *N Engl J Med* 1994;**331**:1414–16.
8 Duke GJ, Briedis JH, Weaver RA. Renal support in critically ill patients: Low dose dopamine or low dose dobutamine? *Crit Care Med* 1994;**22**:1919–25.
9 Duke GJ, Bersten AD. Dopamine and renal salvage in the critically ill patient. *Anaesth Intensive Care* 1992;**20**:277–302.
10 Weisberg L, Kurnik B, Allgren RL. Clinical outcomes in ischaemic and nephrotoxic acute tubular necrosis. *Abstract, J Am Soc Nephrol* 1995;**904**/480.
11 Baldwin J, Henderson A, Hickman P. Effect of post-operative low dose dopamine on renal function after elective major vascular surgery. *Ann Intern Med* 1994;**120**:744–7.
12 Myles PS, Buckland MR, Schenk NJ, Cannon GB, Langley M, Davis BB. Effect of renal dose dopamine on renal function following cardiac surgery. *Anaesth Intensive Care* 1993;**21**:56–61.
13 Hall KA, Wong RW, Hunter GC, *et al.* Contrast induced nephrotoxicity: the effects of vasodilator therapy. *J Surg Res* 1992;**53**:317–20.
14 Dawson JL. Jaundice and anoxic renal damage: protective effect of mannitol. *BMJ* 1964;**i**:810–13.
15 Gubern JM, Sancho JJ, Simo J, Sitges-Serra A. A randomised trial on the effect of mannitol on post-operative renal function in patients with obstructive jaundice. *Surgery* 1988;**103**:39–44.
16 Rahman SN, Kim GE, Mathew AS, *et al.* Effects of atrial natriuretic peptide in clinical acute renal failure. *Kidney Int* 1994;**45**:1731–8.
17 Marbury TC, Rahman SN, Sweet RM, Feneves AZ, Weisberg L, Lafayette RA. A randomised double blind, placebo controlled multi-centre clinical trial of Anatride atrial natriuretic peptide (ANP) in the treatment of ATN. *N Engl J Med* 1997;**336**:828–34.
18 Rahman SN, Butt AR, DuBose TD, *et al.* Differential clinical effects of Anatride atrial natriuretic peptide (ANP) in oliguric and non-oliguric ATN. *J Am Soc Neprhol* 1995;**6**:474.
19 Ding H, Hirschberg R, Cohen A, Kopple JD. Recombinant human insulin-like growth factor-1 accelerates renal recovery and reduces catabolism in rats with acute renal faillure. *J Clin Invest* 1993;**91**:2281–7.
20 Kierdorf H. Continuous versus intermittent treatment: clinical results in acute renal failure. *Contrib Nephrol* 1991;**93**:1–12.
21 McDonald BR, Metha RL. Decreased mortality in patients with acute renal failure undergoing continuous arteriovenous haemodialysis. *Contrib Nephrol* 1991;**93**:51–6.
22 Davenport A, Will EJ, Davison AM. Continuous versus intermittent forms of haemofiltration and/or dialysis in the management of acute renal failure in patients with defective cerebral autoregulation at risk of cerebral oedema. *Contrib Nephrol* 1991;**93**:225–33.

# 17:   The surgical abdomen

M POEZE, J W M GREVE and G RAMSAY

The surgical or "acute" abdomen is classically described as a surgical condition with a rapid onset of abdominal pain requiring early evaluation and surgical intervention.[1] Approximately 16% of patients with abdominal pain presenting to the emergency department have an acute surgical problem.[2] A small proportion of this subgroup may require (on admission or later) intensive care management, for example, patients with acute pancreatitis, a perforated viscus, or postoperative intra-abdominal sepsis.[3] Additionally, critically ill patients admitted to the ICU with unrelated problems may develop surgical abdominal complications.[4] The intensive care clinician must therefore become adept at abdominal examination and diagnosis, particularly as acute surgical conditions may be obscured by critical illness, may be complicating or causing critical illness, and are likely to be fatal if left untreated.

The major decision in a critically ill patient in the ICU who appears to have an abdominal problem is whether and when to treat the problem surgically. This is particularly important in the assessment of secondary (often postoperative) intra-abdominal pathology. A patient in the ICU who, despite apparently adequate therapy, deteriorates following an abdominal operation, has a new, or incompletely treated, abdominal problem until proven otherwise.[5,6] Successful management requires a comprehensive understanding of the incidence and pathophysiology of diseases that cause an acute abdomen, and close cooperation between surgeon and intensivist.

This chapter examines the pathogenesis, early detection, and treatment of disease processes such as pancreatitis, gut ischaemia, abdominal trauma, and abdominal sepsis, with particular emphasis on decision-making, when to (re)operate on patients with acute abdominal problems, and how to prepare them for surgery.

## Evaluation of the acute abdomen in the ICU patient

A careful history and a complete physical examination is required in all patients.[7] However, both elements are often difficult to obtain and interpret in critically ill, sedated patients receiving organ-system support. For example, the hallmark of the acute abdomen, abdominal pain, may be masked by impaired consciousness, the use of opioids or immunomodulatory treatment (corticosteroids), and concurrent diseases.[8] Obtaining a clear history may require contacting family, friends, and the family doctor. The first abdominal examination is the most important because it is usually the most complete and gives the physician a clinical baseline. However, findings are often non-specific, and identifying a change or trend in sequential examinations is important for making correct decisions. Laboratory tests should be used to confirm or refute a clinical diagnosis, but should not be relied on exclusively.[5]

In traumatised patients the initial diagnostic work-up may need to be performed before the patient is admitted to the ICU, to minimise delay in definitive treatment. Following initial assessment and physiological stabilisation, the secondary survey can be completed. A tertiary system survey or routine in-hospital follow-up should be performed to exclude minor, delayed, or missed injuries. Careful documentation and collaborative consultation between trauma surgeon and intensivist are essential.

## Pathophysiology of abdominal sepsis

An abdominal source for infection should always be excluded in a patient with an unexplained systemic inflammatory response. Peritonitis develops when the normal defence mechanisms are overwhelmed, either by the volume of infective material or by impaired host defence.

The visceral and parietal peritoneum is lined by a layer of mesothelial cells which in the diaphragmatic part of the abdomen form intracellular spaces called stomata.[9] These intercellular stomata vary in diameter according to diaphragmatic movement, facilitating transport of fluid and particles through the open stomata[10] and thence into the lymphatics. The diaphragm thus plays an active role in the clearance of material from the peritoneal cavity during peritonitis[11] but, if the bacterial load is high, this system may also promote the systemic spread of bacteria and toxins.[12] Following bacterial or other noxious challenges, several other defence mechanisms are activated. Vasoactive amines and cytokines, released by mast cells and macrophages, cause increased vascular permeability and a subsequent exudation of plasma with fibrin deposition, in order to localize the infection by forming abcesses. If this fails, a diffuse peritonitis will develop.[13] Localised complement activation stimulates opsonisation, chemotaxis, and phagocytosis by a large influx of neutrophils,[14] and a syste mic response stimulated by bacterial absorption through diaphragmatic lymphatics.[15]

## The role of diagnostic tests

When a patient is seen with an obvious acute abdomen, there is rarely an indication for time-consuming diagnostic tests, which should be reserved for cases in which there is uncertainty about the diagnosis, or to clarify anatomy. When indicated, diagnostic tests should be planned so as to minimise risk to the patient and delay in specific operative treatment.

The most commonly used radiological study in patients with acute abdominal problems is the plain abdominal radiograph, which is useful in the diagnosis of perforated viscus (free air on decubitus views), ischaemic bowel (absence of gas), bowel obstruction, or colonic volvulus (gaseous distension).[16] As with any radiological procedure, the diagnostic "yield" will be improved by close collaboration between radiologist, surgeon, and intensivist.

Ultrasound is available, portable, and safe, but its value is dependent on the skill of the radiologist, and the image may be obscured by fat or fluid. It is of particular value in hepatobiliary disease,[17,18] and in the diagnosis of intra-abdominal abcesses; transvaginal or transrectal views may be required in suspected pelvic sepsis.

Contrast-enhanced spiral CT provides detailed views of all structures, and information about organ blood supply,[19] and is the diagnostic modality of choice for the splenic region, pancreas, and retroperitoneum.[21,22] However, the examination is time consuming and requires transporting a critically ill patient to an environment in which monitoring and access are difficult. This is even more of a problem in MRI scanning, for which metal components must also be excluded from equipment. The diagnostic information obtained from CT imaging may be helpful in only a small percentage of critically ill patients.

Gallium scanning for diagnosing intra-abdominal abcesses is not suitable for routine use in critically ill patients, because the patient has to be transported twice, the procedure takes a long time, and the yield is disappointing.[23] Its principal value would be to clarify an inconclusive ultrasound or CT scan in a patient with complex abdominal disease and possible abdominal sepsis. Peritoneal lavage or laparoscopy may be useful for specific indications.[24,25]

## Preoperative assessment and management

A balance must be found between the need for urgent surgery and the demands of physiological stabilisation of a critically ill patient. Significant morbidity may occur during transportation of the patient between the ICU and the operating room. It is of the utmost importance that intensive care management continues during the operative period, and this must be provided by senior intensive care staff or intensive care-trained anaesthetists in close collaboration with the ICU staff, or both. Several studies have demonstrated a reduction in mortality from maximising systemic oxygen delivery in high-risk surgical patients, with intravascular volume expansion and inotropic agents,[26] and this type of approach cannot be provided using an anaesthetic technique designed for elective surgery on fit patients. Full monitoring and organ-system support should be continued during surgery, although in patients with renal failure continuous haemodiafiltration can generally be discontinued.

# Specific conditions

## Pancreatitis

Pancreatitis usually presents as a generalised illness with epigastric or hypochondrial pain, and when severe with abdominal tenderness, fever, tachycardia, and hypotension.[27] Acute pancreatitis is usually associated with alcohol abuse or biliary obstruction from stones, or less commonly with blunt abdominal trauma, drugs, and toxins,[28] and results in severe local inflammation with haemorrhage and extensive tissue necrosis. Massive fluid sequestration and mediator release produce a systemic inflammatory response with progression to multiple organ failure if the patient is not resuscitated sufficiently.[29] Morbidity and mortality risk can be estimated for the individual patient with the use of Ranson's criteria.[30] Optimal fluid resuscitation is essential, with monitoring of arterial and central venous pressure, renal function, and acid–base status, as well as haemoglobin, serum calcium and amylase, and glucose.

Following stabilisation and analgesia, ultrasound and contrast–enhanced CT scanning are necessary to assess the extent of the pancreatitis. CT scanning in patients with acute pancreatitis should be performed in all patients not improving by three days, and in all patients with suspected complications. The CT scan should be performed with intravenous and enteral contrast enhancement,[21,31] which allows assessment of necrosis. If necrosis is suspected, fine needle aspiration should be used to diagnose complicating infection.[32] Infected necrosis requires surgical débridement and weekly CT assessment. Laparotomy should also be considered for patients with severe local and systemic complications despite optimal intensive care treatment lasting more than three days, pulmonary insufficiency, renal failure, shock, sepsis, or suspected intestinal perforation.[33] Surgery is usually not indicated in the first week, because the occurrence of infected necrosis during this period is rare, and a better demarcation of viable and non-viable tissue occurs after one week. Moreover, surgery may convert sterile necrosis into an infected abscess.

The goal of surgical intervention is the débridement of devitalised tissue and drainage of abcesses, with preservation of functional pancreatic tissue. Pancreatic infection differs from other infections, because retroperitoneal necrosis is a self-sustaining process in the presence of pancreatic duct disruption and bacteria. At operation it is important to look for a defined cavity in the necrotic pancreas, because this can be treated with closed irrigation and sump drainage; this removes necrotic tissue and mediators, which seems to reduce overall mortality.[34,35] Open packing and frequent re-operation is probably preferable when no defined cavity is found.[36] The role for less invasive techniques such as percutaneous CT-guided puncture and drainage is very limited.[37]

Systemic complications include shock, acute lung injury, acute renal failure, or disseminated intravascular coagulation.[38] Several therapeutic measures have been proposed to prevent the occurrence of these secondary complications, such as prolonged peritoneal lavage. However, none of the studies has shown improved patient survival.[39] Attention must be paid to adequate nutrition; there is no firm consensus about the best route of administration, although parenteral nutrition may be the only option in patients with an ileus or following laparotomy.

Since 80% of patients dying of acute necrotising pancreatitis do so either because of, or with, infection, systemic antibiotic prophylaxis seems logical. However, no beneficial effects have been found in adequately performed prospective trials. One study of selective decontamination of the digestive tract has shown a significant reduction in mortality,[40] supporting previous animal studies.

Late complications include abscess or pseudocyst formation. Abscesses are uncommon (1–4%) and are usually diagnosed about three to four weeks after the onset of acute pancreatitis. The systemic signs are less pronounced than the original presentation of acute pancreatitis, but the mortality rate is still 20%.[41] CT scanning is the diagnostic modality of choice, and should be accompanied by CT-guided percutaneous drainage. Inadequate drainage or tissue necrosis requires surgery. Pseudocyst formation complicates recovery in 1–8% of patients; spontaneous resolution occurs in about 30% by three weeks. Pseudocysts that persist after six weeks should be treated surgically because of the risk of complications such as bleeding or infection.[42]

## Gut ischaemia

Acute intestinal ischemia can have numerous causes. Occlusive disease of the superior mesenteric artery must be differentiated from non-occlusive disease and venous occlusion.[43] Patients at risk of occlusive disease of the superior mesenteric artery include those over 50 years of age with cardiovascular disease, such as atherosclerosis, diabetes, poorly controlled congestive heart failure, recent myocardial infarction, cardiogenic shock, cardiac arrhythmias, and following abdominal aortic surgery.[1] The signs and symptoms of bowel ischaemia are non-specific, but a characteristic aspect is the discrepancy between the patient's history of abdominal pain and the limited findings on examination. Signs of intestinal necrosis may include a leukocytosis, metabolic acidosis, or blood-tinged fluid on peritoneal lavage, but these may be very variable. Recent work suggests that elevated serum levels of the isomer D-lactate (produced by colonic bacterial fermentation) may indicate gut ischemia.[44,45] Arteriography or contrast-enhanced CT scanning may be required. The diagnosis is often difficult, and requires a high index of suspicion.

Treatment includes active haemodynamic support of blood flow and pressure, and management of treatable underlying disease, while preparing the patient for embolectomy or aortomesenteric bypass[46] if appropriate. Delay in diagnosis usually means that necrotic bowel is often present, and this may be extensive. Attempts should be made before surgery to establish the patient's wishes in the event of gut necrosis incompatible with resumption of enteral nutrition.

## Abdominal sepsis

Early diagnosis is essential for reducing multiple organ failure and the high mortality[47] associated with abdominal sepsis. Once the diagnosis is suspected, broad-spectrum antibiotics and urgent resuscitation should be followed by surgery as soon as possible.[6]

A complete exploratory laparotomy must be performed and all possible foci of sepsis must be removed, including adhesions. Obstructed bowel should be decompressed. If a generalised peritonitis is present, then peritoneal lavage must be performed. Sources of continuing contamination must be eliminated by excision, exteriorisation, or controlled drainage by forming fistulae. Localised abcesses should be drained. Delayed closure either leaving the abdomen open or using a Vicryl mesh is appropriate for faecal contamination, multiple abcesses, or extensive fibrin deposits, when further débridements will be needed.

Acalculous cholecystitis is often diagnosed late, and may consequently present as abdominal sepsis following necrosis and perforation of the gallbladder. It occurs as a co-morbid complication in about 2% of critically ill patients.[48] The aetiology of the disease process is unknown. A high index of suspicion should be maintained in patients on morphine, with an ileus, following abdominal surgery, on total parenteral nutrition, or on ventilatory support, who develop an obstructive pattern on liver function tests. The diagnosis can be confirmed by ultrasound, which will show a thickened gallbladder wall.[49] These patients should be operated upon promptly, or diagnosis should be confirmed by percutaneous drainage which can be used as temporary treatment in the critically ill.

## Postoperative aspects of surgical abdomen in ICU patients

The evaluation of the ICU patient after a laparotomy can be difficult because of the disturbed physical findings. A high index of suspicion is required to detect postoperative bleeding, sepsis, and intestinal ischemia, because these conditions can be difficult to detect and require immediate intervention.[50] Significant bleeding often presents with non-specific signs, such as anxiety and pain. The presentation of hypovolaemic shock with its clinical signs may also occur, but already indicates a large blood loss of over 1 litre, and in those patients immediate surgery is required.

Patients with postoperative intra-abdominal sepsis have a high mortality rate. A difficult aspect of evaluating ICU patients is the assessment of secondary intra-abdominal pathology. In such patients, failure to progress or remote organ failure with no obvious cause are reasons to consider the diagnosis of postoperative intra-abdominal sepsis.[51] This assessment is preferably not performed only by the surgeon who has operated on the patient, in order to avoid doctor bias. A surgeon–intensivist or one fixed surgical consultant can optimally perform this task. In case of an operation with faecal contamination, the surgeon must define whether and at what time point a second-look operation should be performed. It is difficult to give guidance on the use of planned re-laparotomy. Enthusiasts for the approach are usually dealing with specific subgroups of patients. A recent trial has failed to show any benefit for planned re-laparotomy over re-laparotomy only on clinical indication.[52] A re-laparotomy in patients who develop evidence of multiple organ failure should generally be performed only with supporting clinical or radiological findings.

## Developments

The acute abdomen and its complications, such as sepsis and mutiple organ failure, will continue to be the subject of research interest for many years to come. Treatment used in patients with acute abdomen has been mainly directed towards intervention in the causative disease process. Indeed, early mortality has been decreased after these therapeutic modalities have been applied. The importance of prevention of late mortality, by early intervention, has gained attention only recently. For the systemic complications of acute abdomen (for example, pancreatitis complicated by sepsis and multiple organ failure), only supportive measurements, such as aggressive fluid resuscitation and intensive care support, are available. The occurrence of sepsis and multiple organ failure is associated with a high mortality and this has not decreased despite these measures. Current research is focusing on aspects of the pathogenesis of peritonitis and intervention. For the time being, therapy in patients with an acute abdomen must rely on early intervention, fluid resuscitation, appropriate antibiotics, frequent re-evaluation, and if necessary repeated laparotomies.

## Conclusion

- In critically ill patients with a suspected surgical abdominal problem, request surgical consultation early.
- An accurate history and physical examination are essential, even though

both may be difficult to obtain.

- Diagnostic procedures can be valuable, but should be used selectively and by local protocols.
- Complex diagnostic tests are not indicated if a laparotomy is inevitable.
- An exploratory laparotomy may be less harmful than procrastination.

1 Jung PJ, Merrell RC. Acute abdomen. *Gastroenterol Clin North Am* 1988;**17**:227–44.
2 Brewer RJ, Golden GT, Hitch DD. Abdominal pain: An analysis of 1,000 consecutive cases in a university hospital emergency room. *Am J Surg* 1976;**131**:219.
3 Guenther HJ, Trede M. Acute pancreatitis: the role of early surgery. *Baillières Clin Gastroenterol* 1991;**5**:773–86.
4 Aranha GV, Goldberg NB. Surgical problems in patients on ventilators. *Crit Care Med* 1981;**9**:478.
5 Mustard RA, Bohnen JMA, Schouten BD. The acute abdomen and intraabdominal sepsis. In *Principles of intensive care* (Hall JB, Schmidt GA, Wood LDH, eds). New York: McGraw-Hill Inc., 1992:990–9.
6 Johnson DJ, Tonnesen AS. The abdomen as a source of occult sepsis. *Gastroenterol Clin North Am* 1988;**17**:419–31.
7 Bohner H, Yang Q, Franke K, Ohman C. Bedeutung anamnestischer Angaben und klinischer Befunde für die Diagnose der akuten Apppendizitis. Studiengruppe Akute Bauchschmerzen. *Z Gastroenterol* 1994;**32**:579–83.
8 Reines HD. Evaluating the acute abdomen in an ICU patient. In *Critical care* (Civetta JM, Taylor RW, Kirby RR, eds). Philadelphia: JB Lippincott Co., 1992:659–68.
9 Tsilbary EC, Wissig SL. Absorption from the peritoneal cavity: SEM study of the mesothelioma covering the peritoneal surface of the muscular portion of the diaphragm. *Am J Anat* 1977;**149**:127.
10 Tsilbary EC, Wissig SL. Lymphatic absorption from the peritoneal cavity: regulation of patency mesothelial stomata. *Microvasc Res* 1983;**25**:22.
11 Dumont AE, Maas WK, Ilieocu H, *et al.* Increased survival from peritonitis after blockade of transdiaphragmatic absorption of bacteria. *Surg Gynecol Obstet* 1986;**162**:248.
12 Gallinaro RN, Polk Jr HC. Intra-abdominal sepsis: the role of surgery. *Baillières Clin Gastroenterol* 1991;**5**:611–37.
13 van Goor H, de Graaf JS, Kooi K, *et al.* Effect of recombinant tissue plasminogen activator on intra-abdominal abscess formation in rats with generalized peritonitis. *J Am Coll Surg* 1994;**179**:407–11.
14 Redl H, Schlag G, Bahrami S, Davies J, Jochum M, Bengtsson A. Experimental and clinical evidence of leucocyte activation in trauma and sepsis. *Prog Clin Biol Res* 1994;**388**:221–45.
15 Berczi I. Neuroendocrine defence in endotoxin shock (a review). *Acta Microbiol Hung* 1993;**40**:265–302.
16 Flak B, Rowley AA. Acute abdomen: plain film utilization and analysis. *Can Assoc Radiol J* 1993;**44**:423–8.
17 Braley SE, Groner TR, Fernandez MU, Moulton JS. Overview of diagnostic imaging in sepsis. *New Horizons* 1993;**1**:214–30.
18 Shea JA, Berlin JA, Escarce JJ, *et al.* Revised estimates of diagnostic test sensitivity and specificity in suspected biliary tract disease. *Arch Intern Med* 1994;**154**:2573–81.
19 Siewert B, Rastopoules. CT of the acute abdomen: findings and impact on diagnosis and treatment. *AJR* 1994;**163**:1317–24.
20 Norwood SH, Civetta JM. Abdominal CT scanning in critically ill surgical patients. *Ann Surg* 1985;**202**:166.
21 Balthazar EJ. CT diagnosis and staging of acute pancreatitis. *Rad Clin North Am* 1989;**27**:19–37.
22 Adam EJ, Page JE. Intra-abdominal sepsis: the role of radiology. *Baillières Clin Gastroenterol* 1991;**5**:587–609.

23  Reines HD, Khoury N, Spicer KM. The efficacy of gallium scanning for diagnosis and treatment of intra-abdominal abscess. *Am J Surg* 1982;**48**:59.

24  Blazeby JM, Tulloh BR, Adams DCR, Poskitt KR, Bristol JB. Fine-catheter peritoneal cytology in the management of acute abdominal pain. *Br J Surg* 1994;**81**:684.

25  Cuesta MA, Borgstein PJ, Meijer S. Laparoscopy in the diagnosis and treatment of acute abdominal conditions. *Eur J Surg* 1993;**159**:455–6.

26  Boyd D, Grounds RM, Bennett ED. The beneficial effect of supranormalization of oxygenation delivery with dopexamine hydrochloride on perioperative mortality. *JAMA* 1993;**76**:372–6.

27  Büchler M, Uhl W, Beger HG. Acute pancreatitis: when and how to operate. *Dig Dis* 1992;**10**:354–62.

28  Guenther HJ, Trede M. Acute pancreatitis: the role of early surgery. *Baillières Clin Gastroenterol* 1991;**5**:773–86.

29  Steinberg W, Tenner S. Medical progress: acute pancreatitis. *N Engl J Med* 1994; **330**:1198–210.

30  Ranson JHC, Rifkind KM, Roses DF, *et al.* Prognostic signs and the role of operative management in acute pancreatitis. *Surg Gynecol Obstet* 1974;**139**:69–81.

31  Bradley EL III. Prediction of pancreatic necrosis by dynamic pancreaticography. *Ann Surg* 1989;**210**:495–504.

32  Sunday ML, Schuricht AL, Barbot DJ, Rosato FE. Management of infected pancreatic fluid collections. *Am Surg* 1994;**60**:63–7.

33  Beger HG. Surgery in acute pancreatitis. *Hepato-Gastroenterol* 1991;**38**:92–6.

34  Beger HG. Surgical management of necrotizing pancreatitis. *Surg Clin North Am* 1989;**69**:529–49.

35  Beger HG, Büchler M, Bittner R, Block S, Nevelainen T, Roscher R. Necrosectomy and postoperative local lavage in necrotizing pancreatitis. *Br J Surg* 1988;**75**:207–12.

36  Bradley EL, Fulenwider JT. Open treatment of pancreatic abscess. *Surg Gynecol Obstet* 1994;**159**:509–13.

37  Ranson JHC. The role of surgery in the management of acute pancreatitis. *Ann Surg* 1990;**211**:382–93.

38  Büchler M, Beger HG. Surgical strategies in acute pancreatitis. *Hepato-Gastroenterol* 1993;**40**:563–8.

39  Ranson JHC, Berman RS. Long peritoneal lavage decreases pancreatic sepsis in acute pancreatitis. *Ann Surg* 1990;**211**:708–16.

40  Luiten EJT, Hop WCJ, Lange JF, Bruining HA. Controlled clinical trial of selective decontamination for the treatment of severe acute pancreatitis. *Ann Surg* 1995; **222**:57–65.

41  Gliedman ML. Management of unresolved acute pancreatitis. *Contemp Surg* 1990;**36**:67–84.

42  Poston GJ, Williamson RCN. Surgical management of acute pancreatitis. *Br J Surg* 1990;**77**:5–12.

43  Wilson C, Gupta R, Gilmour DG, *et al.* Acute superior mesenteric ischaemia. *Br J Surg* 1987;**74**:279–81.

44  Murray MJ, Gonze MD, Nowak LR, Cobb CF. Serum D(−)-lactate levels as an aid to diagnosing acute intestinal ischemia. *Am J Surg* 1994;**167**:575–8.

45  Poeze M, Froon AHM, Greve JWM, Ramsay G. D-Lactate as an early marker of intestinal ischaemia after ruptured abdominal aortic aneurysm repair. *Br J Surg* 1998;**85**:1221–4.

46  Ottinger LW. The surgical management of acute occlusion of the superior mesenteric artery. *Ann Surg* 1978;**188**:721–6.

47  Fry DE. Multiple system organ failure. In *Multiple system organ failure* (Fry DE, ed.). St Louis: Mosby Year Book, 1992:3–14.

48  Shapiro MJ, Luchtefeld WB, Kurzweil S. Acute acalculous cholecystitis in the critically ill. *Am Surg* 1994;**60**:335.

49  Cornwell EE, Rodriquez A, Mirvis SE, Shorr RM. Acute acalculous cholecystitis in critically injured patients. Preoperative diagnostic imaging. *Ann Surg* 1989;**210**:52–5.

50  Flint LM. Early postoperative acute abdominal complications. *Surg Clin North Am* 1988;**68**:445–55.

211

51 Rogers PN, Wright IH. Postoperative intra-abdominal sepsis. *Br J Surg* 1987; 74:973–5.
52 Hau T, Ohmann C, Wolmershauser A, Wacha H, Yang Q, for the Peritonitis Study of the Surgical Infection Society–Europe. Planned relaparotomy vs relaparotomy on demand in the treatment of intra-abdominal infections. *Arch Surg* 1995;**130**:1193–7.

# 18:  Management of acute hepatic failure

J WENDON

Acute hepatic failure (AHF) is a syndrome associated with the sudden cessation of normal hepatic function. The clinical features are listed in Box 18.1. The rate and mode of progression are variable. There have been several attempts to produce a formal definition based on acuity and encephalopathy. Trey and Davidson proposed an 8-week interval between initial symptoms and the development of hepatic encephalopathy, in the absence of pre-existing liver disease.[1] Gimson *et al* described late-onset hepatic failure as encephalopathy starting 8–24 weeks from the onset of jaundice.[2] Benhamou *et al* used an interval from jaundice to encephalopathy of 2 weeks or less for fulminant liver failure and 2–12 weeks for subfulminant.[3] O'Grady *et al* have suggested the terms hyperacute (encephalopathy within 8 days of the onset of the jaundice), acute (8–28 days), and subacute hepatic failure (4–26 weeks).[4] A high proportion of the patients with hyperacute liver failure will develop grade IV coma and cerebral oedema, but may recover with supportive treatment, whilst the subacute patients will have a lower incidence of cerebral oedema, but more will require liver transplantation. (Paracetamol acetaminophen) toxicity and mushroom poisoning predominate in the hyperacute group and seronegative hepatitis in the subacute group.

There are many causes for AHF (Box 18.2). Chronic liver disease (CLD) is excluded as a cause of AHF by the presence of cirrhosis. However, many of the complications seen are similar to those of AHF, although they are not

---

**Box 18.1** *Clinical features of acute hepatic failure*

- Encephalopathy
- Jaundice
- Coagulopathy
- Renal failure
- Sepsis
- Cardiovascular instability
- Metabolic acidosis
- Cerebral oedema
- Multiple organ failure

complicated by the development of cerebral oedema. The more common causes for decompensation from CLD are sepsis (respiratory, urinary, ascitic fluid), electrolyte imbalance, variceal haemorrhage, development of hepatocellular carcinoma, and dehydration. The clinical diagnosis is usually easy to make, and the management, as with many causes of AHF, is supportive, although some patients with acute alcoholic hepatitis may also benefit from steroid therapy.

## Investigations

By the time of presentation, the liver will already have suffered substantial damage regardless of aetiology, but this should not discourage attempts to define the cause since treatment options may vary. For example, it would be inappropriate to consider liver transplantation in a patient with malignant infiltration, and chemotherapy would be indicated for lymphoma. Investigations and imaging will depend on the clinical situation. The more common are listed in Box 18.3.

## Management

### General aspects

Hypoglycaemia is a consequence of reduced clearance of circulating insulin, impaired gluconeogenesis, and failure to mobilise glycogen stores. It is common and potentially lethal, so blood sugar must be measured frequently. Patients may require 10–50% dextrose as an infusion to maintain euglycaemia. Hypophosphataemia and hypomagnesaemia are also common when urine output is maintained; low levels require intravenous replacement.

A metabolic acidosis carries a very poor prognosis regardless of the aetiology of the AHF and should trigger urgent referral for liver transplantation. Patients at this time may appear surprisingly well but deteriorate very quickly and can be difficult to transfer safely. The aetiology of the acidosis is multifactorial, and includes impaired hepatic lactate clearance as well as tissue hypoxia from inadequate volume resuscitation. Any patient with a low serum bicarbonate (venous blood can be used) should have a central line inserted and be given colloid as dictated by their clinical state. A blood lactate should also be obtained. In some patients the acidosis will resolve with colloid resuscitation, but despite this they are still in a high-risk group and should be discussed with a liver transplant centre as early as possible.

Patients with AHF are at increased risk of bacterial and fungal infections because of impaired neutrophil and Kupffer cell function and deficiency of opsonins. Bacterial infection rates of up to 80% within a few days of

---

**Box 18.2** *Causes of acute hepatic failure*

| | |
|---|---|
| **Toxic agents** | Paracetamol, Ecstasy, mushrooms (*Amanita phalloides* and *Lepiota*), carbon tetrachloride |
| **Viral agents** | Hepatitis A, hepatitis B + D, hepatitis E, seronegative hepatitis (non-A, B, C, D, E); herpes simplex virus, cytomegalovirus and Epstein–Barr virus; haemorrhagic fevers have all been described but are rare causes; adenovirus has been described in children |
| **Drug reactions** | |
| *Microvascular steatosis* | Tetracycline, non-steroidal anti-inflammatory drugs (NSAIDs), sodium valproate |
| *Hepatonecrosis* | Paracetamol, anaesthetic agents (halothane), antiepileptics (phenytoin, carbamazepine), antibiotics (isoniazid, pyrazinamide, rifampicin, nitrofurantoin, ketoconazole), dantrolene, propylthiouracil, NSAIDs, phosphorus, cocaine, herbal teas, Ecstasy, cyproterone |
| *Veno-occlusive disease* | Busulphan, 6-thioguanine, azathioprine, cyclophosphamide, dacarbazine, pyrrolizidine alkaloids (e.g. comfrey) |
| **Other causes** | Wilson's disease, fatty liver of pregnancy, HELLP (**h**aemodialysis, **e**levated **l**iver enzymes, **l**ow **p**latelets), lymphoma, malignant infiltration, sepsis, acute Budd–Chiari syndrome, veno-occlusive disease, ischaemic hepatitis, acute autoimmune hepatitis |

---

admission have been reported. Some centres routinely use prophylactic antibiotics, including systemic antifungal agents, particularly for those patients scheduled for transplantation or those who have developed multiple organ failure. Antimicrobial resistance is an increasing problem. The investigation and management of infections should be based on multidisciplinary unit policies.

The coagulopathy of AHF is not only inherent to the disease process but also one of the most important prognostic indicators. Trends in the international normalised ratio (INR; prothrombin time) are an important guide to deterioration or resolution, and fresh frozen plasma must not be given unless the patient is actively bleeding. Thrombocytopenia should be treated with platelet transfusions.

Gastrointestinal bleeding is uncommon. Either H$_2$-receptor-blocking drugs or sucralfate may be used as prophylaxis. Enteral nutrition should be

---

**Box 18.3** *Investigations for acute hepatic failure*

- Electrolytes, urea and creatinine, and liver function tests
- Full blood count and film (if haemolysis, consider Wilson's disease)
- INR and clotting profile
- Procoagulant screening for Budd–Chiari or veno-occlusive disease
- Blood lactate
- Toxicology screen if clinically indicated
- Blood urate (elevated in fatty liver of pregnancy)
- Wilson's disease: serum copper, ceruloplasmin, and urinary copper pre- and post-penicillamine challenge (500 mg twice daily for 1 day)
- Immunoglobulins
- Autoantibodies
- Virological studies: hepatitis A IgM, hepatitis B (surface Ag and IgM core Ab initially and, if these are positive, Ag and Ab), hepatitis C RNA (although C is a very rare cause of AHF in northern America and Europe), and hepatitis E (IgG only available at present)
- Ultrasound of liver, biliary tree, and portal and systemic circulations

---

started as soon as possible. Care must be taken with fluid balance, particularly in encephalopathic patients in whom fluid overload or rapid shifts in sodium balance may produce fatal brain-stem herniation or central pontine myelinolysis respectively.

Paracetamo toxicity is one of the commonest causes of AHF in the United Kingdom and one for which there is an available and effective antidote in the form of *N*-acetylcysteine. Recent work[5] suggests that *N*-acetylcysteine is effective beyond the previously determined "time window" of 15 hours and in a range of conditions: we now treat most patients with AHF regardless of aetiology and time in their disease process with *N*-acetylcysteine with a loading dose of 150 mg/kg over 30 minutes and thereafter a maintenance dose of 150 mg/kg per day. The agent appears to reduce the incidence of organ failures and improve measures of tissue oxygenation.[6]

### Systemic circulation

The haemodynamic disturbances seen in patients with AHF are similar to those of patients with sepsis, with an elevated cardiac output and hypotension from a low systemic vascular resistance. Relative hypovolaemia secondary to vasodilatation is common, and a pulmonary artery flotation catheter may be required to optimise fluid replacement. Colloid loading is usually needed. Dextrose infusions are required only to maintain a normal blood glucose. Initially the hypotension responds to colloid resuscitation, but vasoconstrictors are usually required in order to maintain an adequate perfusion pressure (particularly cerebral perfusion) and to avoid excessive fluids as patients progress to encephalopathy and cerebral oedema. Noradrenaline should be started at a dose of 0·05 µg/kg per min. Vasoconstrictors may reduce oxygen delivery and hence consumption,[7] and some centres employ N-acetylcysteine or epoprostenol to counteract this. The role of nitric oxide synthase blockade is uncertain at present. Plasmapheresis has also been proposed as a method for improving haemodynamic stability by removing vasorelaxant mediators.[8,9]

## Cerebral dysfunction

Encephalopathy is characteristic of the syndrome of AHF. Patients progress at variable rates from being mildly confused, through aggression, to deep coma, sometimes within 24 hours. Patients with a deteriorating conscious level or a metabolic acidosis should be referred to a specialist unit. They should in general be intubated and electively ventilated before transfer, unless the attendant is sufficiently experienced to be able to do this during transport without risk to the patient. Patients should not be transferred by inexperienced medical staff, and must be physiologically stable before departure.

An increase in brain tissue volume occurs in most patients with grade IV encephalopathy, but improvements in management may have reduced the incidence of cerebral oedema in AHF to 40%.[10] The clinical signs of cerebral oedema (systemic hypertension, decerebrate posturing, and abnormal pupillary reflexes) are generally attributed to brain-stem compression, but experience gained from autopsies suggests that this is now comparatively uncommon, implying that other mechanisms may also be involved. These include increased vascular permeability, intracellular oedema and cytotoxicity, impaired $Na^+/K^+$ ATPase activity, and sodium shifts. Although cerebral hyperaemia may precede or coincide with cerebral oedema on CT scanning, cerebral blood flow (CBF) varies markedly in encephalopathic patients (from 12 to 50 ml/min per 100 g in our studies with radioactive xenon), and contrary to expectations may fall as coma deepens,[11] with increased lactate production in some patients indicating impaired oxygen delivery or use. Substantial increases in CBF can be demonstrated following the infusion of mannitol and N-acetylcysteine, associated with a rise in cerebral oxygen utilisation and a fall in lactate production.

Hypoxaemia and hypercapnia will aggravate cerebral injury. Patients who are progressing to grade III encephalopathy should be intubated and mechanically ventilated in order to protect the airway and the brain. Mild hyperventilation may be used in the short term to reduce intracranial pressure, but it does this by reducing CBF, and the effect is evanescent. Early detection of cerebral oedema is important in order to initiate appropriate management, but many of the normal clinical signs are lost, and treatment decisions must be be made on the basis of systolic hypertension, tachycardia, or pupillary abnormalities. Intracranial pressure monitoring in all ventilated grade IV patients is recommended, but the relative risks (haemorrhage, inaccurate readings) must be weighed against the benefits (early detection). It may not be possible to correct the coagulopathy sufficiently with clotting factors to permit insertion. Extra-dural systems appear to have the lowest incidence of complications.[12]

Intracranial pressure (ICP) monitoring allows calculation of the cerebral perfusion pressure (CPP), which is the mean arterial pressure (MAP) minus the intracranial pressure (CPP = MAP − ICP). An adequate CPP is essential for brain survival. However, there is uncertainty about what constitutes an adequate CPP. Full recovery has been reported despite CPP values <40 mm Hg for more than 24 hours.[13] Jugular bulb catheterisation permits measurement of jugular venous saturation ($Sjo_2$) and lactate, and calculation of arterial jugular lactate difference, providing information about the adequacy of global cerebral oxygen supply. A jugular venous saturation >55% and no arterial jugular lactate difference implies an adequate CBF and CPP. A fall in CPP with a reduction in $Sjo_2$ associated with vasodilatation requires vasoconstrictor therapy, whereas, if the change is caused by a rising ICP, mannitol (0·5 mg/kg) should be given.

Mannitol requires removal of fluid, either by a diuresis or, if the patient is oligo-anuric, by haemofiltration. Plasma osmolarity should be measured, and should not exceed 320 mo/smol. Mannitol should be given immediately to any patient with AHF who develops pupillary abnormalities.

Cerebral function monitoring (CFM) may be used to detect subclinical epileptiform activity. Sensory evoked potentials may also be useful, especially in assessment of outcome and suitability for liver transplantation.

Thiopentone (50 mg boluses followed by an infusion of 50 mg/h for up to 6 hours) may be used for intractable intracranial hypertension. However, it produces arterial hypotension, may interfere with pupillary reactions, and will take many days to clear.

## Renal failure

Renal failure (urine output of <300 ml/24 h and serum creatinine of >300 mmol/l) despite adequate intravascular filling pressures affects up to 70% of patients with AHF. The main causes are acute tubular necrosis from antecedent hypovolaemia, activation of inflammatory mediators of sepsis, and interstitital nephritis from the toxic effects of drugs such as paracetamol. Initial management involves restoration of circulating volume and arterial blood pressure, but despite these measures renal function often continues to deteriorate, and requires renal replacement therapy to control acidosis, hyperkalaemia, fluid overload, and a rising creatinine and urea. Treatment should also be instituted in any patient who is oliguric with signs of cerebral oedema, and in patients with significant hyponatraemia. A continuous technique such as pumped venovenous haemodiafiltration (CVVHD) is the preferred mode of renal replacement therapy in AHF. High-volume haemodiafiltration may also be used, but care must be taken in the choice of replacement fluid, since patients will not be able to metabolise many of the standard solutions in which lactate or acetate is the predominant buffer; bicarbonate-buffered solutions may be better tolerated. Intermittent machine-driven haemodialysis should be avoided because haemodynamic instability adversely affects CPP. Heparin can be used to anticoagulate the extracorporeal circuit, although resistance may occur because of concomitant antithrombin III deficiency. Prostacyclin may be infused at 5 ng/kg per min as an alternative.

## Transplantation

The aim of management in AHF is to reduce the risk of developing other organ failures and to promote spontaneous liver regeneration. Plasmapheresis or extracorporeal liver assist devices have been advocated, but controlled trials are needed. There is currently no real alternative to transplantation for patients deteriorating despite maximal medical therapy. The decision to proceed to transplantation is based on mortality risk using one of two simple clinical models[14,15] with a high sensitivity and specificity.

The Clichy group in Paris have established criteria for a poor outcome in non-paracetamol-induced liver failure, based on the presence of coma or confusion in association with a factor V level <20% of normal for patients <30 years old, or <30% for those aged ≥30 years. The O'Grady criteria separate paracetamol and non-paracetamol patients. The criteria for paracetamol-induced AHF are a pH <7·3 more than 24 hours after ingestion and following resuscitation, or the concurrent findings of prothrombin time >100 s (INR >6·5) + creatinine >300 μmol/l + grade III/IV encephalopathy. In non-paracetamol patients the criteria are prothrombin time >100 s (irrespective of level of encephalopathy) or any three of the following:

- aetiology seronegative hepatitis or drug-induced liver failure;
- age <10 years or >40 years;
- jaundice to encephalopathy time of >7 days;
- prothrombin time >50 seconds;
- serum bilirubin >300 μmol/l.

These models are equally useful, but do not apply to children, Budd–Chiari syndrome, acute Wilson's disease, and fatty liver of pregnancy.

Patients developing AHF should be referred to a liver transplant centre before they satisfy the criteria for transplantation to allow time for assessment and preparation (of family as well as patient), and to allow maximum time for identifying a suitable donor. Eight-year data from Europe (1988–1996) demonstrate a survival rate of 52% for a group of patients with a predicted mortality rate of 90% with medical management. Future developments include auxiliary liver transplantation which may allow immunosuppression withdrawal in patients whose native liver regenerates.

## Conclusion

Acute hepatic failure is a life-threatening illness complicating acute hepatic necrosis from a variety of insults. The main clinical features are an encephalopathy and coagulopathy, and a profound metabolic derangement including hypoglycaemia, hypophosphataemia, and a metabolic acidosis. The majority of patients develop renal failure and hypotension, in association with vasodilatation and a high cardiac output state. Nearly all patients are significantly volume depleted at presentation, and require active and carefully monitored volume resuscitation. Care must be taken with fluids, however, as the mode of death is brain-stem herniation from cerebral oedema. Level of consciousness can change rapidly; an apparently normal conscious state should not encourage a false sense of security. Patients in grade III coma should be electively ventilated to facilitate general treatment and limit the risks of cerebral oedema. Consideration should always be given to the possible need for liver transplantation as this may reduce the mortality rate from 90% with medical treatment alone to around 50%. Early discussion with a regional referral centre is recommended. Transfer should be conducted only by experienced medical staff after the patient has been stabilised.

1 Trey C, Davidson C. *The management of fulminant hepatic failure.* London: Grune & Stratton, 1970.
2 Gimson AE, O'Grady J, Ede LJ, Portmann S, Willis L. Late onset hepatic failure: Clinical, serological and histological features. *Hepatology* 1986;6:288–94.
3 Berneau J, Reuff S, Benhamou JP. Fulminant and subfulminant liver failure: definitions and causes. *Semin Liver Dis* 1986;6:97–106.
4 O'Grady JG, Scholm SIV, Williams R. Acute liver failure: identifying the syndromes. *Lancet* 1993;342:273–5.
5 Keays R, Harrison PM, Wendon JA, Gimson AES, Alexander GJM, Williams R. Intravenous acetylcysteine in paracetamol induced fulminant hepatic failure: a prospective controlled trial. *BMJ* 1991;303:1026–9.
6 Harrison PM, Wendon JA, Gimson AES, Alexander GJM, Williams R. Improvement by acetylcysteine of haemodynamics and oxygen transport variables in patients with fulminant hepatic failure. *N Engl J Med* 1991;324:1852–8.
7 Wendon J, Harrison P, Keys R, Gimson A, Alexander G, Williams R. Effects of vasopressor agents and epoprostenol on systemic haemodynamics on oxygen transport variables in patients with fulminant hepatic failure. *Hepatology* 1992;15:1067–71.
8 Kondrup JAT, Vilstrup H, Tygstrup N. High volume plasma exchange in fulminant hepatic failure. *Int J Artif Organs* 1992;11:669–76.
9 Larsen FSHB Jorgensen LG, Secher NH, *et al.* Cerebral blood flow velocity during high volume plasmapheresis in fulminant hepatic failure. *Int J Artif Organs* 1994;17:353–61.

10 Makin A, Wendon J, Williams R. A 7-year experience of severe acetaminophen induced toxicity (1987–1993). *Gastroeneterology* 1995;**109**:1907–16.
11 Aggarwal SKD, Yonas H, Obrist W, Kang Y, Martin M, Policare R. Cerebral haemodynamic and metabolic changes in fulminant hepatic failure A retrospective study. *Hepatology* 1994;**19**:80–7.
12 Blei A, Olafsson S, Webster S, Levy R. Complications of intracerebral pressure monitoring in fulminant hepatic failure. *Lancet* 1993;**341**:157–8.
13 Davies MH, Mutimer D, Lowes J, Elias E, Neuberger J. Recovery despite impaired cerebral perfusion in fulminant hepatic failure. *Lancet* 1994;**343**:1329–30.
14 Bernuau J, Goudeau A, Poynard T, *et al.* Multivariate analysis of prognosis in fulminant hepatitis B. *Hepatology* 1986;**6**:648–51.
15 O'Grady JG, Alexander GJ, Hallyar KM, Williams R. Early indicators of prognosis in fulminant hepatic failure. *Gastroenterology* 1986;**2**:439–45.

# 19: CNS injuries – cerebral protection and monitoring

P J D ANDREWS and P F X STATHAM

## Acute brain injury

Injury to the nervous system is characterised by a stereotypical pattern irrespective of the *primary injury*, which includes trauma, ischaemia, hypoxia, hypoglycaemia, or subarachnoid haemorrhage. The primary insult initiates a multitude of inflammatory cascades resulting in *secondary brain injury*, the effect of which is at least as important as the primary injury. This period of brain inflammation has a duration of two to three weeks and renders the brain more susceptible to the effects of systemic insults (hypotension, hypoxia, pyrexia) occurring after the primary injury; these are called secondary insults. Recently postmortem examination of patients dying from severe traumatic brain injury revealed that almost 90% had concomitant ischaemic damage.[1] The concept of cerebral protection has been extended to encompass prevention of secondary injury.

Proposed inflammatory mediators contributing to autodestructive tissue damage include excitatory amino acids, free radicals, membrane breakdown products, eicosanoids, platelet-activating factor, serotonin, endogenous opioids, and changes in certain cations. These factors cause an interactive network or cascade resulting in reduced central nervous system (CNS) blood flow, reduced metabolism, and disruption of cell membranes. The investigation of these processes is complicated by the occult nature of neurological cell death, and is dependent on a better understanding of the process of apoptosis.

### Excitotoxicity

Excitatory amino acids, aspartate and glutamate, are released in a threshold manner in response to a reduction in cerebral blood flow (CBF $<20$ ml/100 g per min) and result in rapid cell death (3–5 min) via activation of the $N$-methyl-D-aspartate (NMDA) receptor and associated

---

**Box 19.1** *Sites within the NMDA receptor ion channel complex*

- Competitive antagonists: CGS 19755 and CPPene
- Non-competitive blockade: MK 801, CNS 1102, phencyclidine, ketamine
- Glycine receptor: HA 966, ACEA 1021, kynurenate
- Polyamine site: ifenprodil, eliprodil
- Presynaptic: riluzole
- Ion channel blockade: magnesium sulphate

---

$Ca^{2+}$ ion channel. This receptor-operated ion channel (ROC) permits $Ca^{2+}$ influx and immediate, complete cell death. Slow cell death occurs if excess glutamate is presented to the recognition site at $\alpha$-amino-3-hydroxy-3-methyl-4-isoxasole (AMPA)/kainate receptors and associated $Na^+$ channels. The resultant overwhelming build-up of intracellular $Na^+$ ultimately results in the cell exchanging $Na^+$ for $Ca^{2+}$; cell death occurs by cell shrinkage and DNA laddering (apoptosis). Excitotoxicity may be mediated by an increase in inducible nitric oxide synthase (iNOS) in astrocytes and microglia with NO forming a "super-radical" after interaction with $O_2$ free radicals.[2]

Elevation of extracellular glutamate occurs owing to increased release and impaired uptake into neurons and astrocytes. Pharmacological manipulation can occur at a number of sites within the NMDA receptor ion channel complex (Box 19.1).

*Protection via NMDA receptors*

Opening of the NMDA receptor is voltage and, therefore, user dependent. The effect of non-competitive antagonists is enhanced with increased extracellular glutamate concentrations and reduced competitive antagonists. Non-competitive agents are lipophilic with good CNS penetration, but they are associated with respiratory depression, haemodynamic instability, derangements in learning and memory functions, ataxia, sedation, and anaesthesia at anti-ischaemic doses. In experimental studies, reversible cellular swelling and vacuolisation were noted in areas of the limbic system and are associated with an increase in glucose use. Competitive agents are devoid of such effects at anti-ischaemic dosage, the behavioural effects being evident at 3–10 times such dosage. These side effects limit the usefulness of these agents in stroke where management is in an open ward.

It is now accepted that brain injury can be reduced by blockade of the NMDA receptor ion channel complex, irrespective of species, receptor site, or whether administered before or after injury. These agents are under phase III investigation with many failed or inconclusive studies, and are not yet part of our therapeutic strategy after brain injury.[3]

## Free radicals

Direct biochemical evidence for free radical damage and lipid peroxidation in human CNS injury is hampered by methodological difficulties. However, indirect evidence suggests a key role for oxygen radicals following ischaemia, especially when the self-perpetuating nature of free radicals and the damage they produce are examined. Following CNS injury iron is decompartmentalised from ferritin, transferrin, and haemoglobin, owing to axonal shearing, microhaemorrhage, and subarachnoid haemorrhage. $Fe^{2+}$ catalyses reactions including Fenton and Haber–Weiss reactions to give free radicals. Other sources include catecholamine oxidation, ATP oxidation by xanthine oxidase, acidosis, and eicosanoid metabolism.[4] Of particular importance is the effect of reperfusion and availability of oxygen to fuel free radical formation after ischaemia (Figure 19.1).

### Protection against free radical damage

Superoxide dismutase is a potent free radical scavenger but it has a short half-life. Conjugation with polyethylene glycol (PEG-SOD) has permitted experimental and clinical investigation. Tirilazad mesylate is a lazaroid or 21-aminosteroid which has demonstrated efficacy as a protector against free radicals and oxidant damage. Initial experimental results showed a reduction in one week mortality rate after mouse head injury from 73 to 21%. This has led to subsequent clinical trials in both North America and Europe. The outcome data from a phase II trial in which 104 patients received 2500, 5000 or 10 000 IU PEG-SOD demonstrated a significant reduction in the number of dead or severely disabled patients at six months in the high-dosage group.

Tirilazad works by restoring blood–brain barrier permeability to pre-

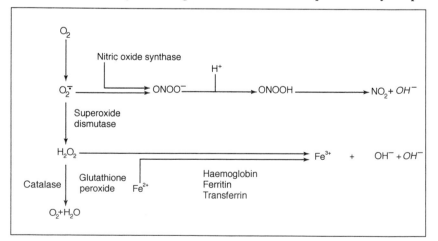

Fig 19.1   The production of free radicals.

injury threshold values, by an ability to scavenge hydroxyl radicals and improve CNS metabolic profile. This cell-protecting agent can act upon subsequent cell death-inducing events preventing apoptosis, even by non-calcium-mediated mechanisms. The mode of action appears similar to that of vitamin E and there is evidence that lazaroids slow vitamin E inactivation and increase its scavenging capacity.[4]

## Eicosanoids

Normal cellular function relies upon transitory activation of enzymes by $Ca^{2+}$. If this $Ca^{2+}$ signal is excessive, dysfunctional activation occurs of phospholipases, non-lysomal proteases, protein kinases, phosphatases, endonucleases, and NO synthase. The activation of phospholipases releases free fatty acids which, in excess, cause increased mitochondrial membrane permeability to protons, and uncouple oxidative phosphorylation. Activation of phospholipase $A_2$ produces excess arachidonic acid (AA), inducing endothelial dysfunction and derangement of the blood–brain barrier. Moreover, the oxidation of AA by cyclo-oxygenase and lipoxygenase pathways results in overproduction of eicosanoids with free radical properties and adverse effects upon the microvasculature. The resultant effect is vasoderegulation, worsening ischaemia, and microvascular thrombosis.

## $\kappa$ Opioid agonists

The neuropeptide dynorphin is an agonist at the $\kappa$ receptor and experimentally causes flaccid paralysis similar to that seen after spinal cord trauma. In vivo dynorphin accumulates at this receptor site after trauma and upregulation of the $\kappa$ receptor is noted. A number of structurally different opioid antagonists improve outcome after experimental traumatic head injury. The effect is stereospecific suggesting an opioid receptor mechanism. $\kappa$-Active and $\kappa$-selective antagonists have an enhanced effect. Receptor subtypes and isoreceptors are responsible for protective and destructive functions, $\kappa_1$ protective and $\kappa_2$ destructive. Nalbuphine is non-selective and currently under phase I investigation in acute spinal cord injury.

## Traumatic brain injury

Traumatic brain injury (TBI) constitutes a major health and economic burden for the country. The incidence is approximately 100–300 hospital admissions per 100 000 population per year, with road traffic accidents accounting for more than half. The majority occur in young males. The overall mortality varies from 15 to 23 per 100 000 per year, including those who die before arrival at hospital. To allow comparison of the effect of

225

treatment and to establish some prediction of outcome, TBI is classified as severe if the Glasgow Coma Score (GCS) is ≤ 8 with no eye opening (in coma), moderate if the GCS is ≤ 12 but not in coma, and mild if the GCS is 13–15. All such examinations should be after non-neurosurgical resuscitation (airway, breathing, and circulation) and further refinement can be made by assessment of pupil response and presence of lateralising signs.

### Referral criteria following traumatic brain injury

Referral guidelines and computed tomography (CT) guidelines have been devised to minimise the potential of unrecognised development of an intracranial haematoma, an important source of preventable morbidity and mortality following TBI.

All patients who have clinical or radiological skull fracture (vault or base) or a decreased level of consciousness persisting after non-neurosurgical resuscitation should have urgent computed tomography. Patients with a suspected penetrating injury or post-traumatic seizure, or those who develop focal neurological signs should have an early CT scan, which should be discussed with and the image transferred to the neurosurgical service. Transfer should occur only after appropriate resuscitation and stabilisation.[6] Neurological intensive care units must have access to 24-hour-a-day CT scanning services. Patients who should be admitted for intensive rather than high dependency care include those:

- in coma (GCS <9 with no eye opening) prior to intubation and ventilation or neurosurgical intervention;
- with multiple injuries including head injury;
- with respiratory impairment, such as aspiration, neurogenic pulmonary oedema, or lung contusion, in association with head injury.

### Intensive care following traumatic brain injury

Neurological intensive care unit (NICU) management following TBI includes prevention of physiological derangements that worsen ischaemic brain damage.[1] It is therefore essential that other organ systems are not neglected. Promotion of maximal neuronal survival will both improve functional recovery and reduce mortality. There is no evidence that high-quality intensive care of severely brain-injured patients reduces mortality rates by increasing the number of patients in the persistent vegetative state. The incidence and importance of disturbed physiology (secondary insults) following TBI have recently been reported: the most significant predictors of mortality at 12 months were the duration of hypotension, pyrexia, and hypoxaemic insults during the intensive care stay. The best predictors of a good outcome were the absence of hypotension during intensive care and preservation of pupillary reflexes on admission.[7]

### Therapeutic goals

Cerebral perfusion pressure (CPP) is the mean arterial pressure (MAP) minus the intracranial pressure (ICP), and is the principal determinant of cerebral blood flow. A reduction in arterial pressure is considerably worse for an individual patient than an increase in intracranial pressure and therefore an arterial pressure-oriented approach to CPP rather than an intracranial pressure-oriented approach is recommended.[7] It is worth noting that most treatments that reduce intracranial pressure do so by cerebrovascular vasoconstriction and may have a deleterious effect upon regional adequacy of oxygen and substrate delivery. Current recommended therapeutic targets are a mean arterial pressure of ≥ 90 mm Hg and a cerebral perfusion pressure of 70 mm Hg,[8] achieved by optimisation of myocardial preload and then noradrenaline infusion. Multimodality monitoring of systemic oxygen delivery variables must consist not only of mean arterial pressure but also of one of its principal determinants, cardiac output. Vasopressor manipulation of the systemic circulation without measurement of cardiac output will be suboptimal.

### Intracranial pressure

Measurement of intracranial pressure has become synonymous with intensive care management of patients following TBI. However, the philosophy behind the management of intracranial pressure has changed with an emphasis on arterial pressure rather than intracranial pressure when manipulation of cerebral perfusion pressure is being considered. Intracranial pressure can be monitored extradurally, subdurally, in the subarachnoid space, in the brain, and by placing a catheter in the lateral ventricle. When measured simultaneously from these sites, pressure gradients throughout the intracranial space are noted. These pressure gradients are physiological and important for resolution of oedema fluid. All ICP measurement systems should be interfaced with a bedside monitor or chart recorder to allow visualisation of the waveform. The shape of the intracranial pressure waveform may be of greater clinical significance than its absolute numerical value as the shape reflects changes in brain elastance.[9] The intracranial pressure wave consists of three successive peaks of diminishing amplitude; however, when the volumetric compensatory mechanisms within the skull are depleted, this changes, with the second and third peaks being larger than the first. A patient with this type of waveform is at greater risk of cerebrovascular decompensation than a patient with a similar magnitude of intracranial pressure but normal waveform and brain elastance.

Intracranial pressure is a valuable monitor of extracranial physiology. A reduction in lung compliance, alteration in blood gases, plasma hypo-osmolality, pyrexia, and neck position will all result in secondary increases in ICP necessitating treatment of the cause but not directly of the intracranial pressure. Thus we have a continuous monitor that will alert us to deviations in normal physiology. The ICP should always be displayed on a polygraph recorder with arterial pressure to aid interpretation of the fluctuations in ICP and their temporal relationship to changes in blood pressure, heart rate, and arterial saturation.

## Intracranial hypertension

Traditionally a staircase approach to increasing ICP has been adopted starting with mild hypocapnia ventilating to a $Paco_2$ between 3·5 and 4·0 kPa, escalating to regular mannitol treatment and CSF drainage, followed by hypnotic coma with barbiturates, $\gamma$-hydroxybutyrate, or propofol, and finally profound hypocapnia to prevent coning. This approach may result in inappropriate therapeutic interventions which should more properly be tailored to individual pathophysiology (Figure 19.2).

Ideally, there should be a coupled reduction in cerebral metabolic rate ($CMRO_2$) and cerebral blood flow, avoiding cerebral hypoperfusion and potential ischaemia. Hypothermia has been demonstrated to reduce morbidity and mortality in the most severely injured patients[10,11] and will reduce both cerebral blood flow and $CMRO_2$ (below the isoelectric point) in a coupled fashion. Hypnotic infusions have similar potential, although they may also cause a reduction in arterial pressure resulting in a critical reduction in cerebral perfusion pressure and cerebral blood flow. Efficacy of these agents depends upon preservation of cerebral electrical activity and $Paco_2$ responsivity. Continuous EEG monitoring is required to prevent unnecessary hypnotic dosage beyond burst suppression.

Agents that reduce plasma viscosity may cause an improvement in regional cerebral perfusion which, in a patient with normal vasoreactivity, results in a compensatory vasoconstriction and a reduction in intracranial pressure. Examples include mannitol, which is also a potent free radical scavenger, and hyperoncotic hyperosmotic solutions (HHS). Controversy still surrounds the mode of action of mannitol with protagonists for compensatory vasoconstriction[5] and osmotic reduction in brain water.[12] An HHS solution which has been used in initial resuscitation of trauma patients is 7·2% saline in 10% Dextran 60. It is uniquely suited to management of the trauma patient with multiple injuries including severe head injury, producing a sustained reduction in ICP while improving intravascular volume.

Indomethacin inhibits cyclo-oxygenase activity and specifically restores cerebral vasoreactivity. It may have a role in reducing ICP pressure in the most severely injured patients when other therapies have failed, provided that cerebral venous oxygen saturation is monitored.

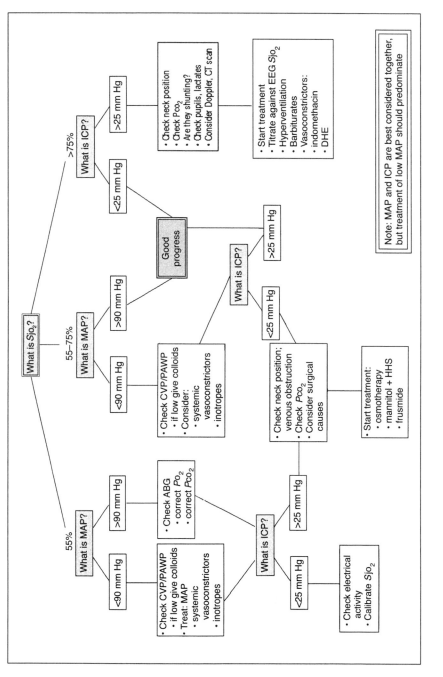

Fig 19.2 Management of severe brain injury by optimisation of cerebral oxygen delivery and reduction of cerebral hypoperfusion. ABG, arterial blood gases; CVP, central venous pressure; PAWP, pulmonary artery wedge pressure; $Sjo_2$, jugular venous oxygen saturation.

Dihydroergotamine (DHE) and profound hypocapnia reduce cerebral blood flow independently of cerebral metabolism, and may be of value in patients with hyperaemia. DHE has precapillary and cerebral venous vasoconstrictor activity, and has been recommended with regular osmotic therapy to improve mortality following head injury.[13] The use of this regimen in association with arterial pressure control with clonidine and metoprolol does not have general acceptance, given the absence in these reports of measures of cerebral blood flow and the small sample size.[14]

**Detection and prevention of cerebral ischaemia**

Following TBI there is often a global imbalance between cerebral metabolic rate and cerebral blood flow. Fibreoptic technology allows continuous assessment of the oxygen saturation of cerebral venous blood. The technique of jugular bulb cannulation has gained increasing popularity, and the availability of continuous monitors allows the detection of isolated, short duration events.[15,16] Provided arterial oxygen saturation and haemoglobin remain constant, the recording of jugular venous oxygen saturation ($Sjo_2$) is proportional to the ratio of cerebral blood flow to cerebral metabolic rate for oxygen (Figure 19.3). The brain compensates for acute reductions in oxygen and substrate delivery by increasing oxygen extraction ratio and reducing $Sjo_2$. Prolonged reductions in oxygen delivery such as with anaemia result in a compensatory increase in cerebral blood

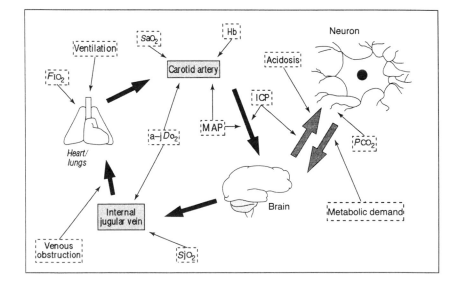

Fig 19.3 The cerebral oxygen delivery cascade: relationship between, and factors affecting, neuronal oxygen and substrate delivery, and $Sjo_2$ and a–$jDo_2$ (arterial–jugular oxygen saturation difference).

flow, so any increase in oxygen extraction ratio and reduction in $Sjo_2$ is of clinical importance and the cause must be investigated. Normal values are between 50 and 75%, with luxury cerebral perfusion occurring above the upper limit and hypoperfusion below the lower limit. Compensated cerebral hypoperfusion can be differentiated from ischaemia by assessment of cerebral arteriovenous lactate content difference. Likewise, luxury cerebral perfusion can be subdivided into an absolute or relative cerebral hyperaemia by measurement of cerebral blood flow. This differentiation is important when considering the prognostic implications of an elevated $Sjo_2$. Continuous assessment of $Sjo_2$ is of great practical importance:

- it allows a continuous monitor of the adequacy of cerebral blood flow;
- it gives a global indication of the effect of rising intracranial pressure on the relationship between cerebral blood flow and metabolism;
- it may be of value in predicting which therapeutic intervention will be of greatest value;
- it provides a continuous monitor of the effect of any therapeutic intervention on adequacy of cerebral oxygenation.

Transcranial Doppler ultrasonography uses a 2 mHz gated probe insonating the cerebral vessels through a temporal bony window. Anterior, middle, and posterior cerebral vessels are all assessable with this device. However, in head injuries usually the middle cerebral artery is assessed bilaterally. Velocities are measured for the systolic component of the envelope, the diastolic component, and a mean velocity is also derived. The dimensionless pulsatility index (PI) is systolic minus diastolic divided by mean. This index is normally less than one but, when the cerebral perfusion pressure is reduced, either by a reduction in mean arterial pressure or an increase in intracranial pressure, diastolic flow velocity decreases and the pulsatility index increases.[8]

## Non-traumatic coma

The aetiology of ischaemic non traumatic coma encountered in the ICU is given in Box 19.2. Management and outcome of metabolic causes of coma are described in other chapters.

Physicians and families of patients in non-traumatic coma face a difficult decision when considering life-extending care and whether it will achieve a desirable outcome. The majority of such patients will not survive two months (69% die), and of those who do survive many will not regain independence (29% suffer severe disability). The most frequent primary causes of coma include cerebral infarction or haemorrhage (36%) and cardiac arrest (31%).[17] Development of out-of-hospital resuscitation and improved training and equipment of paramedical staff has resulted in an increase in the number of patients in coma after cardiac arrest.

231

**Box 19.2** *Aetiology of non-traumatic coma*

*Metabolic*
- Diabetic ketoacidosis
- Hyperosmolar non-ketotic coma
- Hypoglycaemia
- Thyrotoxicosis
- Myxoedema
- Hepatic encephalopathy
- Coma worsened by uraemia
- Hypo- and hypernatraemia
- Hypo- and hypercalcaemia
- Panhypopituitarism
- Addisonian crisis

*Ischaemic*
- Cardiac arrest
- Cerebral infarction
- Intracerebral haemorrhage
- Subarachnoid haemorrhage
- Status epilepticus
- Near-drowning syndrome

*Pharmacological*
- Anaesthetic agents
- Overdose
- Treatment of seizures/pseudoseizures
- Carbon monoxide poisoning
- Heavy metal poisoning

*Infective*
- Sepsis
- CNS infection (encephalitis, meningitis, cerebritis, abscess)
- Miller–Fischer variant of Guillain–Barré syndrome

*Degenerative*
- Alzheimer's disease
- Motor neuron disease – chronic hypoventilation
- Muscular dystrophies – chronic hypoventilation
- HIV dementia
- Inherited/congenital

*Neoplastic*
- Intracranial neoplasm ± haemorrhage into tumour

## Prognosis – clinical and physiological examination

Reliable prognosis can be achieved by clinical and physiological examination of five clinical and physiological variables during the first three days after insult:[17,18]

- abnormal brain-stem responses
- absent withdrawal response to pain
- absent verbal response
- creatinine level $\geq$ 132·6 μmol/l
- age $\geq$ 70 years.

Patients with four or five of these risk factors have a 97% mortality rate at two months. Abnormal brain-stem reflexes and absent motor response are the best predictors of functional outcome. Patients with absent brain-stem reflexes or absent motor withdrawal response to pain have a 96% probability of death or severe disability.

A management protocol similar to that adopted for TBI is appropriate, as the pathophysiology of secondary injuries following the primary insult is similar. There are however, a few important differences. Ischaemic infarction will result in tentorial herniation earlier than in intracerebral haemorrhage because of differences in brain viscoelastic properties. Hydrocephalus must be considered if neurological deterioration is evident in patients following spontaneous subarachnoid haemorrhage. Clinical assessment is confounded by sedative medication given to facilitate intermittent positive-pressure ventilation.

## Prognosis – neurophysiology and functional imaging

Neurophysiological monitoring within the NICU includes assessment of cortical electrical activity and functional integrity by evoked potential measurement. Functional imaging is improving, and quantification of cerebral lactate and *N*-acetylaspartate by magnetic resonance spectroscopy may in future give clues to the severity of CNS injury.

### EEG

Frequency- and time-domain analyses are required to make informed judgments. Continuous monitoring will detect seizures, a source of preventable morbidity, and provide a guide for hypnotic therapy. Prognostically EEG is weak but is improved by serial measures and reactivity to external stimuli.

### Evoked potentials

Sematosensory evoked potentials (SSEPs) have been used to assess severity of injury after traumatic and non-traumatic CNS injury. Following TBI, SSEPs are of value but offer no predictive advantage over clinical assessment when the latter is possible. Injury from cerebral ischaemia results in absent N20 waves in short-latency SSEPs in patients with a poor prognosis.[19,20] The electrical environment within the NICU may result in a low signal-to-noise ratio which makes this type of examination technically challenging.

# Conclusion

- Primary brain injury leads to a stereotypical pattern of secondary brain injury.
- Secondary brain insults, particularly hypotension and pyrexia, adversely affect outcome.
- Cerebral protection can be administered after the primary injury to mitigate the effects of the secondary injury and improve mortality and functional outcome.
- Management of cerebral perfusion pressure should be arterial pressure oriented.
- The most powerful predictors of functional outcome from non-traumatic coma are motor responses and brain-stem reflexes.

1 Graham DI, Ford I, Adams JH, et al. Ischaemic brain damage is still common in fatal non-missile head injury. J Neurol Neurosurg Psychiatry 1989;52:346–50.
2 Choi DW, Koh J-Y, Peters S. Pharmacology of glutamate neurotoxicity in cortical cell culture: Attenuation by NMDA antagonists. J Neurosci 1988;8:185–96.
3 McCulloch J. Excitatory amino acids and their potential for the treatment of ischaemic brain damage in man. Br J Pharmacol 1992;34:106–14.
4 Rice-Evans CA, Diplock AT. Current status of antioxidant therapy. Free Radical Biol Med 1993;25:77–96.
5 Muizelaar JP, Wei EP, Kontos HA, Becker DP. Mannitol causes compensatory cerebral vasoconstriction and vasodilation in response to blood viscosity changes. J Neurosurg 1983;59:822–8.
6 Andrews PJD, Piper IR, Dearden NM, Miller JD. Secondary brain insults during intrahospital transport of head injured patients. Lancet 1990;335: 327–30.
7 Jones PA, Andrews PJD, Midgely S, et al. Measuring the burden of secondary insults in head-injured patients during intensive care. J Neurosurg Anaesthesiol 1994;6:4–14.
8 Chan KH, Miller JD, Dearden NM, Andrews PJD, Midgely S. The effect of changes in cerebral perfusion pressure upon middle cerebral artery blood flow velocity and jugular bulb venous oxygen saturation after severe brain injury. J Neurosurg 1992;77:55–61.
9 Piper IR, Miller JD, Dearden NM, Leggate JR, Robertson I. Systems analysis of cerebrovascular pressure transmission: an observational study in head-injured patients. J Neurosurg 1990;73:871–80.
10 Marion DW, Obrist WD, Carlier PM, et al. The use of moderate therapeutic hypothermia for patients with severe head injuries. J Neurosurg 1993;79:354–62.
11 Shiozaki F, Sugimoto H, Taneda M, et al. Effect of mild hypothermia on uncontrollable intracranial hypertension after severe head injury. J Neurosurg 1993;79:363–8.
12 Ravussin P, Archer DP, Meyer E, Abou Madi M, Yamamoto L, Trop D. The effects of rapid infusions of saline and mannitol on cerebral blood volume and intracranial pressure in dogs. Can Anaesth Soc J 1985;32,506–15.
13 Asgeirsson B, Grande PO, Nordstrom CH. A new therapy of post-trauma brain oedema based on haemodynamic principles for brain volume regulation. Intensive Care Med 1994;20:260–7.
14 Andrews PJD, Dearden NM. Validation of Oximetrix 3 for continuous jugular venous oxygen saturation following severe head injury: comparison with IIL 282 in vitro co-oximeter. Br J Anaesth 1990;64:393.
15 Souter MJ, Andrews PJD. A review of cerebral venous oximetry. Intensive Care Wld, 1996;13:32–8.
16 Andrews PJD. What is the optimal perfusion pressure after head injury? A review of the evidence with an emphasis on arterial pressure. Acta Anesthesiol Scand 1995;39(suppl 105):112–15.

17 Hamel MB, Goldman L, Teno J, *et al.* Identification of comatose patients at high risk for death or severe disability. *JAMA* 1995;**273**:1842-8.
18 Edgren E, Hedstrand U, Kelsey S, Sutton-Tyrell K, Safar P, BRCT I Study Group. Assessment of neurological prognosis in comatose survivors of cardiac arrest. *Lancet* 1994;**343**:1055-9.
19 Berek K, Lechleitner P, Luef G, *et al.* Early determination of neurological outcome after prehospital cardiopulmonary resuscitation. *Stroke* 1995;**26**:543-9.
20 Chiappa KH. Interpretation of abnormal short-latency somatosensory evoked potentials. In *A textbook of clinical neurophysiology* (Halliday AM, Butler RS, Paul R, eds). Chichester: John Wiley & Sons Ltd, 1987.

# 20: Neurological evaluation of the ICU patient

M T E HEAFIELD

Although neurological complications are frequent in critically ill patients, it is often difficult to separate the various contributions of local neurological disease from the systemic illness and those from the effects of drugs and their metabolites. Too often neurologists are called only to confirm a poor prognosis or support withdrawal of treatment. Consequently some neurological disorders are diagnosed late or *post mortem*, when earlier intervention might have improved the outcome.

Neurological assessment in the ICU involves establishing clearly the basic problem requiring investigation, identifying trends in CNS function, and being prepared to re-evaluate the patient regularly.[1] Box 20.1 summarises clinical and historical features, and details the features that should be considered in evaluating altered consciousness in the ICU patient. Laboratory tests (particularly radiology) should be ordered to confirm or refute clinical diagnoses, and not as a substitute for thorough clinical appraisal.

## Terms used to describe features of altered consciousness

- *Consciousness* is the state of awareness of self and environment. The ability to demonstrate awareness of the environment determines the level of consciousness, and may be affected by interruption of several complex pathways (see Recommended reading).
- *Coma* is the exact opposite of consciousness, and includes failure to open the eyes in response to noise, absence of comprehensible words, no response to commands, and no appropriate movement of the extremities to localise or resist painful stimuli.[2]
- *Stupor, obtundation, and delirium* are often used interchangeably and incorrectly. Stupor is akin to sleep or reduced responsiveness and the patient can be aroused. Delirium is a disorder of mental state where the patient is not lucid but may have intermittent periods of improvement. There is commonly a state of detachment and superimposed disordered

perception and hallucinations. Obtundation is the mental blunting that is often subtle and may fluctuate with stupor. It is important to detect rate of alteration in these states as clues to the evolution of central lesions.

## Neurophysiology and neuroanatomy of consciousness

Whereas conscious purposeful behaviour requires hemisphere function integrated by the thalamic and brain-stem subcortical nuclei, alertness or arousal depends on the activity of the brain-stem reticular activating pathways and their projection to the hypothalamic and other diencephalic

---

**Box 20.1** *Assessment of the intensive care patient with altered consciousness or focal neurological deficit*

*History*
- Date and time of onset of neurological lesion
- Witnessed events, e.g. cardiopulmonary resuscitation, trauma, surgery
- Preceding neurological function: seizures, rate of development of focal signs, "awareness"
- Preceding systemic illness: cardiac, respiratory, e.g. bronchiectasis, stroke, metabolic, infective
- Evidence for drug or alcohol misuse: right heart murmurs, venous access sites
- Immunosuppression: pharmacological or as a feature of systemic disorder

*Clinical examination*
- ABC + blood glucose, current serum sodium, acid–base status
- Presence of recent sedation or paralysing agent
- Skin appearance, bruising, needle marks, rashes, cyanosis, jaundice
- Respiration: rate, rhythm, depth, regularity (spontaneous respiration if ventilated); odour of exhaled breath
- Level of consciousness
- Eye opening
- Best motor response: particular relevance of extensor or asymmetrical posturing
- Trunk and limb posture:
  - neck rigidity: meningeal irritation (establish exclusion of cervical injury)
  - spontaneous movements: myoclonus, seizures, tremor, stimulus-sensitive movements
  - involuntary movements: hiccoughs, yawning, chewing, grimacing
- Ocular movements: evoked or spontaneous, roving, dys/conjugate, oculocephalic reflexes, corneal reflexes
- Deep tendon reflexes: presence and symmetry
- Plantar responses: extensor responses and symmetry

*Place neurological disease in context* (e.g. resolving sepsis, other organ system dysfunction)
*Exclude structural disease and raised ICP*
*Exclude seizures, particularly* subclinical status epilepticus
*Put likely outcome in context*

---

nuclei. One of the specific properties of the human CNS which differentiates other mammalian responses is the presence of highly developed language skills. A significant weakness of measurement of consciousness in humans is the necessity to rely on speech and response to commands, these responses being disturbed excessively when dominant hemisphere function is disturbed.

## Pathological anatomy of lesions causing coma

The pupils are controlled by the parasympathetic and sympathetic nervous system (PSNS). The pupilloconstrictor fibres are the most important in differentiating structural from metabolic coma. PSNS fibres run through the midbrain around the cerebral aqueduct and pupillary constriction occurs when they are stimulated. Pupillary dilatation should be taken to imply failure of PSNS supply and therefore disturbance in the efferent pathway through the midbrain, along the third cranial nerve and to the sphincter pupillae. A laterally situated mass lesion will displace the medial temporal hippocampus and uncus causing uncal herniation, with pressure on the ipsilateral third nerve, posterior cerebral artery, and the peduncular pathways. This stretches the midbrain and pons producing ischaemic lesions. In metabolic coma the pupils are almost invariably small and reactive, although prior injury or surgery and drugs (particularly opioids, atropine, and barbiturates) must be excluded.

Box 20.2 shows the neuroanatomical features and areas of assessment appropriate in coma and those that should be re-evaluated. The finding of asymmetry is most important, as is the interpretation of respiratory and

---

**Box 20.2** *Describing brain-stem reflexes*

*Pupillary signs*
- Normal/abnormal
- Regular/irregular
- Reactive/unreactive
- Symmetrical/asymmetrical

*Motor signs*
- Grasp response/frontal release
- Paratonia
- Obeying commands
- Localising pain
- Flexing to pain
- Decorticate
- Decerebrate
- No motor response
- Symmetry

*Eye movements*
- Primary position
- Conjugate/dysconjugate/divergent
- Nystagmus
- Spontaneous movements
- Roving
- Bobbing/upversion/down
- Horizontal

*Respiratory signs*
- Sighing/Cheyne–Stokes
- Central neurogenic hyperventilation
- Cluster/apneustic breathing
- Sighing/gasping/ataxic breathing

---

haemodynamic disturbances. There is a caudal to rostral hierarchy of increasing sophistication in movement, respiratory function, and pupillary and ocular disturbance, which determines the site of a neurological lesion. Common sites and causes include the following:

- *Supratentorial mass lesions* must be bilateral to cause coma, or exert bilateral effects through midline shift or oedema. A unilateral hemisphere lesion might give rise to the syndrome of uncal herniation described above.
- *Infratentorial lesions* will affect the ascending pathways of the reticular activating system, which in the brain stem are close together, so coma is common, and signs usually symmetrical. Pontine haemorrhage produces pinpoint pupils, oculomotor, respiratory, and autonomic features, and quadriparesis.
- *Global disorders* are commonly metabolic in origin. The commonest cause is hypoxic–ischaemic injury following cardiorespiratory arrest. The cerebral metabolic rate is temperature dependent, and hypothermic (exposure, myxoedema) and hyperthermic (psychoactive drugs, stimulants) syndromes are often overlooked. Other causes include hyper- and hypo-osmolar states, alterations of sodium balance, hypoglycaemia, hypercalcaemia, hepatorenal dysfunction, and endocrine and cofactor deficiency states, all of which may present with various focal or non-focal neurological signs.

Seizures usually present with classic tonic–clonic motor activity, but they may also resemble fluctuating encephalopathies with disturbances of consciousness and be difficult to diagnose. In the critically ill patient without an antecedent history of epilepsy, the commonest causes are vascular lesions, intracranial infection, metabolic disorders, and hypoxia;[4] other causes include mass lesions, hypertension, and vasculitides such as systemic lupus.

## Brain metabolism and autoregulation

Cerebral blood flow is regulated to match the metabolic needs of the brain. In adults 15% of cardiac output goes to an organ that represents only 2% of the total body weight. The brain is primarily dependent on glucose, and consumes 75% of the glucose produced by the liver. During high metabolic rates, amino acids and ammonia may also be used. Metabolism is coupled to flow by the vasodilator effect of locally produced hydrogen ions referred to as autoregulation. Conditions that produce an acidosis such as hypoxia, hypercapnia, and ischaemia produce cerebrovascular dilatation and increased flow, which may be harmful if intracranial pressure is increased. In cerebral injury, metabolic autoregulation may be impaired, flow becomes more pressure dependent (often referred to as pressure passive as described in Chapter 19), and there is the potential for further neuronal ischaemia. Some areas of the brain are particularly susceptible to ischaemic necrosis: the hippocampus, the occipital cortex, and cerebellar Purkinje cells. Hypothalamic injury, which may accompany a transtentorial pressure cone, and the vasodilatation that may occur may, additionally, limit the potential cerebral perfusion and add to a cycle of neuronal injury.

In the most common metabolic encephalopathy, namely hypoxic–ischaemic injury, cerebral metabolism before, during, and after cardiac arrest determines outcome. If cerebral blood flow is reduced to 15 ml/100 g per min (one third or less of normal), membrane function fails with leak of potassium, influx of calcium, loss of ATP production, membrane peroxidation, and progressive neuronal death. The EEG becomes isoelectric and evoked potentials cannot be elicited. If blood flow is restored, a period of hyperaemia with reperfusion injury occurs, followed later by reduced blood flow.

## Metabolic encephalopathies

These (often poorly understood) conditions are usually multifactorial in origin, and the clinical signs may be multifocal, including confusion, stupor, or coma, and a range of disturbances of brain-stem function. Metabolic lesions which may present in the ICU are shown in Box 20.3. The diagnosis may be one of exclusion, and it is essential that specific remedial causes are identified, such as sedative drug metabolites, intra-cranial sepsis, and vascular lesions producing pressure effects within the cerebral hemispheres. Common causes of lesions that may mimic metabolic encephalopathy are listed in Box 20.4.

The most important aspect of management is to keep an open mind about the diagnosis, and to identify reversible causes, or new neurological complications, such as a cerebral infection in an immunosuppressed transplant recipient with an encephalopathy related to cyclosporin, renal failure, hyponatraemia, and systemic sepsis.

Certain tests may be of value to exclude reversible causes of encephalo-pathy. The EEG may help to distinguish seizures, hypoxic–ischaemic injury, or encephalitis. Brain-stem evoked potentials may provide prognostic information. EEGs cannot easily be interpreted in the presence of certain hypnotic agents, particularly benzodiazepines, propofol, and thiopentone, and care must be taken to exclude persisting effects from opioid and benzodiazepine metabolites. CT or MRI scanning may show ischaemic or mass lesions. Cerebrospinal fluid should be taken only after excluding raised intracranial pressure and coagulopathies; it is of particular value to exclude infection in immunosuppressed patients with neurological signs.

The prognosis in encephalopathies depends on both the underlying disease and the accuracy of diagnosis.[1,4,5] Tests of brain-stem function and motor and verbal responses are the best validated clinical measures. Important factors are the cause, depth, and duration of coma, and the presence or absence of brain-stem reflexes. In metabolic coma associated with infection, multiple organ failure, or metabolic/biochemical abnormalities, up to 35% may recover. Hypoxic–ischaemic injury has a poor prognosis: only 11% make a quality recovery, falling to 7% in those patients with cerebral infarction and coma. In a study of 500 patients with non-traumatic coma, no patient survived who had absent corneal reflexes at 24 hours or a motor response worse than withdrawal.[2] Patients who at 24 hours demonstrate roving eye movements, speech, nystagmus on caloric

---

**Box 20.3** *Disorders resembling metabolic encephalopathies which may be associated with raised ICP and seizures*

*Structural lesions*
- Primary and secondary tumours (with accompanying oedema)
- Hydrocephalus

*Vascular lesions*
- Cerebral haemorrhage (subarachnoid, intracerebral)
- Cerebral arterial infarction (especially proximal middle cerebral)
- Cerebral venous infarction (venous sinus thrombosis)

*Intracranial sepsis*
- Cerebral abscess (bacterial, mycobacterial, fungal, protozoal)
- Meningitis (venous cortical infarction, cerebral toxic oedema)
- Encephalitis (herpes, cytomegalovirus)
- Systemic septic emboli (endocarditis, central catheter)

*Systemic metabolic lesions*
- Fulminant hepatic failure
- Hyperammonaemia (Reye-like syndromes)
- Diabetic ketoacidosis
- Hypertensive encephalopathy (including eclampsia)
- Hypoxic–ischaemic encephalopathy (cardiac arrest)
- Drug overdose (secondary hypoxic/metabolic insults)
- Central pontine myelinolysis (sodium shifts)
- Porphyrias and metabolic myopathies with acid–base imbalance

*Trauma*
- Diffuse axonal injury
- Focal extra-axial haemorrhage
- Focal haemorrhagic contusion
- Fat embolism

*Status epilepticus*
- Subconvulsive
- Late overt status epilepticus

---

---

**Box 20.4** *Common causes of metabolic encephalopathies in the intensive care unit*

| *Hypoxic–ischaemic* | *Systemic disorders* | *Toxic/poisoning* |
|---|---|---|
| • Cardiac arrest | • Sepsis | • Alcohol |
| • Hypoventilation | • Focal infection | • Opioids |
| • Respiratory disorders | • Renal impairment/ failure | • Benzodiazepines |
| • Severe anaemia | • Hepatic impairment/ failure | • Phenothiazines |
| • Hypotension | • Nutritional failure (thiamine) | • Butyrophenones |
| • Cardiac arrhythmia | • Hyperglycaemia/ Hypoglycaemia | • Heavy metals: lead, lithium |
| • Hyperviscosity | | |
| • Hypotension | • Hyperosmolar syndromes | • Hypnotics |
| • Hypertension | • Acid–base imbalance | • Penicillin |
| • Cerebral infarction | • Electrolyte/fluid imbalance | • Cephalosporins |
| • Pulmonary infarction | • Pancreatitis | • Phenytoin |
| • Hyperthermic syndromes | • Paraneoplastic syndromes | • Corticosteroids |
| | • Systemic vasculitis | |
| | • Thyroid dysfunction | |

---

testing, and eye opening to pain or better, have a 25% chance of a good recovery. A proportion of patients with severe hypoxic–ischaemic injury, often accompanied by trauma, may fulfil the criteria for persistent vegetative state (PVS).[3]

## Peripheral neuropathies

These may present initially as disorders of airway maintenance, sputum clearance, respiration or gas exchange, or circulatory disturbances from autonomic involvement or thromboembolic disease in immobile patients. The mode of presentation may be acute, subacute, or chronic paralysis of voluntary and involuntary musculature. Causes are listed in Box 20.5 in an anatomical format.

The intensivist encounters these patients either on the wards as respiratory failure complicating a neuropathy or after an intervention such as surgery, or in the ICU after prolonged sepsis, respiratory failure, and prolonged use of neuromuscular blocking drugs. These last agents may be associated with a specific myopathy with vacuolation and loss of muscle fibres, elevated creatine phosphokinase levels, and fasciculation detectable by electromyography (EMG); the syndrome has been reported more

**Box 20.5** *Differential diagnosis of limb, trunk or respiratory paralysis*

*Spinal cord disorders*
- Spinal cord trauma
- Epidural structural lesions (primary or secondary tumours, haematoma)
- Epidural sepsis
- Spinal arteriovenous malformation
- Inflammatory cord lesions (unusual causes of respiratory weakness)
- Primary cord infections (herpes/varicella)

*Neuromuscular junction disorders*
- Myasthenia gravis
- Lambert–Eaton myasthenic syndrome
- Botulism
- Organophosphate poisoning

*Myopathic/myositic disorders*
- Polymyositis/dermatomyositis
- Neuroleptic malignant syndrome
- Familial dyskalaemic periodic paralyses
- Toxic myopathies (drug-induced)
- Anterior horn cell disease (MND)
- Inherited myopathies
- Enzyme deficiencies
- Rhabdomyolysis/myoglobinuria syndromes

*Neuropathic disorders* (i.e. affecting the lower motor neuron)
- Acute inflammatory demyelinating polyneuropathy
- Chronic inflammatory demyelinating polyneuropathy
- Acute myelomeningoradiculopathy
- Poliomyelitis
- Porphyria
- Diphtheria
- Heavy metal intoxication (lead, mercury, thallium, *cis*-platinum)
- Tick-bite encephalomyeloradiculoneuropathy

frequently with the steroidal relaxants used in conjunction with systemic corticosteroids.

## Clinical approach to progressive limb, trunk, or respiratory weakness

The history and examination should identify the rate of onset and any preceding neurological deficit, and distinguish between toxic, post-infectious, and myasthenic weakness. Foreign travel or trauma may suggest infectious causes. Vomiting followed by constipation, oropharyngeal paresis, and oculomotor signs may suggest the toxin of *Clostridium botulinum*, in which respiratory muscle weakness is more marked than limb weakness. Lower motor neuron facial weakness and autonomic signs suggest

Guillain–Barré syndrome, whereas ptosis and fatiguable weakness indicate myasthenia gravis. Porphyria should be excluded in patients with altered mentation and encephalopathy, and lead poisoning in those with abdominal pain.

The principles of early management include attention to the ABC of resuscitation, the exclusion of potentially reversible causes such as cord compression or ischaemia, and the prevention of secondary complications including inhalation of gastric contents, sputum retention, dysrhythmias, venous thrombosis, and pulmonary emboli. Early warning of respiratory complications includes a poor cough impulse, inability to clear secretions or saliva, and a forced vital capacity (FVC) of 25 ml/kg. Tachypnoea and respiratory distress are late signs, and respiratory support should be provided before hypoxaemia or hypercapnia develops. Ward staff must be told to document trends in respiratory function, including forced expiratory volume in 1 second ($FEV_1$), respiratory rate, and $Spo_2$.

## Guillain–Barré syndrome (GBS)

*History and epidemiology*

Octave Landry described this syndrome in 1859, and Georges Guillain, Jean Barré, and Andre Strohl described the cerebrospinal fluid (CSF) changes in 1916. The description of GBS as a war illness in the paper by Guillain and Barré in 1920, "travaux neurologiques de guerre", made their names the preferred eponyms. In the United Kingdom the disease peaks in spring and late autumn, with an overall incidence of 1·7:10 000 per year, and a mortality rate of up to 18%. The largest population-based study reported[6] that 33% required ventilation and 3% died. At 12 months, 7% were severely disabled, 14% were unable to walk, and 13% had died.

*Cause*

The cause is uncertain, but the pathophysiology suggests an immune cell-mediated destruction of peripheral and cranial nerve myelin, associated with a preceding infection which may be viral, bacterial, or mycobacterial. Glycolipid antibodies may be responsible, produced after a wide range of community-acquired infections. *Borrelia burgdorferi* (Lyme disease) produces an inflammatory CSF with > 50 cells/mm³, and should be suspected in the UK in patients from wooded areas harbouring ticks in the deer and sheep population. A variant of Guillain–Barré syndrome may also occur in HIV-infected individuals, and following the use of attenuated viral vaccines containing myelin proteins.

*Clinical presentation*

This is variable,[7] and includes the extremes of isolated motor, sensory, or autonomic involvement, a paraparesis, or the Miller–Fischer variant of ataxia and ophthalmoplegia. Commonly the pattern is mixed. Essential features are progressive motor weakness of more than one limb, and reduced or absent tendon reflexes in two or more limbs. Weakness may range from minimal leg weakness with ataxia to a flaccid quadriparesis. Other features that support the diagnosis include rapid progression of weakness to a nadir at three to four weeks, symmetry, mild sensory symptoms or signs (dissociation of sensory loss or level are against GBS), bilateral facial weakness (50%) and bulbar weakness, and autonomic dysfunction.

*Laboratory investigations*

Examination of the CSF and nerve conduction studies are mandatory. The CSF classically shows an elevated protein (up to 2 g/l) with a leukocytosis of < 50 cells per high power field. In one third of cases the CSF protein may be normal at presentation, falling to 18% at two weeks. Neurophysiological abnormalities include proximal conduction block, progressing to slowing of conduction velocities and distal conduction block. There is little correlation with these findings and the clinical features.

*Management*

This involves identifying the patient at high risk of requiring respiratory support, preventing complications, and providing specific treatment.[8] Adverse prognostic factors are: being bedbound at four days, very low distal motor amplitudes on EEG, advanced age, and mechanical ventilation. Criteria for ventilation include an $FEV_1$ of < 15 ml/kg, sputum retention with pulmonary collapse or consolidation, loss of protective airway reflexes, and deteriorating gas exchange. However, intubation and ventilation should not be delayed until hypoxaemia and hypercapnia have occurred. Patients will be understandably frightened, and full discussion of what intensive care involves and the likelihood of a complete recovery (75% return to independent life) should be discussed with the patient and relatives long before ICU admission. Prophylactic care must include appropriate monitoring to detect respiratory and autonomic deterioration early on, and patients may require admission to intensive or high-dependency care to facilitate this. Continuous positive airway pressure (CPAP) should not be delivered in an ordinary ward. Heparin, antiembolism stockings, and physiotherapy are essential. Nasogastric feeding should be implemented for patients who cannot swallow.

Specific therapies include plasmapheresis ($6 \times 3.5$ litre exchanges) or intravenous $\gamma$-globulin (0·4 g/kg per day for 5 days).[9] Plasmapheresis may cause hypotension from fluid shifts and autonomic involvement, and should be performed in a properly monitored environment by skilled staff.

The ICU mortality rate in ventilated patients is around 7%, usually from preventable complications. The most serious of these are pulmonary colonisation and sepsis, acute lung injury from aspiration, dysrhythmias, hypotension, and cardiac arrest from altered vasomotor control in response to relatively minor stimuli, such as tracheal suction, venous thrombosis and pulmonary emboli, and hyponatraemia. Early tracheostomy may help to reduce lung sepsis by improving oropharyngeal hygiene. Enteral feeding should be started immediately on admission to ICU, if this has not been initiated earlier, and might help to reduce stress ulceration.

## Myasthenia gravis

### Pathology and epidemiology

Myasthenia gravis is an autoimmune disease in which circulating IgG antibodies to nicotinic acetylcholine receptors prevent neuromuscular transmission at the motor end-plate, causing weakness and muscle fatigue.[10] There is complement-mediated destruction and loss of receptors. The disease usually affects women aged 15–30 years or older men (>65 years). The pathology is associated with other autoimmune disorders such as systemic lupus, pernicious anaemia, autoimmune thyroid disease, and autoimmune platelet disorders. Thymic hyperplasia or thymic malignancy is associated with myasthenia in up to 15% of patients although, even after thymectomy, acetylcholine receptor antibodies persist.

### Clinical features

The disease presents with exertional weakness (fatigue), diplopia or ptosis, facial weakness, bulbar signs (dysarthria, dysphagia), and respiratory muscle failure often out of proportion to limb weakness. This presentation is described as the myasthenic crisis. Cholinergic crises occur with overtreatment, causing excessive acetylcholine stimulation, muscle weakness and cramps, salivation, and sweating.

### Diagnosis

Diagnosis is made on the basis of the clinical features, a response to a test dose of anticholinesterase, and the detection of acetylcholine receptor antibodies. The Tensilon (edrophonium) test involves premedication with atropine 0·6 mg i.v., both as the placebo arm of the test and to counteract the muscarinic effects of edrophonium, which blocks acetylcholinesterase systemically for up to 5 minutes, increasing acetylcholine concentrations at the motor end-plate. Bronchospasm, bradycardia, and gastrointestinal muscle cramps may occur. The Tensilon test in a patient with incipient respiratory failure is potentially risky and should be performed either in the ICU or with ICU staff available. Several objective measures of muscle power should be employed before and after, in order to evaluate the response. A video camera may be a helpful adjunct.

### Management

Box 20.6 details an approach to the emergency management of myasthenia gravis. Myasthenic crises may occur following surgery or as part

---

**Box 20.6** *Emergency management of myasthenic crisis*

- Correct positioning
- Administer oxygen and monitor $Spo_2$
- Prevent aspiration/pass fine-bore nasogastric tube
- Perform Tensilon test: continue with pyridostigmine, steroids, and immunosuppression
- Blood tests: exclude hypokalaemia, hypomagnesaemia
- Treat infection
- Anticipate need for mechanical ventilation
- Arrange plasma exchange (5–8 exchanges of 1–2 litres)

---

of an intercurrent illness, and patients may require admission to the ICU or high-dependency unit (HDU) for monitoring, or following thymectomy. The general principles of care are similar to those for GBS. Specific treatment[11] in addition to the routine anticholinesterase includes corticosteroids (which may cause an initial deterioration), azathioprine or methotrexate, and plasmapharesis. Several drugs worsen myasthenia: aminoglycoside antibiotics, anticonvulsants with membrane-stabilising effects, verapamil, and penicillamine. Failure to respond to conventional treatment may indicate concurrent hypothyroidism.

### Critical illness polyneuropathies and myopathies

Patients who fail to wean from mechanical ventilation, particularly those recovering from systemic sepsis, may have a critical illness polyneuropathy (CIP).[12] Although neurophysiological testing shows that the sensory system is also affected, clinically the most obvious feature is distal muscle weakness and wasting with arreflexia. Nerve conduction studies show denervation of muscles with fibrillation potentials and reduction in both sensory and motor compound action potentials. The CSF is normal. Nerve biopsy shows axonal loss. In the absence of sensory involvement, it may be appropriate to perform a muscle biopsy to exclude a muscle relaxant-induced myopathy. In some patients, a septic myopathy and septic encephalopathy may coexist with CIP.

Because of sedation and severity of illness, the diagnosis is usually made late, during the recovery phase from the acute illness, but it is possible to identify patients at risk earlier and detect development of the syndrome. With nerve conduction studies, the incidence may be as high as 60% in mechanically ventilated patients with multiple organ failure and sepsis, and in those receiving aminoglycoside antibiotics and long-term neuromuscular blockade. In most instances the prognosis is good, with recovery over weeks, but patients with axonal polyneuropathy may require respiratory support for months.[13]

It is important to rule out the other common causes of flaccid muscle weakness including hypokalaemia and hypophosphataemia, drug effects, and paraneoplastic syndromes. Muscle weakness alone is very common in the critically ill as a consequence of immobility, catabolism, and suboptimal nutrition, and this will contribute to the apparent severity of the neuropathy.

# Status epilepticus

### Epidemiology and aetiology

Status epilepticus is a medical emergency. The estimated UK incidence is around 18–28 per 10 000[14] and the condition largely occurs in children. Of those other lesions associated with epilepsy, the most epileptogenic seem to be associated with frontal structural lesions. Otherwise status epilepticus is associated with established epilepsy and its complications: 5% of adults with epilepsy may present at some time in status. Other common causes include cerebral infection, trauma, cerebrovascular disease, cerebral tumour, metabolic disturbance, and febrile illnesses, particularly in young children.

---

**Box 20.7** *Management of status epilepticus[a]*

*Immediate management*
- Ensure that you have adequate assistance
- Airway: establish and protect
- Breathing: oxygenation
- Cardiovascular assessment
- Intravenous access
- Anticonvulsant: diazepam (if receiving chronic anticonvulsants, take blood sample to check levels; consider additional bolus)

*Followed by*
- Blood tests
  - sugar (give thiamine with dextrose boluses)
  - electrolytes: $Na^+$, $K^+$, $Ca^{2+}$, $Mg^{2+}$, and osmolality
  - FBC, platelets, clotting and fibrinogen
- Neurological examination: establish a working diagnosis and appropriate interventions
- Transfer to a high dependency area
  - oxygen saturation monitoring
  - arterial blood gas analysis (particularly $P$a$CO_2$ and base deficit)
  - record temperature (treat hyperpyrexia)
  - blood and CSF cultures as appropriate
  - EEG and ECG
  - CT scan when patient stabilised

[a] Status = fitting for > 1 min, or second seizure without recovery of consciousness.

---

## Assessment, classification, and management

Although status epilepticus is usually defined as two or more seizures within 30 minutes without recovery of consciousness, this is an inappropriately loose definition since many patients may develop very severe complications and organ compromise within this time period, and require early intervention.

In the early stage which may last minutes to hours, many discrete generalised tonic–clonic seizures may occur. As time passes, clonic activity ceases and the patient may become deeply unconscious with compromised airway, breathing, and circulation. Autonomic disturbances, with hyper- and hypotension and cardiac dysrhythmias may occur. A compensatory phase develops, with increased cerebral metabolism and blood flow, and a lactic acidosis. Other signs include hyperpyrexia, sweating, bronchorrhoea, salivation, and vomiting. If uncontrolled, this progresses to multiple organ failure.

---

**Box 20.8** *Established status epilepticus[a]*

*Transfer to ICU*
- Intubation and ventilation
- If inadequate response to diazepam/lorazepam or chlormethiazole, give:
  - thiopentone 5 mg/kg over 30 seconds (infusion to establish a "flat EEG") or
  - propofol 2 mg/kg bolus, plus infusion (infusion to establish a "burst suppression EEG")
- Establish EEG monitoring; neurophysiological advice
- Maximise therapeutic levels of chosen anticonvulsants
- Establish the cause: history, examination

*Monitoring and investigations in addition to those listed above*
- Intra-arterial cannula; arterial blood gases
- CVP monitoring and drug access
- Continuous EEG monitoring

*Second-stage anticonvulsants*
- Phenytoin: 10–15 mg/kg by i.v. infusion (*caution*: hypotension and arrhythmia; most adult men will require 1·25 g, women 0·75 g); maintenance at least 300 mg/day
- Sodium valproate: 400–800 mg by i.v. infusion over 5 minutes, then 400 mg hourly until seizures stop to a maximum of 2·4 g; maintenance at least 200 mg 8 hourly
- Alternatives: paraldehyde 10–20 mg deep i.m. injection, *or* chlormethiazole 0·8% 1 ml/kg i.v. bolus (maximum), followed by 10 ml/min infusion

[a] Fitting for > 60 min: neurological deficit, hypotension, acidosis, compromised airway/respiration.

---

Management involves immediate attention to the ABC of resuscitation, followed rapidly by control of fitting and the prevention of complications (Box 20.7). Intensive care staff should be involved at the earliest possible opportunity. Careful records should be kept of the timing of events, interventions, drugs and doses, and the response to treatment. In the early stages, anticonvulsants such as diazepam, midazolam, or clonazepam are suitable (alternatives include chlormethiazole or paraldehyde), but should be accompanied by longer-term control using phenytoin. Care should be taken to determine chronic drug treatment, if any, and the time of the last dose. In established status epilepticus,[15] phenytoin, sodium valproate, or phenobarbitone may be required. In refractory status epilepticus it may be necessary to anaesthetise the patient with thiopentone or propofol while establishing a therapeutic level of a long-term anticonvulsant.

Treatment may fail because of inadequate drug dosage, inadequate physiological stabilisation, or failure to correct the underlying cause. Care should be taken to exclude (using EEG monitoring) subclinical non-convulsive status epilepticus which may result in permanent neurological morbidity. Appropriate investigations are given in Box 20.8, and should be arranged according to the clinical circumstances and urgency. The prognosis[16] may be very poor, particularly for patients suffering complications.

1 Bates D. The management of medical coma. *J Neurol Neurosurg Psychiatry* 1993; **56**:589–98.
2 Levy DE, Bates D, Caronna JJ, *et al*. Prognosis in non-traumatic coma. *Ann Intern Med* 1981;**94**:293–301.
3 Howard RS, Miller DH. The persistent vegetative state. *BMJ* 1995;**310**:341–2.
4 Bleck TP. Neurological complications of critical medical illnesses. In *Neurological and neurosurgical intensive care*, 3rd edn (Ropper AH, ed.). New York: Raven Press, 1993.
5 Bleck TP, Smith MC, Pierre-Louis SJ-C, *et al*. Neurological complications of critical medical illnesses. *Crit Care Med* 1993;**21**:98–103.
6 Asbury AK, Cornblath DR. Assessment of current diagnostic criteria for Guillain–Barré syndrome. *Ann Neurol* 1990;**27**(suppl):S21–24.
7 Winer JB, Hughes RAC, Osmond CA. A prospective study of acute idiopathic neuropathy. 1. Clinical features and their prognostic value. *J Neurol Neurosurg Psychiatry* 1988; **51**:605–12.
8 Ng KKP, Howard RS, Fish DR, *et al*. Management and outcome of severe Guillain–Barré syndrome. *Q J Med* 1995;**88**:243–50.
9 Ropper AH. Critical care of Guillain–Barré syndrome. In *Neurological and neurosurgical intensive care*, 3rd edn (Ropper AH, ed). New York: Raven Press, 1993.
10 Drachman DB. Myasthenia gravis. *N Engl J Med* 1994;**330**:1797–810.
11 Richman DP, Agius MA. Myasthenia gravis:pathogenesis and treatment. *Semin Neurol* 1994;**14**:106–10.
12 Raps EC, Bird SSJ, Hansen-Flaschen J. Prolonged muscle weakness after neuromuscular blockade in the intensive care unit. *Crit Care Clin* 1994;**10**:799–813.
13 Leijten FSS, Joukje E, Harinck de Weerd MD, *et al*. The role of polyneuropathy in motor convalescence after prolonged mechanical ventilation. *JAMA* 1995;**274**:1221–5.
14 Shorvon S. Tonic clonic status epilepticus. *J Neurol Neurosurg Psychiatry* 1993;**56**:125–34.
15 Jordan KG. Status epilepticus. A perspective from the neuroscience intensive care unit. *Neurosurg Clin North Am.* 1994;**5**:671–86.

16 Jagoda A, Riggio S. Refractory status epilepticus in adults. *Ann Emerg Med* 1993; **22**:1337–48.

## Recommended reading

Plum F, Posner JB. *The diagnosis of stupor and coma*, 3rd edn. Philadelphia: FA Davis Co., 1982.
Ropper AH. *Neurological and neurosurgical intensive care*, 3rd edn. New York: Raven Press, 1993.
Ropper AH, Wijdicks EF. *Guillain–Barré syndrome*. Philadelphia: FA Davis Co., 1991.

# 21: Antimediator therapies

J HILL

Tissue injury activates an inflammatory response. In self-limiting tissue injury, the inflammatory response serves to repair the damaged tissue. This necessitates a carefully coordinated interaction between the cellular components and circulating mediators shown in Figure 21.1. There is considerable evidence that, following extensive tissue injury, the inflammatory response may become systemic and uncontrolled. This has been termed the systemic inflammatory response syndrome and is thought to be responsible for the death of many critically ill patients. It can be initiated by endotoxin, Gram-positive organisms and fungal infections and non-infective insults such as ischaemia–reperfusion, burns, and pancreatitis.

Whilst most of the important mediators of systemic inflammation have probably been identified, a much better understanding of the temporal events, local versus systemic interactions, and relative importance of different mediators in different injury states is required. This will increase the likelihood of effective antimediator therapies being developed for the heterogeneous population of critically ill patients.

## Endotoxin

Endotoxin is released during lysis of Gram-negative bacteria. It has three components: the lipid A moiety, the O-side chain, and the core antigen. The lipid A moiety, responsible for most of the toxic effects of endotoxin, binds to receptors on monocytes and macrophages leading to cytokine release. Natural endotoxin inhibitors do exist and these may offer some protection against endotoxin. They include bactericidal/permeability increasing protein (BPI) and endogenous antiendotoxin core antibody (EndoCAb). BPI is released by leukocytes during infections, binds endotoxin, and prevents cytokine release. BPI has been beneficial in experimental settings and clinical trials are anticipated. The importance of EndoCAb is suggested by a recent clinical study of intensive care patients with sepsis which demonstrated that significant depletion of EndoCAb levels is associated with high circulating endotoxin levels and significantly increased mortality.[1]

Whilst the potential benefits of "blocking" endotoxin are considerable, it is important to appreciate that one half of all infections in the intensive care

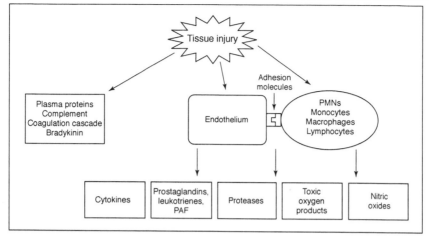

Fig 21.1   Activated host defence mechanisms following tissue injury. PAF, platelet-activating factor; PMNs, polymorphonuclear leukocytes.

unit are caused by Gram-positive organisms and fungi. A variety of antibodies directed against endotoxin has now been developed. In 1991, Ziegler *et al* using a monoclonal antibody (HA-1A) to the lipid A moiety of *Escherichia coli* endotoxin reported a 39% reduction in the mortality of patients with Gram-negative bacteraemia.[2] However, there was no overall survival benefit for all patients treated with the antibody, and the subgroup of patients who benefited from treatment with the HA-1A antibody could only be identified retrospectively from blood culture results. As endotoxin is an initiator of the systemic inflammatory response syndrome, anti-mediator therapy needs to be instituted as early as possible, and before blood culture and endotoxin results are available; thus all patients with suspected Gram-negative sepsis need to be treated. Further clinical studies have raised concerns about the toxicity of HA-1A in patients without Gram-negative sepsis and the antibody has recently been withdrawn. Anti-endotoxin strategics continue to be pursued and other antibodies to endotoxin have been developed. In 1995 Bone *et al* reported the results of a clinical study using E5, a murine monoclonal antibody directed against endotoxin in the treatment of Gram-negative sepsis.[3] As in Ziegler's study there was no overall reduction in mortality, although the antibody did seem to lead to greater resolution of organ failure in patients with Gram-negative sepsis.

## Tumour necrosis factor α

Until the 1980s the widely held belief was that bacteria and endotoxin were directly toxic to host tissues and that the reticuloendothelial system

253

---

**Box 21.1** *Effects of TNFα*

- Hypotension
- Metabolic acidosis
- Focal hepatic necrosis
- Hypoglycaemia
- Hyperkalaemia
- Pulmonary inflammation with increased lung permeability
- Acute renal tubular necrosis
- Intestinal ischaemia
- Intravascular fibrin deposition
- Death

---

acted only to minimise the host's pathophysiological response to injury or infection. Recent experiments indicate that the cytokines tumour necrosis factor $\alpha$ (TNF$\alpha$) and interleukin-1 (IL-1) mediate most endotoxin-induced injury. For example, C3HeJ mice which are unable to manufacture TNF$\alpha$ are resistant to endotoxin. The effects of an intravenous injection of TNF$\alpha$ (in quantities similar to those produced endogenously in response to sepsis) are as indicated in Box 21.1. These changes occur within a matter of hours and are nearly indistinguishable from those induced by endotoxin or septic shock. TNF$\alpha$ antibodies are able to reduce the mortality from experimental endotoxaemia and septic shock.[4]

Although an excess of TNF$\alpha$ may be injurious, the gene encoding TNF$\alpha$ is highly conserved in mammals, suggesting that it confers a significant survival advantage. Experimentally, a low dose of TNF$\alpha$ administered 24 hours before a lethal dose of TNF$\alpha$ or endotoxin significantly reduces mortality rates. Cytokines trigger local production of collagenases, eicosanoids, acute phase proteins, catecholamines, ACTH, glucagon, and growth factors, including granulocyte–macrophage colony-stimulating factor, platelet-derived growth factor, and transforming growth factor, and activate endothelium and neutrophils, all of which may aid tissue destruction and remodelling during inflammation.

Tumour necrosis factor $\alpha$ causes tissue injury in part by its effects on vascular endothelium and neutrophils. It activates endothelium to express adhesion molecules which increase neutrophil adherence to endothelium. It induces endothelial procoagulant activity making the endothelium more thrombogenic. This may then lead to capillary thrombosis and inadequate tissue perfusion. TNF$\alpha$ increases neutrophil superoxide production and is a neutrophil chemoattractant. It stimulates neutrophils to synthesise and release other inflammatory mediators such as thromboxane $A_2$, leukotriene $B_4$, and platelet-activating factor. Prostaglandins are probably important in mediating some of the effects of TNF$\alpha$, as inhibition of prostaglandin production with ibuprofen or indomethacin prevents the acidosis, changes in blood glucose, and leukocyte killing, and reduces mortality following an injection of TNF$\alpha$.

Tumour necrosis factor $\alpha$ is produced in nearly all organs containing mononuclear cells (liver, kidney, lung, and spleen) including circulating blood mononuclear cells, and in response to a large number of stimuli. These include endotoxin, Gram-positive organisms, C5a, interleukin-1, interferon-$\gamma$, and viral antigens. Endotoxin is a particularly potent stimulus, with low doses inducing elevated TNF$\alpha$ levels within minutes in human volunteers.[5] TNF$\alpha$ has a half-life of only 14–18 minutes in the circulation. As tissue-fixed macrophages exist near effector cells in numerous organs, cytokines derived from these tissue macrophages may exert important local paracrine influences, and local tissue levels may be of greater importance than circulating levels.

Given the weight of experimental and clinical evidence for an important role of TNF$\alpha$ in mediating the effects of Gram-negative and Gram-positive infections, clinical trials using antibodies to TNF$\alpha$ have been disappointing. A large-scale phase III clinical trial using two doses of TNF$\alpha$ monoclonal antibodies (7·5 mg/kg and 15 mg/kg) has now been carried out. In septic shock patients who received the antibody, there was a significant reduction in mortality three days after treatment, but neither dose resulted in any increase in overall survival at 28 days.[6] Recently, soluble TNF$\alpha$ receptors have been identified, which represent shed portions of cell surface receptors released into the circulation during the inflammatory process. They have some biological activity and may inhibit free circulating TNF$\alpha$. Soluble TNF$\alpha$ receptors have been found in high concentrations in patients with sepsis, in 300 to 1000-fold higher concentrations than those of TNF$\alpha$ itself, and they are predictive of mortality.[1] This may explain in part why clinical trials using soluble TNF$\alpha$ receptors have also been unable to demonstrate survival benefit. Indeed, one trial demonstrated increased mortality in septic patients treated with soluble TNF$\alpha$ receptors.

The importance of tissue-associated TNF$\alpha$ is supported by the fact that pretreatment with antibodies to TNF$\alpha$ has been necessary in all animal studies to date in order to ameliorate tissue injury. This suggests that access to tissue sites is necessary rather than simple antibody/antigen neutralisation in the circulation. A further possible explanation of the failure of these clinical trials is that in the majority of cases TNF$\alpha$ neutralisation therapy was administered after the septic illness was established. If TNF$\alpha$ is an early mediator of the inflammatory response, this may have been too late.

## Interleukin-1

Interleukin-1 has a wide spectrum of biological effects. Metabolic effects are increased acute-phase protein synthesis, decreased albumin synthesis, increased insulin production, and increased sodium excretion. IL-1 has direct inflammatory effects, causing monocyte and basophil histamine release. Haematological effects include stimulation of haematopoietic progenitors and induction of a neutrophilia. IL-1 induces fever and the production of other cytokines including IL-1, IL-2, IL-6, TNFα, and interferon-γ.[7]

Interleukin-1 induces prostaglandin $E_2$ (PGE$_2$), prostacyclin (PGI$_2$), and platelet-activating factor release from human endothelial cells, and also thromboxane $A_2$ release by neutrophils. A principal effect on endothelium is to increase neutrophil adherence by upregulation of endothelial adhesion proteins. IL-1 also increases endothelial cell surface procoagulant activity and production of plasminogen-activator inhibitor which initiates thrombin formation and clotting.

The production of IL-1 has been demonstrated in nearly all organs that contain mononuclear phagocytes including the liver, lung, and spleen, and also by peritoneal and circulating blood mononuclear cells. Endothelial cells, smooth muscle cells, and several other non-phagocytic cells also produce IL-1. Mononuclear cells are able to produce large amounts of IL-1 and secrete it more efficiently than other cells, and are therefore an important source. IL-1 production is stimulated by bacterial products, complement components, and inflammatory agents such as leukotriene $B_4$.

In vitro studies indicate that up to 80% of mature IL-1 produced is retained intracellularly, so this too may act mainly as a cell-associated mediator. IL-1 was detected in the circulation of only 29% of patients with severe sepsis and was detected more frequently in patients with shock.[1]

An interleukin-1 receptor antagonist protein (IL-1ra) has recently been purified and cloned.[8] IL-1ra appears to be a pure antagonist, binding completely to the IL-1 receptor and blocking the action of IL-1 while exhibiting no detectable agonist activity.[8] In sepsis circulating concentrations of IL-1ra are several thousand times greater than circulating levels of IL-1.[1] How does IL-1 continue to have a biological effect despite such high circulating IL-1ra levels? IL-1 receptor occupancy of only 5% produces a cellular response and IL-1ra might not get access to tissue sites where IL-1 is being produced.

IL-1ra increases survival after lethal endotoxaemia and injection of live *E. coli* in experimental models.[9] Early results using this receptor antagonist in treating sepsis in humans were encouraging[10] but, as with other trials of anticytokine therapy, ultimately proved disappointing.

## Other cytokines

Interleukins IL-6 and IL-8 are proinflammatory cytokines which probably also contribute to the systemic inflammatory response syndrome. IL-6 activates T cells to produce IL-2, IL-4, IL-13, interferon-γ, and granulocyte–macrophage colony-stimulating factor. IL-8 is a chemoat-tractant to polymorphonuclear leukocytes.

Interleukins IL-4, IL-10, and IL-13 inhibit the production of the proinflammatory cytokines IL-1, IL-6, TNF$\alpha$, and IL-8. IL-10 also increases production of IL-1ra and IL-10 treatment has been shown experimentally to prevent death following endotoxin administration. It thus has a potential therapeutic role in systemic inflammation.

## Endothelial–neutrophil interaction

To patrol the body effectively for infectious organisms, cells of the immune system must both circulate as non-adherent cells in the blood and lymph, and migrate as adherent cells through tissues to sites of infection or inflammation. Evidence accumulating over the last ten years indicates that signals are generated at inflammatory sites that activate circulating phagocytes and the adjacent endothelium. Circulating mediators such as the cytokines may produce more generalised endothelial activation. It has become clear that endothelial activation is complex, there are multiple separate but also probably overlapping states of endothelial activation, and not all activated endothelial cells behave in the same way.[11]

Activation of endothelium and circulating phagocytes leads to one or both cell types becoming more adhesive. This results initially in loose adherence via specific membrane adhesion molecules, the selectins. This is then followed by stronger adhesion by another group of adhesion molecules, the $\beta_2$-integrins. Selectins and integrins are located on the surface of the neutrophil and mediate adherence with adhesion molecules ICAM-1 and ICAM-2 on the endothelial surface. Stimulation of neu-trophils by circulating mediators such as C3a, C5a, platelet-activating factor, thromboxane, and leukotriene $B_4$ causes initial neutrophil adhesion via the selectins. Under appropriate conditions such as cytokine activation, this is followed by $\beta_2$-integrin binding of the leukocyte to endothelium, mediated via CD11b/CD18, which also results in cellular activation with generation of oxygen free radicals and proteases. CD18-mediated adhesion is followed by diapedesis, degranulation, and superoxide release. Injury may occur while the neutrophils are adherent to the luminal surface of the endothelial cell. If there is a chemotactic gradient across the endothelium, phagocytes move between the junctions of endothelial cells, emigrate through the subendothelial matrix, and participate in the inflammatory reaction.

The role of neutrophils in inflammation is now considered to be two-fold:

- they control vascular permeability, phagocytose bacteria, and contribute to tissue healing during self-limiting inflammation when there is no inappropriate tissue damage;

- in certain circumstances, such as the systemic inflammatory response syndrome, activated neutrophils may inappropriately damage endothelial cells, leading to excess permeability and tissue damage.

In an animal model of haemorrhagic shock, treatment with adhesion molecule CD18 resulted in smaller volumes of resuscitation fluid to maintain blood pressure and haematocrit, and significantly increased survival.[12,13] An anti ICAM-1 MoAb has been shown to reduce lymphocyte sequestration and acute graft rejection following renal transplantation in primates. However, full knowledge of the effects of antileukocyte adhesion antibodies on the immune system is still in its infancy. Adhesion molecules are important in neutrophil emigration at sites of infection, and "anti-adhesion" therapy has been shown to increase susceptibility to infection.

## Complement

Complement consists of 20 different enzymatic proteins which are activated in an amplifying cascade by various stimuli including antigen–antibody reactions. Complement is important in inflammation, chemotaxis, and phagocytosis. C3a, C4a, and C5a are anaphylatoxins derived from their inactive precursors C3, C4, and C5, respectively. C5a in particular is a highly potent mediator of inflammation. These peptides are hormone-like messenger molecules which bind to specific cell-surface receptors with high affinity. Cells responding to these peptides are polymorphonuclear leukocytes, macrophages, mast cells, basophils, and smooth muscle cells. The cellular responses to complement stimulation are release of arachidonic acid metabolites, platelet-activating factor, histamine, serotonin, and oxygen free radicals. The binding of C5a to the surface of a neutrophil produces profound changes in the cell, including stimulation of the oxidative burst, degranulation and chemotaxis, and enhanced adherence of neutrophils to each other. Complement activation also causes direct cell damage when the membrane attack complex C5b-9 is inserted into the cell membrane, forming a cylinder-like structure with loss of cell membrane integrity. The cell cannot maintain its osmotic equilibrium, swells, and then bursts.

Complement may have a role in the systemic inflammatory response syndrome. Systemic complement activation with zymosan induces characteristic haemodynamic changes similar to those seen in the progressively deteriorating stages of sepsis with hepatic and renal hypoperfusion. C5a induces transcription of both TNFα and IL-1, known mediators of sepsis. Endotoxin and pancreatitis activate intravascular complement and are risk factors for acute lung injury, and elevated levels of C5a have been found to predict the onset of this syndrome.

In 1991, a specific complement inhibitor, human soluble complement receptor type 1(sCR1) became available. This suppresses complement activation by reversibly binding to the C3b or C4b (or both) subunits of the bi- and trimolecular complexes that are the convertases of the two complement pathways.[14] The inhibitor sCR1 has been reported to decrease the size of infarcted myocardium following myocardial ischaemia and reperfusion.[14] Neutrophil accumulation at the site of the injury was significantly reduced and sCR1 was demonstrated to reduce endothelial binding of C3 and C5b-9. This molecule is currently being used to investigate the role of complement in several models of inflammation, and clinical trials in burn injury patients are anticipated.

## Nitric oxide

Abnormalities of nitric oxide (NO) metabolism are found in many acute and chronic inflammatory conditions and NO has also been suggested to have a role in mediating the systematic inflammatory response syndrome.[15] It is formed constitutively by many tissues, particularly vascular endothelium. Upregulation of the inducible nitric oxide synthase occurs in response to a variety of stimuli, particularly sepsis. Monocytes, macrophages, and neutrophils are all potential sources of NO and its production is interrelated with that of the cytokines and oxygen free radicals.

In the setting of acute inflammation, NO causes vasodilatation and reacts with oxygen free radicals to form compounds that increase blood vessel permeability. Elevated levels have been found in septic and burn patients. In endotoxic shock, it may have a direct negative inotropic effect and cause increased venous pooling, both of which lead to hypotension and organ hypoperfusion. NO also reduces platelet activation and adhesion to endothelium and inhibits neutrophil activation and adhesion. NO is thought to act late in the inflammatory pathway, so blocking excessive production of NO offers a potential advantage over blocking cytokines or endotoxin. Clinical studies are under way examining inhibitors of NO in sepsis. It has been suggested that NO blockade may keep a patient alive long enough for the systemic inflammatory response to resolve through standard treatment. Preliminary results are not, however, encouraging.

## Conclusion

Clinical studies using antimediator therapies have demonstrated that no single agent is of benefit to all patients with critical illness. These studies have also highlighted the difficulties of studying the heterogeneous group of patients in ICUs. Further difficulties arise in early detection of critical illness and identifying the precise causative agent. Attempts are being made to stratify patients according to such parameters as underlying disease and severity of disease. Whilst this may make for better comparisons of different treatment strategies, much more knowledge is required of the different inflammatory mediators in different clinical settings, particularly the interaction of pro- and anti-inflammatory mediators, temporal relationships, and circulating versus paracrine effects. Improved methods of detection of endotoxaemia and bacteraemia may enable earlier and more precise treatment with antiendotoxin or anticytokine therapies. Multiple treatments may also be necessary, with blockade of more than one agent at the same time or blockade of different inflammatory mediators at different stages of a patient's illness. This complex area requires continued clinical and basic science research.

1 Goldie AS, Fearnon KCH, Ross JA, et al. Natural cytokine antagonists and endogenous antiendotoxin core antibodies in sepsis syndrome. JAMA 1995;274:172–7.
2 Ziegler EJ, Fischer CJ Jr, Spring CL. Treatment of Gram negative bacteremia and septic shock with HA-1A human monoclonal antibody against endotoxin – a randomised, double blind, placebo-controlled trial. N Engl J Med 1991;324:429–36.
3 Bone RC, Balk RA, Fein AM, et al. A second large controlled clinical study of E5, a monoclonal antibody to endotoxin: results of a prospective, multicenter, randomized, controlled trial. Crit Care Med 1995;23:994–1006.
4 Tracey KJ, Fong Y, Hesse DG, et al. Anti-cachetin/TNF monoclonal antibodies prevent septic shock during lethal bacteraemia. Nature 1987;330:662–4.
5 Michie HR, Manogue KR, Spriggs DR, et al. Detection of circulating tumor necrosis factor after endotoxin administration. N Engl J Med 1988;318:1481–6.
6 Abraham E, Wunderlink R, Silverman H et al. Efficacy and safety of monoclonal antibody to human tumor necrosis factor-$\alpha$ in patients with sepsis syndrome: a randomised, controlled, double blind, multicentre clinical trial. JAMA 1995;273:934–41.
7 Dinarello CA. Interleukin-1 and interleukin-1 antagonism. Blood 1991;77:1627–52.
8 Carter DB, Deibel MR, Dunn CJ, et al. Purification, cloning, expression and biological characterization of an interleukin-1 receptor antagonist protein. Nature 1990;344:633–8.
9 Wakabayashi G, Gelfand JA, Burke JF, Thompson RC, Dinarello CA. A specific receptor antagonist for interleukin-1 prevents Escherichia coli-induced shock in rabbits. FASEB J 1991;5:338–43.
10 Fischer CJ, Dhainaut JF, Opal SM, et al. for the Phase III rhIL-1ra Sepsis Syndrome Study Group. Recombinant human interleukin-1 receptor antagonist in the treatment of patients with sepsis syndrome: results of a randomised, double blind, placebo-controlled trial. JAMA 1994;271:1836–43.
11 Springer TA. Adhesion receptors of the immune system. Nature 1990;346:425–34.
12 Vedder NB, Winn RK, Rice CL, Chi EY, Arfors KE, Harlan JM. A monoclonal antibody to the adherence-promoting leukocyte glycoprotein, CD 18, reduces organ injury and improves survival from hemorrhagic shock and resuscitation in rabbits. J Clin Invest 1988;81:939–44.
13 Mileski WJ, Winn RK, Vedder NB, Pohlman TH, Harlan JM, Rice CL. Inhibition of CD18-dependent neutrophil adherence reduces organ injury after haemorrhagic shock in primates. Surgery 1990;108:206–12.
14 Weisman HF, Bartow T, Leppo MK, et al. Soluble human complement receptor type 1: In vivo inhibitor of complement suppressing postischemic myocardial inflammation and necrosis. Science 1991;249:146–51.
15 Davies MG, Fulton GJ, Hagen P-O. Clinical biology of nitric oxide. Br J Surg 1995;82:1598–610.

# 22: Coagulopathies and anticoagulation

A WEBB and I MACKIE

## The coagulation mechanism

There is a complex interaction between blood cells, plasma factors, and the vascular endothelium to ensure that blood remains in a fluid state. A fine balance exists between procoagulant and anticoagulant mechanisms which favours coagulation when the vascular endothelium is breached. Following trauma to the endothelial surface, there is formation of a platelet plug that is stabilised rapidly by cross-linking fibrin strands. The processes leading up to this are limited and localised by a number of control mechanisms. It is convenient to divide them into functional areas:

- platelet function
- the coagulation enzyme cascades (intrinsic and extrinsic pathways)
- contact activation
- natural anticoagulants
- the endothelium
- fibrinolysis.

### Platelet function

Platelets can be activated by many stimuli and respond by:

- adhesion (sticking to surfaces)
- aggregation (sticking together)
- granular secretion
- providing a surface on which procoagulant reactions take place.

Platelets will not normally adhere to intact vascular endothelium but adherence is rapid where the subendothelium is exposed or a foreign surface is encountered.

### The coagulation cascade

The coagulation cascade is rather artificially divided into an intrinsic and extrinsic system (Figure 22.1). Both consist of a series of enzyme systems

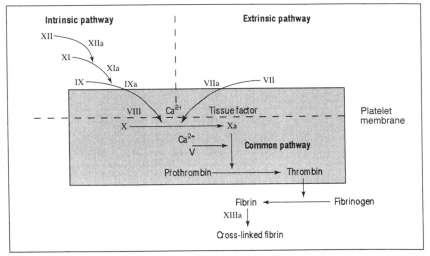

Fig 22.1   The coagulation cascade.

that result in the formation of a stable fibrin clot. They are designed to amplify signals and, by a series of negative and positive feedback loops, to facilitate their own control. The intrinsic system can be initiated either by contact activation (see below) or by the direct activation of factor XI on the surface of activated platelets. The extrinsic system is activated when tissue damage exposes the tissue factor thromboplastin.

## Contact activation

Contact activation refers to the activation of plasma factor XII (Hageman factor). As well as subendothelial collagen and smooth muscle, certain proteases and endotoxin can activate Hageman factor.[1] Hageman factor sits at the hub of a web of enzyme cascades, including intrinsic and extrinsic coagulation, fibrinolysis, kinin generation, and complement activation. Control of the contact system is exerted by a series of protease inhibitors. The most important of these is C1 esterase inhibitor (C1-INH), which accounts for 90% of the factor XII inhibitory capacity.

## Natural anticoagulant mechanisms

Antithrombin III (AT-III) is a serine protease inhibitor that can inhibit thrombin, factors Xa, IXa, XIa, and XIIa, and kallikrein.[2] This action is greatly potentiated by heparin. Thrombin generation is limited by the protein C/protein S system. Thrombin binds to a receptor on the vascular endothelium, thrombomodulin, allowing activation of protein C. Protein C inactivates factors Va and VIIIa in reactions catalysed by protein S.

### The vascular endothelium

The normal vascular endothelium is both anticoagulant and anti-thrombotic. It synthesises key anticoagulant molecules and binds both them and exogenously derived molecules on its luminal surface, thus localising anticoagulant and fibrinolytic pathways.

### Fibrinolysis

Dissolution of fibrin clots depends on the presence of plasminogen activators and the subsequent conversion of plasminogen to plasmin. Endothelial cells synthesise and release inactive precursors of the plasminogen activators tissue plasminogen activator (t-PA) and urinary plasminogen activator (u-PA).

## Disorders of coagulation

Coagulation disorders affecting critically ill patients may be congenital or acquired. They may lead to minor bleeding (e.g. at puncture sites) or severe haemorrhage. Such bleeding may be spontaneous or may occur after trauma (with up to six hours' delay). Bleeding associated with congenital coagulation defects may promote intensive care admission and require treatment with blood products as well as management of the blood loss. Coagulation defects occurring as a result of critical illness or treatment are, however, a more common cause of bleeding in the ICU.

### Massive blood transfusion

Rapid transfusion of more than one blood volume (< 5 litres) dilutes platelets and coagulation factors. In addition citrate, used as an anticoagulant for stored blood, binds circulating $Ca^{2+}$ ions. Correction of dilutional coagulation defects should be based on laboratory assessment of platelet counts, prothrombin times, and activated partial thromboplastin times (APTT). Calcium replacement is required for transfusions of > 10 units.

### Disseminated intravascular coagulation

Disseminated intravascular coagulation (DIC) is characterised by acute or chronic intravascular consumption of platelets and coagulation factors with microvascular thrombosis, fibrinolysis, and haemorrhage. Some causes of DIC are listed in Box 22.1.

The hallmark of DIC is unequivocally raised fibrin degradation products with thrombocytopenia, prolonged coagulation times, and evidence of secondary fibrinolysis. Management requires correction of the cause, replacement of coagulation factors and platelets, and, if fibrinogen levels are < 1 g/l, cryoprecipitate.

263

---

**Box 22.1** *Causes of disseminated intravascular coagulation*

*Endothelial damage*
• Shock and hypoxaemia
• Hyperthermia
• Chronic infection
• Vascular malformations

*Activation of the extrinsic pathway*
• Obstetric emboli
• Circulating tumour cells
• Trauma
• Intravascular haemolysis
• Transfusion reactions

*Mixed pathway activation*
• Bacterial sepsis
• Malignancy
• Pre-eclampsia
• Snakebite

---

### Vitamin K deficiency

Vitamin K depletion may be due to malabsorption, inadequate supplementations or inhibition (e.g. warfarin, aspirin). Intravenous vitamin K may be used if malabsorption is the cause or if bleeding is severe.

### Liver disease

Coagulation defects in liver disease relate to failed synthesis or vitamin K malabsorption.

### Renal disease

Uraemic platelet dysfunction is the main cause of bleeding associated with renal disease.

## Anticoagulation

### Heparin

Heparin is a mucopolysaccharide that was discovered by McLean in 1916.[3] In addition to potentiation of naturally occurring AT-III, platelets and proteins in the cell wall are also affected. Unfractionated heparin reduces the adhesion of platelets to injured arterial walls,[4] probably by maintaining vessel wall electronegativity. Heparin is known to increase clotting time by affecting several coagulation factors simultaneously, leading to occult blood loss and haemorrhagic complications.[5]

In 1983 Larm *et al*[6] covalently bonded heparin to surfaces containing amine groups. The technique is now used commercially to produce a biologically active surface on the blood surface of circuits, catheters, and membranes (Carmeda, Stockholm, Sweden). The surface heparin coating acts as a catalyst, accelerating the effects of circulating AT-III to inhibit thrombin binding to the surface actively.

Recent work with chemically depolymerised low-molecular-weight heparin (LMW heparin) has suggested that the recognised side effects of high dose or continuous unfractionated heparin administration may be avoided. LMW heparin appears to influence factor Xa activity specifically; its simpler pharmacokinetics allow for a smaller (around two thirds) dose to be administered to the same effect although the lack of neutralisation by protamine limits its advantages.

## Anticoagulant prostanoids

The effects of the prostanoids depend on the balance between thromboxane $A_2$ ($TxA_2$) and prostacyclin ($PGI_2$). At a wounded endothelial surface the effects of $TxA_2$ predominate, allowing platelet activation, aggregation, and plugging of the vessel wall. There is also local vasoconstriction to reduce blood flow into the wounded area. If $PGI_2$ is infused into an extracorporeal circuit the opposite effect is achieved, since $TxA_2$ levels would be very low. $PGI_2$ is generally used with heparin for anticoagulation of extracorporeal circuits. In the critically ill a reduced risk of bleeding with $PGI_2$ therapy is a particular advantage. The major disadvantage of $PGI_2$ is the potential for hypotension as a consequence of peripheral vasodilatation. This effect can be minimised by careful attention to volume status. The prostaglandins $PGE_1$ and $PGE_2$ have similar effects to $PGI_2$ but they are less potent by up to five times. They are also metabolised in the lungs so that systemic vasodilatation effects should be minimal. This may be an important advantage in the shocked patient.

## Sodium citrate

Sodium citrate chelates ionised calcium. For extracorporeal use citrate has advantages over heparin in that it has no known antiplatelet activity, is readily filtered by a haemofilter (reducing systemic anticoagulation), and is overwhelmed and neutralised when returned to central venous blood. The large sodium load requires a reduction of the sodium content of haemofiltration replacement fluids. In addition metabolic alkalosis has been described. Careful assessment of the serum ionised calcium level is vital to avoid myocardial depression. Additional infusion of calcium may be necessary.

## Warfarin

Warfarin produces a controlled deficiency of vitamin K-dependent coagulation factors (II, VII, IX, and X). Warfarin is given orally and requires 48–72 h to develop its effect.

## Fibrinolytics

Fibrinolytics activate plasminogen to form plasmin that degrades fibrin; they are used in life-threatening venous thrombosis and pulmonary embolus, acute myocardial infarction, and to unblock indwelling vascular access catheters. In acute myocardial infarction they are of most value when used within 12 hours of the onset. They may require adjuvant therapy (e.g. aspirin with streptokinase or heparin with rt-PA) to maximise the effect in acute myocardial infarction. The major side effect is bleeding, particularly from invasive procedures, and embolisation from pre-existing clot as it is broken down. Alteplase (rt-PA) is said to be clot selective and is therefore useful where a need for invasive procedures has been identified. There is also no risk of allergy where there has been previous thrombolysis.

## Serine protease inhibitors

The role of serine protease inhibitors is complicated due to their effects at other points in the coagulation pathway. Aprotinin is a naturally occurring, non-specific, serine protease inhibitor with an elimination half-life of about 2 hours.[7] The effects of aprotinin on the coagulation cascade are dependent on the circulating plasma concentrations (expressed as kallikrein inactivation units – kiu/ml) since the affinity of aprotinin for plasmin is significantly greater than that for plasma kallikrein.[8] At a plasma level of 125 kiu/ml, aprotinin inhibits fibrinolysis and complement activation. Inhibition of plasma kallikrein requires higher doses to provide plasma levels of 250–500 kiu/ml.[9] Plasma kallikrein inhibition will reduce blood coagulation mediated through contact with anionic surfaces and, in the critically ill patient, improve circulatory stability by reduced kinin activation. A further important effect of aprotinin is the prevention of inappropriate platelet activation. High-dose aprotinin (loading dose of $2 \times 10^6$ kiu followed by 500 000 kiu/h), given during cardiopulmonary bypass procedures, has been shown to reduce postoperative blood loss dramatically. More recently the same dose regimen of aprotinin has been used to arrest bleeding associated with prolonged extracorporeal $CO_2$ removal.[10] Prevention of systemic bleeding with aprotinin does not promote coagulation within extracorporeal circulations and may even contribute to the maintenance of extracorporeal anticoagulation. This serine protease inhibitor is therefore a potentially useful adjunct to the management of the extracorporeal circulation.

## Drug dosages

*Heparin*

Dose requirement is variable to produce an APTT of 1·5–3 times the control. This usually requires 500–2000 iu/h with an initial loading dose of 3000–5000 iu.

## LMW heparin

For deep vein thrombosis (DVT) prophylaxis give 2500 iu every 12 hours subcutaneously for 5 days. For anticoagulation of an extracorporeal circuit a bolus of 35 iu/kg is given intravenously followed by an infusion of 13 iu/kg. The dose is adjusted to maintain anti-factor Xa activity at 0·5–1 iu/ml (or 0·2–0·4 iu/ml if there is a high risk of haemorrhage).

## Anticoagulant prostaglandins

It is usual to infuse 2·5–10 ng/kg per min. If used for an extracorporeal circulation the infusion should be started 30 min prior to commencement.

## Sodium citrate

Infused at 5 mmol/l of extracorporeal blood flow

## Warfarin

Start at 10 mg/day orally for 2 days then 3–9 mg/day according to the international normalised ratio (INR). For DVT prophylaxis, pulmonary embolus, mitral stenosis, atrial fibrillation, and tissue valve replacements, the INR should be maintained between 2 and 3. For recurrent DVT or pulmonary embolus and mechanical valve replacements, the INR should be kept between 3 and 4·5.

## Alteplase (rt-PA)

The dose schedule for acute myocardial infarction is 10 mg in 1–2 min, 50 mg in 1 h, and 40 mg over 2 h intravenously.

## Anistreplase

This drug is advantageous in that a single intravenous injection of 30 units over 4–5 min is required in acute myocardial infarction. Anaphylactoid reactions have been reported.

## Streptokinase

This is used in acute myocardial infarction ($1·5 \times 10^6$ units over 60 min) or in severe venous thrombosis (250 000 units over 30 min followed by 100 000 units/h for 24–72 h). Anaphylactoid reactions are not uncommon and patients should not be exposed to streptokinase twice.

*Urokinase*

Used mainly for unblocking indwelling vascular catheters where 5000–37 500 iu are instilled. For thromboembolic disease 4400 iu/kg is given over 10 min followed by 4400 iu/kg per h for 12–24 h.

# Correcting coagulation

### Fresh frozen plasma

A unit (150 ml) of fresh frozen plasma is usually collected from one donor and contains all coagulation factors including 200 units factor VIII, 200 units factor IX, and 400 mg fibrinogen. Fresh frozen plasma is stored at $-30°C$.

### Platelets

Platelet concentrates are viable for three days when stored at room temperature. If they are refrigerated, viability decreases. They must be infused quickly via a short giving set with no filter. Indications for platelet concentrates include platelet count $<10 \times 10^9/l$, platelet count $<50 \times 10^9/l$ with spontaneous bleeding, or, to cover invasive procedures, spontaneous bleeding with platelet dysfunction. They are less useful in conditions associated with immune platelet destruction (e.g. idiopathic thrombocytopenic purpura, ITP).

### Cryoprecipitate

A 15 ml vial of cryoprecipitate contains 100 units factor VIII, 250 mg fibrinogen, and some factor XIII and von Willebrand's factor. It is stored at $-30°C$ and used in haemophilia, von Willebrand's disease, and fibrinogen deficiency. In haemophilia, cryoprecipitate is given to achieve a factor VIII level $>30\%$ of normal.

### Factor VIII concentrate

Contains 300 units factor VIII per vial. In severe haemorrhage owing to haemophilia, 10–15 units/kg are given every 12 hours.

### Factor IX complex

Rich in factors II, IX, and X, this is used in haemorrhage from vitamin K deficiency, e.g. oral anticoagulant overdose, liver disease, Christmas disease. It is formed from pooled plasma, so fresh frozen plasma is preferred.

### Vitamin K

Vitamin K is used to reverse a prolonged prothrombin time as a result of malabsorption, oral anticoagulant therapy, $\beta$-lactam antibiotics, or critical illness. The effects of vitamin K are prolonged so it should be avoided where patients are dependent on oral anticoagulant therapy. A dose of 10 mg is given orally or by slow intravenous injection daily. In life-threatening haemorrhage, 5 mg is given by slow intravenous injection with other coagulation factor concentrates. If INR >7 or in less severe haemorrhage, 0·5–2 mg may be given by slow intravenous injection with minimum lasting effect on oral anticoagulant therapy.

## Protamine

Although this is used to reverse the effects of heparin, it has an anticoagulant effect of its own in high doses. Protamine 1 mg neutralises 100 iu unfractionated heparin if given within 15 min. Less is required if given later, since heparin is excreted rapidly. Protamine should be given by slow intravenous injection according to the APTT. Total dose should not exceed 50 mg. Protamine injection may cause severe cardiovascular depression.

## Tranexamic acid

This has an antifibrinolytic effect by antagonising plasminogen. It reduces bleeding from raw surfaces and is particularly useful in bleeding from prostatectomy or dental extraction, or as a result of fibrinolytic excess. The usual dose is 1–1·5 g every 6–12 hours orally or by slow intravenous injection.

# Monitoring anticoagulation

The basic screen consists of a platelet count, prothrombin time, APTT, and thrombin time. Close attention to blood sampling technique is very important for correct interpretation of coagulation tests. Drawing blood from indwelling catheters should, ideally, be avoided since samples may be diluted or contaminated with heparin. The correct volume of blood must be placed in the sample tube to avoid dilution errors. Laboratory coagulation tests are usually performed on citrated plasma samples. The prothrombin time is prolonged with coumarin anticoagulants, and in liver disease and vitamin K deficiency. The APTT is prolonged by heparin therapy, DIC, severe fibrinolysis, or deficiencies of von Willebrand's factor, factor VIII, factor XI, or factor XIII. The thrombin time is prolonged by fibrinogen depletion, e.g. fibrinolysis or thrombolysis and heparin through AT-III-dependent interaction with thrombin.

## Platelets

Correct interpretation of platelet counts requires blood to be taken from a venepuncture (not capillary blood). Thrombocytopenia is due to decreased platelet production (bone marrow failure, vitamin $B_{12}$ or folate deficiency), or decreased platelet survival (ITP, thrombotic thrombocytopenic purpura, infection, hypersplenism, heparin therapy, DIC). Platelets may also aggregate in vivo giving an apparent thrombocytopenia; this should be checked on a blood film. Spontaneous bleeding is associated with platelet counts $< 20 \times 10^9$/litre and platelet cover is required for procedures or traumatic bleeds at counts $< 50 \times 10^9$/litre.

### Fibrin degradation products (FDPs)

Fibrin fragments are released by plasmin lysis. FDPs can be assayed by an immunological method; they are often measured in the critically ill to confirm DIC. A level of 20–40 µg/ml is common postoperatively, in sepsis, trauma, renal failure, and DVT. Raised levels do not distinguish fibrinogenolysis and fibrinolysis. Assay of the d-dimer fragment is more specific for fibrinolysis, e.g. in DIC, since it is only released after fibrin is formed.

### Coagulation factor assays

Assays are available for all coagulation factors and may be used for diagnosis of specific defects. Heparins inhibit factor Xa activity. Factor Xa assay is therefore the most specific method of controlling LMW heparin therapy. Since this assay is not dependent on contact system activation, factor Xa assay also avoids the effects of aprotinin when monitoring heparin therapy.

### Antithrombin III assay

Antithrombin III is essential for the anticoagulant activity of heparin. It may also prevent some of the vascular damage occurring in multiple organ failure. Levels are often depressed in critically ill patients; assay may allow appropriate replacement therapy.

## Conclusion

Blood coagulation is dependent on platelet function, coagulation enzymes, contact activation, the effects of natural anticoagulants, endothelial function, and the effects of fibrinolysis.

Critically ill patients may be affected by congenital and acquired coagulation defects although the latter are more common. These include dilution effects of massive blood transfusion, DIC, vitamin K deficiency, and hepatic and renal disease.

Anticoagulation of critically ill patients is required for a variety of reasons (e.g. prevention and treatment of thromboembolic disease, maintenance of extracorporeal circulations). Heparin is the mainstay of anticoagulant treatment for critically ill patients, although anticoagulant prostanoids have found increasing use, particularly in shocked patients.

Coagulation defects require correction of factor and platelet deficiencies with blood product therapy. Drug therapies include specific reversal agents (e.g. vitamin K and protamine) but these are rarely useful alone.

Management of coagulation and anticoagulation problems in intensive care depends on appropriate monitoring of the intrinsic pathway (APTT), the extrinsic pathway (prothrombin time), platelet count, and fibrinolytic pathways (FDPs). Specific factor assays are rarely required.

1 Schmaier AH, Silverberg M, Kaplan AP, Colman RW. Contact activation and its abnormalities. In *Hemostasis and thrombosis* (Colman RW, Hirsh J, Marder VJ, Salzman EW, eds). Philadelphia: Lippincott, 1987:18–38.
2 Harpel PC. Blood proteolytic enzyme inhibitors: their role in modulating blood coagulation and fibrinolytic enzyme pathways. In *Haemostasis and thrombosis* (Colman RW, Hirsh J, Marder VJ, Salzman EW, eds). Philadelphia: Lippincott, 1987:219–34.
3 McLean J. The thromboplastic action of cephalin. *Am J Physiol* 1916;**41**:250.
4 Gregorius FK, Rand RW. Scanning electron microspcopy of the rat common carotid artery. III. Heparin efect on platelets. *Surgery* 1976;**79**:583–9.
5 Koch KM, Bechstein PB, Fassbinder W, Kaltwasser P, Schoeppe W. Occult blood loss and iron balance in chronic renal failure. *Proc EDTA* 1975;**12**:681–4.
6 Larm O, Larsson R, Olsson P. A new non-thrombogenic surface prepared by selective covalent binding of heparin via a modified reducing terminal residue. *Biomater Med Dev Artif Organs* 1983;**2**:161-73.
7 Royston D. The serine antiprotease aprotinin (Trasylol): a novel approach to reducing postoperative bleeding. *Blood Coag Fibrinolysis* 1990;**1**:55–69.
8 Fritz H, Wunderer G. Biochemistry and applications of aprotinin, the kallikrein inhibitor from bovine organs. *Arzneimittelforschung* 1983;**33**:479–94.
9 Philipp E. Calculations and hypothetical considerations on the inhibition of plasmin and plasma kallikrein by Trasylol. In *Progress in chemical fibrinolysis and thrombolysis* (Davidson JF, Rowan RM, Samama MM, Desnoyers PC, eds). New York: Raven Press, 1978:291-5.
10 Brunet F, Mira JP, Belghith M, *et al.* Effects of aprotinin on hemorrhagic complications in ARDS patients during prolonged extracorporeal $CO_2$ removal. *Intensive Care Med* 1992;**18**:364-7.

# 23: Carriage, colonisation, and infection

H K F VAN SAENE, A P TOMETZKI,
S J FAIRCLOUGH, J H ROMMES, and A J PETROS

## Definitions

Clinical microbiology is an integral part of medicine in the intensive care unit (ICU), requiring a strict set of definitions[1] in order to guarantee uniformity of approach between the many disciplines involved in the care of the critically ill patient, and to facilitate research.

### Carriage or carrier state

When the same strain of a potential pathogen is isolated from at least two consecutive surveillance samples in any concentration over a period of at least one week, the ICU patient is considered to be in a carrier state.[2] Samples include saliva, gastric fluid, faeces, and a throat or rectal swab. If one surveillance sample is positive for a potential pathogen that differs from previous isolates, the patient is considered to have acquired a potential pathogen. Thus carriage refers to the persistent presence of a micro-organism in the oropharynx and gut and on the skin. An acquired potential pathogen is only transiently present in an otherwise healthy host.

### Overgrowth

Overgrowth of a micro-organism in the digestive tract is defined as $>10^5$ colony-forming units (CFU) of a potential pathogen/ml or gram of saliva, gastric fluid, or faeces. Overgrowth almost invariably occurs in the throat and gut in the critically ill ICU patient with impaired gut motility, and is distinct from low-grade carriage, which is defined as $<10^5$ CFU of a potential pathogen/ml or gram of digestive tract secretions.

### Colonisation

Colonisation is the presence of a potential pathogen in an internal organ that is normally sterile. Diagnostic samples from lower airway secretions, wound fluid, and urine yield $<10^5$ CFU of potential pathogens/ml of diagnostic sample.

272

# Infection

Infection is a microbiologically proven clinical diagnosis of inflammation. This includes not only clinical signs but also the presence of $> 10^5$ microbes/ml in diagnostic samples obtained from an internal organ or the isolation of a micro-organism from a blood culture. Sepsis is the syndrome of clinical signs of generalised inflammation caused by micro-organisms and/or their products. Septicaemia is sepsis combined with a positive blood culture.

# Samples

Diagnostic samples are obtained from sites that are normally sterile, such as the lower airways, bladder, and blood, and are obtained when clinically indicated to find a microbiological cause for the clinical diagnosis of inflammation.[3]

Surveillance samples are defined as samples from body sites where potential pathogens are carried, that is, the digestive tract. A set of surveillance samples consists of throat and rectal swabs taken on admission to the ICU and twice weekly thereafter (e.g. Monday and Thursday). The aim of surveillance samples is to determine the level of carriage of potential pathogens.

Surface samples are defined as swabs from the skin of the axilla, groin, and umbilicus, and from the nose, eye, and ear; they are generally not useful as surveillance samples because surface samples yielding potential pathogens reflect the oropharyngeal and rectal carrier state.

# Normal versus abnormal flora

We all carry micro-organisms in the oropharynx, gut, and vagina, and on the skin.[4] Secretions from the lower airways, sinuses, middle ear, lacrimal glands, and urinary tract are normally sterile. Micro-organisms that are carried by all healthy people constitute the indigenous flora and include anaerobes and aerobes. Saliva contains $10^8$ CFU of anaerobic micro-organisms, e.g. *Veillonella* species and peptostreptococci, as well as $> 10^6$ aerobic viridans streptococci/ml of saliva. Higher concentrations of micro-organisms are present in the large bowel. More than 95% of the gut flora are anaerobic, e.g. *Bacteroides* spp. ($10^{12}$ CFU/g of faeces), *Clostridium* spp. ($10^6$ CFU/g of faeces). Enterococci and *Escherichia coli* are aerobes present in a concentration of $10^3$–$10^6$ CFU/g of faeces. Vaginal flora are basically faecal flora including $10^8$ CFU of anaerobic and $10^3$ CFU of aerobic micro-organisms/ml of vaginal fluid. The aerobic coagulase-negative staphylococci, e.g. *Staphylococcus epidermidis* ($10^5$ CFU/cm$^2$) and the anaerobic *Propionibacterium acnes* ($10^3$ CFU/cm$^2$), are carried by people in and on the skin. Community organisms, including *Streptococcus pneumoniae*, *Haemophilus influenzae*, and *Moraxella catarrhalis*, are carried in the oropharynx by about half of the healthy population. *Staphylococcus aureus* and *Candida albicans* are carried in both the oropharynx and gut in 20–40% of healthy individuals.

Oropharyngeal and gastrointestinal carriage of hospital bacteria is uncommon in healthy people. The hospital bacteria that are clinically most important include *Klebsiella, Proteus, Morganella, Enterobacter, Serratia, Acinetobacter,* and *Pseudomonas* spp. The carriage of epidemic micro-organisms, e.g. salmonellae or *Neisseria meningitidis*, is rare.

The carriage of "normal" flora should therefore be distinguished from "abnormal" flora. We regard both the indigenous and the community flora as normal. The critically ill patient commonly carries abnormal hospital flora, also referred to as opportunistic or nosocomial flora (Table 23.1).

Supercarriage is defined as carriage of hospital bacteria acquired in the ICU, often after the eradication of community micro-organisms by the commonly used antibiotics.

## Mechanisms of carrier state in health and disease

The carrier state of either community or hospital potential pathogens is determined by the severity of the disease process that required ICU admission, surgical interventions, and the patient's background state of health. Fit individuals will tend to carry community potential pathogens and indigenous flora, whereas those with underlying chronic diseases such as diabetes, alcoholism, or chronic obstructive pulmonary disease are likely to demonstrate hospital ("nosocomial") bacteria in oropharyngeal and gastrointestinal secretions.[5] Indigenous flora are still present in high concentrations in oropharyngeal and intestinal secretions.

Although the shift from normal to abnormal flora is determined by severity of both acute and chronic illness,[6] the underlying mechanism for the change from carriage of "community" to "hospital" potential pathogens is not clear. Theories have included inflamed oral mucosae predisposing to *Klebsiella*,[7] "sick mucosal cells" resulting from the underlying disease,[8] low intramucosal pH,[9] and mucosa denuded of fibronectin.[10] Fibronectin is a large glycoprotein produced by the liver, and subsequently excreted on to mucosal surfaces of the oropharynx and gut. It forms a protective layer on mucosal cells and has attachment sites for "community" micro-organisms, including *Strep. pneumoniae* and *Staph. aureus*. Leukocyte activation, resulting in the release of elastase in saliva, bile, and mucus, denudes the mucosal cells of their protective layer of fibronectin, exposing receptor sites for the "hospital" bacteria. Increased adherence of the abnormal potential pathogens *Klebsiella* spp., *Enterobacter* spp., and *Pseudomonas aeruginosa* has been associated with the loss of fibronectin from the surface of digestive tract mucosae as a result of the damaging inflammatory response. Impairment of gastrointestinal mucosal perfusion in critical illness has been associated with pH changes in the mucosa of the digestive tract, leading to intramucosal acidosis ($pH_i < 7.35$) and the promotion of abnormal carriage. Conversely, in patients making a good recovery abnormal carriage of "hospital" bacteria declines rapidly, and approaches control levels within four weeks.[11]

## Mechanisms of colonisation and infection

Carriage of potential pathogens in the gastrointestinal tract often progresses to colonisation and infection of otherwise sterile organs in patients who are admitted to the ICU for three or more days. There are three basic mechanisms: migration, transmural migration, and absorption of endotoxin.

Table 23.1 Classification of micro-organisms using the carrier state as criterion

| | Site | Organism | Intrinsic pathogenicity | Flora |
|---|---|---|---|---|
| Indigenous flora | Oropharynx | Peptostreptococci, *Veillonella* spp., Viridans streptococci | Low pathogenic | "Normal" |
| | Gut | *Bacteroides*, *Clostridium* spp., Enterococci, *Escherichia coli* | | |
| | Vagina | Peptostreptococci, *Bacteroides* spp., Lactobacilli | | |
| | Skin | *Propionibacterium acnes*, Coagulase-negative staphylococci | | |
| "Community" micro-organisms | Oropharynx | *Streptococcus pneumoniae*, *Haemophilus influenzae*, *Moraxella catarrhalis* | Potentially pathogenic | |
| | Gut | *Escherichia coli* | | |
| | Oropharynx and gut | *Staphylococcus aureus*, *Candida* spp. | | |
| "Hospital" micro-organisms | Oropharynx and gut | *Klebsiella*, *Proteus*, *Morganella*, *Enterobacter*, *Citrobacter*, *Serratia*, *Pseudomonas*, *Acinetobacter* spp. | | "Abnormal" |
| "Epidemic" micro-organisms | Oropharynx | *Neisseria meningitidis*, salmonellae | Highly pathogenic | |
| | Gut | | | |

275

Migration is defined as the movement of live potential pathogens from one place, i.e. throat and gut where potential pathogens are present in overgrowth, to other sites, in particular the normally sterile internal organs. The oropharynx is linked with the lower airways via aspiration, the sinuses via the ostia, and the middle ear through the eustachian tube, and the gut is linked with the bladder via the perineum. Migration is the main mechanism by which micro-organisms cause colonisation/infection in the patient with $>100 \times 10^6$ neutrophils/l, that is, most ICU patients. The classic example is oropharyngeal potential pathogens that migrate from the throat into the tracheal site and, subsequently, into the lower airways within a few days.[12,13] The severity of underlying disease causing impairment of clearance of the aspirated saliva, which results from failure of the cilia, is the main factor promoting colonisation of the lower airways. The presence of the plastic endotracheal tube as a foreign body is invariably associated with mucosal lesions, which further enhances colonisation. The progress towards infection, whether tracheitis, tracheobronchitis, bronchopneumonia, or pneumonia, is dependent on the immune status or defence capacity of the patient.

Transmural migration ("translocation") is defined as the ingress of oropharyngeal or gastrointestinal potential pathogens through the mucosal lining of the alimentary canal into gut-associated lymphoid tissue (GALT), which includes macrophages in the mesenteric lymph nodes, liver, spleen, and blood. The GALT macrophages are effective in killing intestinal micro-organisms that are translocating, but they may release the bacterial cell walls which then act as a source of endotoxin, possibly leading to systemic inflammation. Live micro-organisms can reach the blood stream in neutropenic patients[14] with $<100 \times 10^6$ neutrophils/l and in preterm neonates of very low birthweight (VLBW).[15]

In addition to endotoxin release from translocating bacteria killed by macrophages, intestinal endotoxin (1 mg/g of faeces) produced by abnormal hospital bacteria may also be absorbed. Absorption of endotoxin is thought to occur as an end-stage event in patients with gut ischaemia. Splanchnic ischaemia is not uncommon in patients who are critically ill. In its mildest, but most common form, the ischaemia is transient and reversible, in particular in patients undergoing elective cardiac and abdominal aortic operations. The most severe form of transmural gut infarction is the principal finding *post mortem* in 3% of all patients who die in hospital.[16]

## Measuring and reporting carriage, colonisation, and infection

Surveillance samples of throat and rectal swabs are processed qualitatively and semiquantitatively, to detect the level of carriage.[2,17] Three solid media – MacConkey, staphylococcal, and yeast agar – are inoculated using the four-quadrant method combined with brain–heart infusion broth. Each swab is streaked onto the three solid media, then the tip is broken off into 5 ml of enrichment broth. All cultures are incubated aerobically at 37°C. The MacConkey plate is examined after one night and the staphylococcal and yeast plates after two nights. In addition, if the enrichment broth is turbid after one night's incubation it is then inoculated onto the three media. A semiquantitative estimation is made by grading growth density on a scale of 1 + to 5. Standard methods for identification, typing, and sensitivity patterns are used for all micro-organisms. All data are entered onto a database. A simple program enables the intensivist to generate a microbiological overview chart of each long-stay patient on a bedside monitor. A printout of this chart is often more useful than a disjointed series of laboratory reports to be filed in the notes, because it provides a clear view of trends, such as the biphasic pattern of early infection versus late superinfection, and allows these to be correlated with other clinical events and antimicrobial treatment.[17]

## Interaction between carriage, colonisation, and infection

This structured approach which combines data from surveillance and diagnostic samples allows us to categorise micro-organisms and infections into different groups.

### Classifying micro-organisms according to pathogenicity

The ratio between the number of ICU patients infected by a particular micro-organism and the number of patients carrying that organism in the throat or gut is defined as the intrinsic pathogenicity index (IPI) for a particular micro-organism. Indigenous flora, including anaerobes and viridans streptococci, rarely cause infections despite being carried in high concentrations, with an IPI of between 0·01 and 0·03. Enterococci and coagulase-negative staphylococci are also carried in the oropharynx in high concentrations by a substantial percentage of ICU patients, but are unable to cause lower airway infections. These are low-level pathogens, whilst high-level pathogens such as salmonellae have an IPI approaching 1.

There are about 14 potential pathogens with IPIs between 0·1 and 0·3. These include the six "community" micro-organisms already described, present in previously healthy individuals, and the eight "hospital" bacteria carried by patients with an acute or chronic condition. About 30% of ICU patients develop infections with potentially pathogenic micro-organisms (PPMs) during their ICU stay, determined mainly by the patients' illness severity.[18] The IPI of particular micro-organisms therefore varies depending on clinical circumstances. *Staph. epidermidis* is a low-level pathogen in trauma patients, but a PPM in VLBW neonates admitted to the neonatal intensive care unit (NICU). Neonates are culture negative on admission, but acquire *Staph. epidermidis* from the staff, with oropharyngeal and gastrointestinal carriage rates of this nosocomial bacterium being as high as 85% at day 5 of life.[19] They are predisposed to this by parenteral nutrition and antimicrobials that inhibit the establishment of indigenous normal flora.[20] Another PPM of concern is methicillin-resistant *Staph. aureus* (MRSA) with an IPI of 0.3. Again, the degree of underlying disease was significantly higher in patients who carried MRSA compared with patients who did not have MRSA.

## The predictable pattern of ICU infections

### Primary endogenous infections

Primary endogenous infections are the most frequent; they are caused by both "community" and "hospital" PPMs carried in the throat and gut on admission (Table 23.2).[17, 21, 22] These episodes of infection generally occur early during the ICU stay. Examples include lower airway infection in a previously healthy individual caused by *Strep. pneumoniae*, or "hospital"-type organisms such as *Klebsiella* sp. in patients with prior chronic diseases, e.g. obstructive pulmonary disease. The incidence of primary endogenous infections will be reduced by prophylactic parenteral antibiotics.

### Secondary endogenous infections

Secondary endogenous infections are caused by nosocomial PPMs appearing late in the ICU stay. These PPMs are acquired first in the oropharynx, followed by the stomach and gut. One third of ICU infections are secondary endogenous.[17, 22] Significantly, in antibiotic-free patients on admission, almost all such infections develop only in those patients who have had a primary endogenous infection, i.e. a subset of critically ill patients develop more than one infection during their stay in the ICU. Only

Table 23.2   Classification of infections occurring in the ICU using the carrier state as the criterion

| Type of infection | Definition | Causative PPM | Time of onset | Frequency (%) |
|---|---|---|---|---|
| Primary endogenous | Infection caused by a PPM carried in throat and/or gut on admission to ICU | "Community" "Hospital" | "Early" | About 50 |
| Secondary endogenous | Infection caused by a PPM not carried on admission but acquired in the ICU followed by carriage | "Hospital" | "Late" | About 35 |
| Exogenous | Infection caused by a PPM not carried at all during ICU stay | "Hospital" | Any time during ICU stay | About 15 |

the topical application of non-absorbable antimicrobials as part of selective digestive decontamination (see below) have been shown to control secondary endogenous infections.

### Exogenous infections

Exogenous infections are less common (around 15%) but may occur throughout the patient's stay in the ICU and are caused by "hospital" PPMs in particular, *Acinetobacter* spp, *Pseudomonas* spp and MRSA without previous carriage.[17, 21] Typical examples are lower airway infections caused by *Acinetobacter* spp. after the use of contaminated ventilation equipment, cystitis with *Pseudomonas* spp. from urinometers, and tracheobronchitis due to MRSA in patients with tracheostoma. A high level of hygiene is required to control exogenous infections.

Health care providers are considered to be the main vehicle for the transmission of micro-organisms between ICU patients. Saliva or faeces from critically ill patients contain high concentrations of micro-organisms ($>10^8$ CFU/g), and after contact with a critically ill patient hand contamination often exceeds $10^5$ CFU/cm$^2$ of finger surface area. Hand washing with 0·5% chlorhexidine in 70% alcohol effectively clears micro-organisms from the hands, but only if the contamination level is $<10^4$ CFU.[23] Thus, a rigid enforcement of handwashing can only be expected to reduce transmission, not completely abolish it.[22] Transmission may lead to true nosocomial infections comprising of secondary endogenous and exogenous infections only.

## Calculating ICU infection rates

In general, patients requiring three or more days of mechanical ventilation will develop at least one infection during their ICU stay. The incidence of infected patients should be distinguished from the incidence of infection episodes, and should include all nosocomial infection episodes. In a three-month study of critically ill adults undergoing mechanical ventilation for at least three days[22], 8 (38%) of 21 patients developed 12 infection episodes. Half of these were primary endogenous infections and the rest were secondary endogenous.

## Antimicrobials to prevent or treat carriage, colonisation, or infection

The choice of antimicrobial agent is determined by the micro-organism, its pathogenicity, and the site of isolation, as well as drug factors such as toxicity, side effects, interactions, route of administration, the need for drug monitoring, and the cost.

A relatively limited number of antimicrobial agents control almost all ICU micro-organisms. They include the $\beta$-lactams (penicillins and cephalosporins), the aminoglycosides (gentamicin, tobramycin), the polymyxins (polymyxin E, colistin), the glycopeptides (vancomycin), and the polyenes (amphotericin B). The polymyxins, glycopeptides, and polyenes have a rapid action on the microbial cell membrane. The $\beta$-lactams interfere with the cell-wall synthesis, a slower mechanism of action. The aminoglycosides inhibit the synthesis of proteins but still kill microbes in the rest phase. These differences in mechanism of action may explain why aminoglycosides and polyenes are more toxic to the ICU patient compared with $\beta$-lactams when parenterally administered.

A minimal bactericidal concentration (MBC) can be determined for the 14 community and hospital PPMs listed in Table 23.1. The MBC of an antimicrobial agent is defined as the amount of the antimicrobial (mg/l) required to establish irreversible inhibition in the test tube, without the killing activity of leukocytes. Antimicrobial agents with an MBC of $\leq 1$ mg/l for PPM are in general suitable for clinical use. Non-toxic antibiotics such as the $\beta$-lactams are ideal for systemic administration and high doses (50–150 mg/kg per day) can be given. The more toxic agents such as the polymyxins and the polyenes can be safely applied topically in high doses. Polyenes can also be given parenterally in limited dose, although the newer liposomal formulations allow higher and more effective doses to be tolerated without toxicity. Aminoglycosides and glycopeptides, although toxic, are administered systematically in lower doses (5–25 mg/kg per day).

# Potentially pathogenic micro-organisms

### Prophylaxis and treatment of colonisation and infection of internal organs

This requires parenteral antimicrobials. The modern $\beta$-lactams are most widely used because they cover both "community" and "hospital" PPMs. Individual ICUs should establish antimicrobial policies with their microbiologists (see below), but some guidance can be obtained from Table 23.3. Colonisation or infection with "community" PPMs can in general be managed with the use of one antimicrobial agent ("monotherapy"). A combination of a $\beta$-lactam and an aminoglycoside is preferred for colonisation or infection by "hospital" PPMs. Several "hospital" PPMs, such as *Enterobacter* spp., are able to produce $\beta$-lactamase, an enzyme that opens and destroys the $\beta$-lactam antibiotic ring. Most abnormal hospital PPMs release endotoxin, and the newer aminoglycosides such as tobramycin are resistant to $\beta$-lactamases, and bind and neutralise endotoxin. Synergism has been described between $\beta$-lactams and amino-

Table 23.3 Antibiotic dose guide

| Antibiotic/indication | | Total daily dose (mg/kg) | |
|---|---|---|---|
| | Neonate >7 days | 1 month to 12 years | >12 years |
| **1 β-Lactams** | | | |
| 1.1 Cefotaxime: | | | |
| Moderate infection | 50 | 100–150 | 3 g |
| Serious infection with high level pathogen, e.g. *Neisseria meningitidis* | 150–200 | 200 | 6–12 g |
| 1.2 Cephradine | | | |
| Viridans streptococci | 20–50 | 50 | 2–4 g |
| Colonised/infected with *Staph. aureus* | 100 | 100 | 4–8 g |
| 1.3 Ceftazidime | | | |
| *Pseudomonas aeruginosa* | 90 | 100–150 | 6–9 g |
| 1.4 Benzylpenicillin | | | |
| *Strep. pneumoniae* | 45 | 50–100 | 2–4 g |
| Severe infection including *N. meningitidis* | 60–90 | 300 | 12 g |
| 1.5 Ampicillin | | | |
| Enterococci | 50–100 | 50–100 | 2–4 g |
| **2 Aminoglycosides** | | | |
| 2.1 Tobramycin | 4 | 7·5 | 3–5 |
| 2.2 Gentamicin | | | |
| Blind treatment of sepsis with cefotaxime | 6 (>1·5 kg) | 7·5 | 3–5 |
| 2.3 Netilmicin | | | |
| Prophylaxis in cardiac surgery | 6 (>1·5 kg) | 6 | 6 |
| **3 Glycopeptides** | | | |
| 3.1 Vancomycin | | | |
| Staphylococci, streptococci | 15 single dose then 30 | 45 | 2 g |
| 3.2 Teicoplanin | | | |
| Prophylaxis in cardiac surgery | 16 single loading dose then 8 | 10, 12-hourly ×3 doses then 6 daily | 400, 12-hourly ×3 doses then 200 daily |
| **4 Quinolones** | | | |
| 4.1 Ciprofloxacin | | | |
| Salmonellae | | 25×3/7 then 12·5 ×2/7 | 800 |
| **5 Others** | | | |
| 5.1 Rifampicin | | | |
| Eradication of *N. meningitidis* | <1 year: 10 per day | 1–12 years: 20 per day ×2/7 | 1200 |

Table 23.1   Continued

| | Neonate >7 days | Total daily dose (mg/kg) 1 month to 12 years | >12 years |
|---|---|---|---|
| Eradication of *H. influenzae* | <3 months 10 per day ×4/7 | >3 months 20 per day | 600 |
| 5.2 Metronidazole Anaerobes | 22·5 | 22·5 | 1·5 g |
| **Antifungal indication** | | | |
| **6 Polyenes** 6.1 Amphotericin B (start at lowest dose and increase gradually): *C. albicans* | 0·1–0·5 | 0·25–1·5 | 0·25–1·5 |
| 6.2 Lipophilic amphotericin B | Start at 1 | 1–3 per day | 1–3 per day |
| **7 Pyrimidine** 7.1 Flucytosine *C. albicans* | 100 | 200 | 200 |

Note: dosage adjustments may be required in renal/hepatic impairment and in elderly people.

glycosides in the killing of "hospital" PPMs. Colonisation or infection with *Candida* sp. may be prevented or treated with the polyene amphotericin B. Infection with *Aspergillus* spp. always requires amphotericin, still the most potent antifungal agent. Some units combine amphotericin with flucytosine.

## Prevention and eradication of PPM carriage

Oropharyngeal and gastrointestinal carriage of PPMs can be abolished only by topical application of antimicrobials. The mixture of polymyxin E, tobramycin, and amphotericin B (PTA regimen) has been intensively studied[24] and its application is known as selective digestive decontamination (SDD). All three antimicrobials are non-absorbable, and produce high antimicrobial concentrations in saliva, gastric fluid, and faeces. Inactivation of this PTA mixture does occur but only to a moderate extent. An adequate contact time between PPMs and antimicrobial agents is essential for eradication of carriage. The aim of SDD is the conversion of the abnormal carrier state into normal carriage, using PTA. SDD is a prophylactic strategy designed to prevent or minimise the impact of both endogenous and exogenous infections caused by the more common PPM. When properly used, SDD significantly reduces overall mortality by 20% and pneumonia by 65%.[25] In practical terms, only five patients need to be treated with SDD to prevent one pneumonia and only 23 patients to prevent one death on ICU.

# High-level pathogens

### Treatment of infection

High-level pathogens such as *Neisseria meningitidis* and salmonellae cause primary endogenous infections in children, but are less common in adult ICUs. Cefotaxime and penicillin are effective against *N. meningitidis*. The target cell of salmonellae is not the enterocyte, but the GALT macrophage, after translocation through the mucosal lining. Salmonella cells survive within macrophages, but $\beta$-lactams and aminoglycosides do not penetrate into macrophages, which may explain why these antimicrobials fail in systemic salmonella infections. Fluoroquinolones such as ciprofloxacin are excreted via the mucus into the faeces, and sterilise GALT macrophages while on their way to the intestinal lumen; they are the first choice for salmonella infections.

### Eradication of carriage of high-level pathogens

Parenteral penicillin or cefotaxime will usually eradicate the oropharyngeal carrier state of *N. meningitidis*; in some cases rifampicin is required for effective clearance of throat carriage (Table 23.3). It is obvious that the non-absorbable SDD regimen will fail if the mucosal barrier has been breached and translocation has occurred. PTA must then be combined with ciprofloxacin which sterilises the mucosal lining via blood and mucus. Fluoroquinolones do not, however, neutralise endotoxin released by salmonellae. PTA is a potent endotoxin-neutralising regimen because both polymyxin E and tobramycin possess anti-endotoxin properties.[26]

# Antimicrobial policies in the ICU

Every ICU should have clear policies for the use of antimicrobial agents and the control of infection. Policies are important because they facilitate timely treatment of potential pathogens (particularly in the absence of definitive microbiological laboratory results), they allow to monitor emergence of resistant strains, and subsequent outbreaks, help to reduce costs, and improve audit. Antibiotic policies should employ a small number of well-established antimicrobial agents which are associated with a minimum of side effects, but which also allow the control of the three patterns of ICU infections caused by the 14 community and hospital pathogens listed in Table 23.1. Antibiotic prescribing should generally be controlled by senior staff, in close cooperation with clinical microbiologists and pharmacists, who should visit the ICU daily.

The following points should be considered when selecting agents for inclusion in an antimicrobial policy. First, spare the indigenous flora that contribute to physiology rather than infection. Most broad-spectrum antibiotics in particular the most recent ever-more potent antimicrobials affect the beneficial normal flora as well as the 14 PPMs. Broad-spectrum therapy predisposes to yeast overgrowth and candidal superinfection. Second, antimicrobials with anti-endotoxin or anti-inflammatory properties may be beneficial. Aminoglycosides and glycopeptides have been shown recently to possess anti-inflammatory properties, whilst treatment with $\beta$-lactams may increase endotoxin levels and subsequent cytokine production. Third, limit the emergence of resistance, which is encouraged by the routine use of broad-spectrum agents. Resistance to multiple agents including the newer antibiotics is of particular concern.

Surveillance cultures are an essential component of an antimicrobial policy. They distinguish between primary endogenous, secondary endogenous, and exogenous infections, each of which requires a different infection control measure. They help to identify patients with resistant microorganisms as soon as possible, and they are necessary for monitoring the efficacy of antibiotic regimens, such as the SDD regimen. A critical observation emerged from the most recent SDD meta-analysis published in the $BMJ$[25] that – besides the significant 20% survival benefit – there was a virtual absence of any major resistance problems, superinfection or outbreak. The package of surveillance, SDD, respect for ecology and hygiene seems to us to provide a more coherent strategy to control resistance compared with the current traditional approach.[27]

1  Bone RC. Let's agree on terminology. *Crit Care Med* 1991;**19**:973–6.
2  Murray AE, Mostafa SM, van Saene HKF. Essentials in clinical microbiology. In: Stoutenbeek CP, van Saene HKF, eds, *Infection and the anaesthetist. Baillière's clinical anaesthesiology*, vol 5. London: Baillière Tindall, 1991: 1–26.
3  Damjanovic V, van Saene HKF, Weindling AM, *et al*. The multiple value of surveillance cultures: an alternative view. *J Hosp Infect* 1994;**28**:71–4.
4  Rosebury TH. *Microorganisms indigenous to man*. New York: McGraw-Hill, 1962.
5  Mackowiak PA, Martin RM, Smith SW. The role of bacterial interference in the increased prevalence of oropharyngeal Gram-negative bacilli among alcoholics and diabetics. *Am Rev Respir Dis* 1979;**120**:589–95.
6  Kerver AJH, Rommes JH, Mevissen-Verhage EAE, *et al*. Colonisation and infection in surgical intensive care patients – a prospective study. *Intensive Care Med* 1987;**13**:347–51.
7  Bloomfield AL. The mechanism of the *Bacillus* carrier state. *Am Rev Tuberc* 1921;**4**:847–55.
8  Johanson WG, Pierce AK, Sanford JP. Changing pharyngeal bacterial flora of hospitalized patients: emergence of gram-negative bacilli. *N Engl J Med* 1969;**281**:1137–40.
9  Gys T, Hubens A, Neels H, *et al*. Prognostic value of gastric intramural pH in surgical intensive care patients. *Crit Care Med* 1988;**16**:1222–4.
10 Dal Nogare AR, Toews GB, Pierce AK. Increased salivary elastase precedes Gram-negative bacillary colonization in postoperative patients. *Am Rev Respir Dis* 1987;**135**:671–5.
11 Ketai LH, Rypka G. The course of nosocomial oropharyngeal colonization in patients recovering from acute respiratory failure. *Chest* 1993;**103**:1837–41.
12 van Uffelen R, van Saene HKF, Fidler V, Lowenberg A. Oropharyngeal flora as a source of bacteria colonizing the lower airways in patients on artificial ventilation. *Intensive Care Med* 1984;**10**:233–7.

13 A'Court CHD, Garrard CS, Crook D, *et al*. Microbiological lung surveillance in mechanically ventilated patients using non-directed bronchial lavage and quantitative culture. *Q J Med* 1993;**86**:635–48.

14 Tancrede CH, Andremont AO. Bacterial translocation and gram-negative bacteremia in patients with hematological malignancies. *J Infect Dis* 1985;**152**:99–103.

15 Damjanovic V, van Saene HKF. Coagulase-negative staphylococcal sepsis in preterm neonates. *Lancet* 1995;**346**:51.

16 Rocke DA, Gaffin SL, Wells MT, *et al*. Endotoxemia associated with cardiopulmonary bypass. *J Thorac Cardiovasc Surg* 1987;**93**:832–7.

17 van Saene HKF, Damjanovic V, Murray AE, de la Cal MA. How to classify infections in intensive care units – the carrier state, a criterion whose time has come? *J Hosp Infect* 1996;**33**:1–12.

18 Dilworth JP, White RJ, Brown EM. Oropharyngeal flora and chest infection after abdominal surgery. *Thorax* 1991;**46**:165–7.

19 D'Angio CT, McGowan KL, Baumgart S, *et al*. Surface colonisation with coagulase-negative staphylococci in premature neonates. *J Pediatr* 1989;**114**:1029–34.

20 Pierro A, van Saene HKF, Donnell SC, *et al*. Microbial translocation in neonates on long-term parenteral nutrition. *Arch Surg* 1996;**131**:176–9.

21 Stoutenbeek CP, van Saene HKF, Liberati A. Prevention of respiratory tract infections in intensive care by selective decontamination of the digestive tract. In: Niederman MS, Sarosi GA, Glassroth JWB, eds, *Respiratory infections*, 1st edn. Philadelphia: Saunders Co., 1994: 579–94.

22 Murray AE, Chambers JJ, van Saene HKF. Infections in patients requiring ventilation in intensive care: application of a new classification. *Clin Microbiol Infect* 1998;**4**:94–102.

23 Nystrom B. Optimal design/personnel for control of intensive care unit infection. *Infect Control* 1983;**4**:388–90.

24 Baxby D, van Saene HKF, Stoutenbeek CP, Zandstra DF. Selective decontamination of the digestive tract: 13 years on, what it is and what it is not. *Intensive Care Med* 1996;**22**:699–706.

25 D'Amico R, Pifferi S, Leonetti C, Torri V, Tinazzi A, Liberati A. Effectiveness of antibiotic prophylaxis in critically ill adult patients: systematic review of randomised controlled trials. *BMJ* 1998;**316**:1275–85.

26 van Saene JJM, Stoutenbeek CP, van Saene HKF, Matera G, Martinez-Pellus AE, Ramsay G. Reduction of the intestinal endotoxin pool by three different SDD regimens in human volunteers. *J Endotoxin Res* 1996;**3**:337–43.

27 Nardi G, Di Silvestre A, Fairclough SJ, van Saene HKF. Antibiotic policy in the intensive care unit. In: van Saene HKF, Silvestri L, de la Cal MA, eds, *Infection Control in the Intensive Care Unit*, 1st edn. Milan: Springer, 1998:170–94.

# 24:  Organ donation

T MCLEOD and T H CLUTTON-BROCK

Organ transplantation plays an important role in the management of patients with end-stage disease of many major organ systems. Despite advances in surgical technique and postoperative management, transplantation remains a limited option because of the poor supply of transplantable organs. The vast majority of organ donors originate from the intensive care unit (ICU). The principles of organ donation include early donor recognition, accurate diagnosis of brain-stem death, physiological maintenance of the donor, support and considerate handling of the patient's family, and coordination with the local organ procurement team.

It is important to be clear about the relationship between brain-stem death tests and the diagnosis of death. The concept of brain death or *coma depasse* was first described by the French as recently as 1959. Testing is not an invention by transplant surgeons to justify the harvest of organs from beating heart donors, although of fundamental importance in this respect. Traditionally death must be certified by a medical practitioner by establishing that there is irreversible cessation of cardiopulmonary function. This does not infer the death of every cell in the body but implies the death of the patient as a whole being. In a similar way, brain-stem death implies the death of a patient as a whole even though other organ systems may continue to function.

## Consent to organ donation

The legal and moral aspects of organ donation are not always mutually exclusive. For example, after death the body is legally owned by either the hospital administrator or the coroner but it may be morally unacceptable for them to give consent for donation of organs against the wishes of grieving relatives. Consent may have been granted prior to death, this being recorded on either a donor card or register of potential donors (opting in). If this is the case then there is no legal requirement to discuss consent with the relatives, although it is usually recommended practice to do so.

The question of timing requires a degree of tact and much groundwork should have taken place during earlier discussion with the relatives as to the patient's prognosis. Ideally, the subject of organ donation should first be broached after completion of the first set of brain-stem death tests, if the relatives have not already raised the subject. At this time the concept of brain death and the beating heart donor should be fully explained to avoid misunderstanding and later distress.

If there are no relatives, the hospital administrator may grant permission for donation of organs, provided the nature of death does not need reporting, in which case consent from the coroner needs to be obtained. The coroner may require that a representative of his office be present during the retrieval operation. Consent for donation is usually obtained by a senior member of the medical team looking after the patient as they will have developed a relationship with the relatives concerned.

The practice of "opting in" described above refers to the present situation in the United Kingdom and differs from that in other countries. In France it is a requirement that a person not wishing to donate organs after death must register this wish on a central computer and that failure to do so automatically implies that consent is granted. Some American state laws stipulate that physicians must discuss all potential donors with the local transplant team and that it is the transplant team who approaches the relatives. There is no evidence to show that either of these strategies increases the supply of donor organs. It is of interest to note that there are no religious groups who are fundamentally opposed to the concept of organ donation.

## Legal considerations

The present legal situation in the United Kingdom is the subject of Health Department written guidance. The procurement of organs from a donor for transplantation occurs in line with the Human Tissue Act 1961 and the Human Tissue Act (NI) 1962[1] and may be allowed only "after his death". There is no definition of death. In 1976 following a conference held by the Medical Colleges and their Faculties[2] a set of guidelines for the establishment of brain-stem death was laid down. An additional memorandum was produced in 1979 which concluded that "the identification of brain death means that the patient is dead, whether or not the function of some organs, such as the heart beat, is still maintained by artificial means". This implies that the time of death is that at completion of the second set of tests. Another memorandum in 1981 further clarified matters by stating that "there may be circumstances in which it is impossible or inappropriate to carry out every one of the tests – and it is for the doctor at the bedside to decide when the patient is dead". Recommendations as to who should perform the tests and their timing were also provided at this time.

The criteria for organ donation are listed in Box 24.1. These are only guidelines, the interpretation of which may be somewhat flexible depending on the urgency with which transplantable organs are required.

## Brain-stem death

As previously mentioned, brain-stem death implies death of the patient as a whole. As such, continued support in the form of mechanical

---

**Box 24.1** *Criteria for organ donation*

*General*
- Free from transmissible disease:
  - bacterial, viral, fungal, and protozoal
  - hepatitis B antigen negative
  - HIV antibody negative
- Absence of carcinoma other than primary brain tumour
- Absence of trauma or chronic disease in the organ to be transplanted.
- No history of intravenous drug abuse
- Absence of widespread atherosclerosis

*Organ specific*
- Kidneys: < 70 years; urine output > 0·5 ml/kg per h; normal plasma urea and creatinine
- Heart: < 50 years; no ischaemia or other cardiac disease, normal ECG and chest radiograph; no prolonged cardiac arrest or significant inotropic support
- Heart/lung: as above plus artificial ventilation for < 24 h if possible and good gas exchange at $F_{IO_2}$ < 0·3
- Liver: < 55 years; no alcohol abuse, normal liver function tests
- Pancreas: < 50 years; no family history of diabetes mellitus; normal plasma amylase

---

ventilation is futile and may be a source of continued stress for the relatives and staff of the ICU, while placing a further burden on already stretched intensive care resources. In this context it may be seen that the diagnosis of brain death and the decision to cease mechanical ventilation are unrelated to the need for organ donation. Continued ventilation of the brain-dead patient may, however, be justified for a limited period – usually less than 24 hours – on the basis of the need for transplantable organs.

### Diagnosis of brain-stem death

In the United Kingdom, diagnosis of brain-stem death can be made only provided rigid criteria laid down by the Medical Colleges 1976 (revised 1983) have been met. These criteria are based on clinical findings and do not include EEG examination or cerebral blood flow measurements which are mandatory in some other countries. Once certain preconditions and exclusions have been met, the clinical tests themselves are conducted by two clinicians of at least senior registrar grade of whom one must be a consultant. The tests are repeated by the same clinicians usually within 24 hours. They must be clinically independent and unconnected with the transplant team. The criteria are summarised in Box 24.2.

*Essential preconditions*

The diagnosis must be certain, the patient having sustained severe irreversible brain damage of known aetiology and being totally dependent

---

**Box 24.2** *Summary of the criteria for brain-stem death*

- Essential preconditions
  - patient must be unresponsive and ventilator dependent (apnoeic coma)
  - the cause must be irremediable structural brain damage
- Necessary exclusions
  - drug intoxication
  - hypothermia – temperature <35°C
  - metabolic and/or endocrine disturbances
- Clinical tests
  - pupils fixed and dilated
  - absent corneal reflex
  - absent vestibulo-ocular reflex
  - absent motor response in cranial nerve distribution
  - no gag reflex or response to tracheal suction
  - apnoea test

---

on artificial ventilation. If any doubt occurs at this stage, no further steps towards diagnosing brain death should be taken.

*Necessary exclusions*

Hypothermia, metabolic, and endocrine abnormalities must be excluded. Prolonged action of CNS depressants including alcohol must be considered and can be ruled out only by the passage of time. Plasma concentrations of sedative drugs correlate poorly with central effects and should not be relied upon. Some people support the use of specific antagonists such as flumazenil or naloxone but, if their use is even considered, then further testing should not be performed. In addition, their use in brain-injured patients may prove deleterious. A peripheral nerve stimulator should be used to exclude prolonged neuromuscular blockade especially if renally excreted drugs have been used in the presence of renal insufficiency.

Conditions that may mimic brain death include ventral pontine infarction (locked-in syndrome), Guillain–Barré syndrome, and brain-stem encephalitis. All these conditions differ from the common causes of brain death – head injury, intracranial haemorrhage, cerebral hypoxia – in that there is no irremediable structural brain damage as stipulated in the essential preconditions. In addition, careful history-taking and examination will reveal that the patients do not fulfil the criteria on other counts.

*Clinical tests*

1. Pupils must be of fixed diameter and unresponsive to sudden changes in the intensity of incident light. Pupils must not respond directly or consensually.

289

2. Absent corneal reflex – no response to direct corneal stimulation bilaterally.
3. Absent vestibulo-ocular reflex – no eye movement during or following slow injection of 20 ml ice-cold water into each external auditory meatus, clear access to the tympanic membrane having been established by direct inspection through an auroscope.
4. No motor response within the cranial nerve distribution – absence of grimacing or facial movement in response to both cranial and peripheral painful stimulation.
5. No gag reflex or response to tracheal stimulation by a suction catheter passed down the trachea.
6. Apnoea testing – no respiratory movement when the patient is disconnected from the ventilator, provided that the $Pa\text{CO}_2$ is high enough to stimulate respiration and there is no hypoxaemia. The $Pa\text{CO}_2$ level required is a minimum of 6·7 kPa (50 mm Hg) and hypoxia is prevented by administration of 100% oxygen prior to disconnection followed by 6 l/min via a catheter in the trachea during the apnoeic episode. The results should be documented by means of arterial blood gas analysis 10 minutes after disconnection.

Diagnosis of brain-stem death is made on completion of the second set of tests, provided all the preconditions and exclusions are met and all the tests are negative.

## Pathophysiology following brain death

Only after the diagnosis of brain-stem death has been established does the emphasis of management change from patient maintenance, with specific cerebral protection, to optimisation of donor organ function. Maintenance of the multiple organ donor is complicated by the fact that different organ systems may have different requirements. In order to provide organs in an optimal state, an understanding of the pathophysiology following brain death is essential. The brain stem is the central regulator of body mechanisms and its death causes dysfunction of many organ systems.

### Cardiovascular system

The primary and most common problem in the brain-dead patient is hypotension which has a multifactorial aetiology. Paralysis of the vasomotor system results in profound vasodilatation and relative hypovolaemia. Previous management strategies aimed at cerebral protection, such as fluid restriction and diuretic therapy, will compound this. Depression of myocardial contractility occurs owing to an inability to replenish myocardial energy stores which may be related to endocrine abnormalities, including sudden falls in insulin, triiodothyronine ($T_3$), thyroxine, ($T_4$), and cortisol levels. Bradycardia may occur owing to the loss of sympathetic drive and damage to the nucleus ambiguus in the brain-stem which abolishes resting vagal tone; hence it is more likely to respond to treatment with sympathomimetics than with atropine. Other arrhythmias such as supraventricular or ventricular tachycardia, ST segment, and T-wave changes may occur as a result of neurological damage or acid–base or electrolyte imbalance.

## Fluid balance

Specific dehydration therapy is aggravated by diabetes insipidus, glycosuria as a result of steroid therapy, or hyperthermia prior to brain death.

## Temperature control

Extensive brain damage causes loss of centrally controlled thermoregulation, and the body becomes poikilothermic (adopts environmental temperature). Vasodilatation increases heat loss and heat production is concurrently diminished. Hypothermia in itself affects other organ systems, causing bradycardia, coagulopathy, reduced glomerular filtration rate, left shift of the oxygen dissociation curve, and pancreatitis.[3]

## Endocrine failure

Posterior pituitary failure is associated with a fall in secretion of antidiuretic hormone (ADH) and onset of diabetes insipidus.[4] As a result, large volumes of dilute urine are produced in association with hyperosmolality, hypernatraemia, hypermagnesaemia, hypokalaemia, hypophosphataemia, and hypocalcaemia. Hyperglycaemia may be present as a result of falling insulin production, increased plasma catecholamine levels secondary to endogenous production or exogenous administration, and treatment with dextrose-containing intravenous fluids. Anterior pituitary damage has been demonstrated in animals though its relevance in humans has yet to be proven.[5]

## Hypoxaemia

Brain-stem death itself is not a primary cause of hypoxaemia but does necessitate artificial ventilation with its attendant problems of atelectasis, infection, and aspiration. Pulmonary oedema may be evident either as a result of poor cardiac function (cardiogenic) or as a result of increased pulmonary capillary leak which can occur after brain death (neurogenic).

291

# Physiological maintenance of the multi-organ donor

## Maintenance of blood pressure and cardiac output

Ideally a systolic blood pressure of 90–100 mm Hg should be the goal. Good peripheral venous access is required initially, along with a central venous cannula for drug administration and measurement of intravascular pressure. An arterial line and urinary catheter must be placed with strict attention to aseptic technique. Initial management consists of fluid loading using arterial and central venous pressure (CVP), urine output, and core–peripheral temperature gradient as guides of adequacy. A haematocrit of approximately 30% is most appropriate to maintain oxygen delivery and should be achieved with transfusion if necessary. Modified gelatins are the most commonly used intravenous fluids for resuscitation and continued administration should take into account plasma glucose and electrolyte concentrations.

Indications for placing a pulmonary artery flotation catheter are as follows:

- sustained hypotension despite fluid loading to a CVP of 15 mm Hg;
- severe renal dysfunction;
- high positive end-expiratory pressure (PEEP) requirement to maintain oxygenation.

Despite rehydration some patients will require inotropic support, usually in the form of dopamine 2–10 μg/kg per min or dobutamine < 15 μg/kg per min. Vasoconstrictors such as adrenaline and noradrenaline may seem logical choices in the face of vasodilatation and are used in some centres, though this may be at the expense of tissue blood flow.[6] The dose of inotropes should be kept to a minimum to avoid catecholamine receptor depletion (down-regulation) which has been implicated in impaired myocardial performance in the recipient.

## Fluid balance

Regular monitoring of plasma electrolyte concentrations is an important part of donor management. Deficits resulting from diabetes insipidus need replacing with 5% dextrose and added potassium or a solution based on urinary electrolyte losses. Replacement on a volume for volume basis is optimal. The use of vasopressin or desmopressin (DDAVP) is controversial as either may reduce renal and hepatic blood flow. Intramuscular, subcutaneous, and intranasal administration are associated with variable absorption. If treatment for excessive urine output is deemed necessary, a controlled intravenous infusion of vasopressin is probably best. A dose of 2–10 μg/kg per min is used to achieve a urine output of 1·5–3 ml/kg per h.

Oliguria (urine output < 0·5 ml/kg per h) in the face of adequate fluid resuscitation may respond to treatment with mannitol 0·5 g/kg or frusemide 80–100 mg.

## Hypothermia

Heat loss can be reduced by nursing the patient in a warm ambient temperature and covering the patient as far as is possible. The use of a space blanket, heat/moisture exchanger in the breathing system, and warmed intravenous fluids is also beneficial. Active warming with a heat blanket may be helpful if one is available.

## Arrhythmias

Correction of electrolyte imbalance, in particular hypocalcaemia, hypo-kalaemia, hypophosphataemia, and hypomagnesaemia, is important, along with adjustment of ventilation to maintain normal acid–base balance and oxygenation. Development of tachyarrhythmias may be due to inadequate volume resuscitation or excessive inotrope administration both of which may need to be reviewed. Bradycardia may respond to treatment with dopamine. Arrhythmias can be persistent and lead to cardiac arrest, in which case full cardiopulmonary resuscitation is not contraindicated.

## Ventilation

Prior to affirmation of brain-stem death, hyperventilation may have been instituted as a measure to reduce intracranial pressure. After certification, ventilation should be gradually reduced to raise the $P\text{aco}_2$ to 5·3–5·6 kPa without causing significant acidosis. The inspired oxygen concentration should be set to achieve a $P\text{ao}_2$ of 9–13 kPa. Modest levels of PEEP (2·5–7·5 cm $H_2O$) may be useful in preventing alveolar collapse, and higher levels avoided in order to minimise barotrauma and detrimental effects on cardiac output. An aseptic technique must be used for suctioning the trachea.

## Hormone therapy

Mild to severe hyperglycaemia is not uncommon and may require treatment with insulin, preferably by continuous intravenous infusion on a sliding scale.

Animal work has shown that anterior pituitary hormone replacement therapy by way of $T_3$, insulin, and hydrocortisone infusions can reduce the incidence of cardiac and renal abnormalities in brain-dead potential donors.[7] Although some units have adopted this practice, data thus far are conflicting and advice from the recipient team should be sought.

Physiological maintenance of the donor should be continued right up until actual procurement, transport to the operating room being a time for potential instability. Multiple organ retrieval is a complex and lengthy surgical procedure and careful management of the donor is required throughout. Spinal reflexes are preserved in brain-stem death, and neuromuscular blockade will usually be required to facilitate surgical access.

Retrieval teams often come from different transplant centres and previously agreed protocols and procedures should be used to avoid conflicts of interest and confusion.

## Conclusion

In view of the limited supply of transplantable organs, it is the duty of the ICU clinician to optimise organ function in the brain-dead patient. It is important to remember that, until the diagnosis of brain-stem death has been established, the patient must be managed according to the pathophysiology relating to the presenting condition. Whilst intensive care necessitates preservation of all organ systems, specific therapies aimed at optimising function solely with transplantation in mind should not be instituted until after certification of death.

Further research is needed into the management of the donor and the preservation of organ function prior to donation. Current predictors of post-transplantation function are limited in their use and improvements in this area along with better organ preservation should improve the success of organ transplantation.

Compassionate communication between clinicians, nursing staff, relatives, and the procurement team can at least potentially salvage some good from personal disaster as the death of one patient may provide a new lease of life for several others.[8]

1 Health Department of Great Britain and Northern Ireland. *Cadaveric organs for transplantation: a code of practice including the diagnosis of brain death.* London: HMSO, 1983.
2 Honorary Secretary of the Conference of Medical Royal Colleges and their faculties in the United Kingdom. Diagnosis of brain death. *BMJ* 1976;**ii**:1069–70.
3 Reuter JB. Hypothermia: Pathophysiology, clinical settings and management. *Ann Intern Med* 1978;**89**:519–27.
4 Bjorn JD, Hans P, Smitz S, Legros JJ, Kay S. Syndrome of inappropriate secretion of antidiuretic hormone after severe head injury. *Surg Neurol* 1985;**23**:383–7.
5 Novitsky D, Witcomb WN, Cooper DKC, Rose AG, Fraser RC, Barnard CN. Electrocardiographic, haemodynamic and endocrine changes occurring during experimental brain death in the chacma baboon. *J Heart Transplant* 1984;**4**:63–9.
6 Nishimura N, Sugi R. Circulatory support with sympathetic amines in brain death. *Resuscitation* 1984;**12**:25–30.
7 Novitsky D, Cooper DKC, Reichart B. Hemodynamic and metabolic responses to hormonal therapy in brain dead potential organ donors. *Transplantation* 1987;**43**:852–4.
8 Morton JB, Leonard DRA. Cadaver nephrectomy: an operation on the donor's family. *BMJ* 1979;**i**:239.

# Further reading

Bodenham A, Park GR. Care of the multiple organ donor. *Intensive Care Med* 1989; 15:340-8.

Soifer B, Gelb AW. The multiple organ donor: identification and management. *Ann Intern Med* 1989;10:815-23.

# 25: Assessment and management of the trauma patient

G McMAHON and D W YATES

Trauma is the leading cause of death in males and females under the age of 35 years in both developed and most developing countries. In the United Kingdom it is surpassed only by ischaemic heart disease and carcinoma as a leading cause of death in all ages. Approximately 18 000 injured people die every year. One third are a result of road crashes and almost one third occur in the home.

The tragedy of sudden death in young people is enormous, resulting in major emotional and financial losses to both families and society. The financial cost is estimated to be approximately 2.2 billion pounds per year or 1% of the gross national product (WHO estimation).

The first peak in mortality occurs at, or shortly after, the time of injury. Unfortunately, most of these patients have suffered major neurological or vascular injuries and are unsalvageable. It is estimated, however, that primary prevention could reduce this peak by 40%. A second peak has been described, with patients often dying unnecessarily from airway obstruction or cardiorespiratory problems. This "golden hour" of opportunity to resuscitate the patient is of central importance to intensivists and emergency physicians. The distinction between the first and second phases of deaths and the duration of the "golden hour" have recently been challenged. However, it remains clear that there is an opportunity to intervene, and that speed and coordination are critical. Finally there are a number of deaths that occur days to weeks later, predominantly caused by multiple organ failure, sepsis, and acute respiratory distress syndrome (ARDS). It should be appreciated that these three peaks are interdependent. Inappropriate management at the scene may cause fatalities in the emergency department and inadequate resuscitation on arrival at hospital may lead to death on the intensive care unit (ICU). The quality of survival can be sensitively influenced.

This chapter begins with a description of the biomechanics of injury, followed by a structured and systematic approach to the initial assessment and management of the trauma patient.

296

# Mechanism of injury

Paramount to the assessment and management of the injured patient is an understanding of the mechanism of injury. Trauma can be divided into three broad categories: blunt, penetrating, and blast, depending on the mechanism. Blunt injury is by far the most common in Britain accounting for more than 90% of all injuries.

## Blunt trauma

Blunt trauma gives rise to three types of forces:

- Shearing results from two forces acting in opposite directions. Shear injury to skin tends to cause irregular damage and is associated with more underlying tissue injury than a simple laceration. Consequently there is a higher incidence of infections. Shear injury to the abdomen has maximal effect where organs are tethered, e.g. duodenojejunal flexure, spleen, renal vasculature, etc.
- Tension occurs when force hits a tissue surface at an angle of < 90°. This gives rise to flap formation together with similar but more severe tissue injury than that from shearing force.
- Compression results when a force hits the tissue at a 90° angle. The site of impact may be identified by the presence of contusions, haematoma, and possible breech in surface tissue. Surface changes may, however, take several hours to develop and, if the injuring agent is diffuse, the skin may be undamaged (e.g. airbag). This type of force may also lead to rupture of gas-filled organs, such as the gut, in the "closed loop phenomenon".

Blunt injury is, however, usually a combination of these forces working together rather than in isolation. Typically multiple injuries occur; as a general principle, if there are evident injuries to the lower body and to the head there is usually an occult injury to the trunk. A history of fatalities at the scene heightens suspicion of serious injuries in the survivors, as it reflects the amount of force involved in the accident.

There are common patterns of injury resulting from different mechanisms of trauma. For example, an unrestrained driver may produce a "bull's-eye" fracture of the windscreen, together with a collapsed steering column and indented dashboard. This signifies a high-velocity blunt trauma; the typical injuries include serious head and facial injuries, with associated obstructed airway. The potential for cervical spine injury is also extremely high. Blunt injury of the chest wall from the steering column may result in serious thoracoabdominal injuries. Indentations in the dashboard draw attention to potential posterior hip dislocations and pelvic fractures. A fall from a height landing on the feet is associated with painful fractures of the os calci but also with less painful, less obvious, but potentially more serious injuries to the tibial plateau, hips, posterior pelvic ring, and retroperitoneal structures.

## Penetrating trauma

Penetrating trauma is divided into two categories: stab wounds and gunshot wounds.

### Gunshot

The amount of damage to tissues is dependent on the kinetic energy (KE) of the weapon and the consistency of the tissue itself:

$$\left[ KE = \frac{mv^2}{2} \right].$$

where $m$ is the mas and $v$ the velocity. Therefore a bullet object travelling at high velocity will impart a significant amount of KE to the tissues. This is compounded by the coexistence of dirt from outdoor clothing and skin that is dragged deep into the wound. Hence the risk of serious infective complications is high. With high-energy transfer, neighbouring tissues are pushed away from the missile track leaving a temporary cavity. This can reach 30–40 times the diameter of the missile. As the energy wave dissipates the tissues rapidly retract to leave a permanent cavity. Damage to vessels is particularly insidious. Internal damage may occur leading to delayed occlusion without any initial evidence of external injury on inspection. High-velocity gun shot damage to the brain is particularly devastating.

In contrast, shotgun or rifle and some handgun injuries are more localised. The bullet path is, however, often unpredictable and many tissues are usually damaged.

### Stab wound

An incision, produced by low-energy penetrating trauma (e.g. a stab wound), results in a localised wound with little oedema or inflammation. However, a small wound may disguise a deep penetrating injury. Consequently the significance of stab wounds is dependent upon its site and the type and extent of the organs involved.

## Blast injuries

A bomb explosion results in a sudden rise in pressure in the surrounding air – the "blast wave". This moves in all directions from the epicentre at a rate that is faster than the speed of sound. As it spreads out it gets progressively weaker. Pressure gradients are greater in enclosed spaces.

Behind this "blast wave" comes the "blast wind" which is movement of the air itself. As this moves out from the epicentre it carries fragments of the bomb and surrounding debris with it. Many of these fragments can produce "high-energy transfer" wounds because of the velocity at which they are travelling.

The blast wave or shock front primarily affects air-containing organs such as the lung, bowel, and ears. Its magnitude and rate of onset are the main determinants of the extent of tissue damage. If the pulmonary changes are extensive, a ventilation–perfusion mismatch develops, resulting in significant hypoxia. High-pressure blast injuries may also cause air emboli with the potential of sudden death if these obstruct cerebral or coronary perfusion.

Injuries secondary to the "blast wind" are usually caused by the "missile" effect of fragments blown at high velocity. Other injuries may result simply from falling debris and fires. Management will be compromised if, as often occurs, the blast has caused patient deafness.

A basic understanding of the biomechanics of injury aids the early identification of injuries, which in turn leads to a reduction in problems resulting from delayed diagnosis.

## Approach to the multiply injured patient

Management of major trauma has improved significantly over the past 20 years because of the introduction of a number of initiatives. Central to these is the concept of a trauma system and the coordinated management of the patient by a team working to rehearsed, evidence-based guidelines. The Advanced Trauma Life Support course, introduced by the American College of Surgeons in 1978, espouses these ideals and has been widely adopted. Some advocates have, perhaps, been too rigorous in demanding absolute adherence to protocols, but more people are realising that the basic concepts of ATLS are sound and will provide the best care to most patients in most situations.

The concepts behind the ATLS course are simple. The initial assessment and management of the trauma patient must be prioritised on the basis of treating the greatest threat to life first. This approach differs from the standard approach to a non-urgent medical patient, in which a detailed history is followed by a detailed head-to-toe examination. This is not appropriate in the management of the trauma patient.

"Primary survey" and "resuscitation" phases of care are described in the ATLS course. These are usually carried out simultaneously. It is only when all acutely life-threatening problems of the airway, breathing, circulation, and neurological system are assessed and stabilised that it becomes appropriate to take a detailed history and perform the more detailed "secondary survey". It is during this phase that both the potentially life-threatening and the functionally disabling injuries are identified.

### The team approach

Observational studies have established that the trauma patient is more efficiently managed by a well-trained trauma team working to a pre-determined plan.

Once the emergency department is notified of the impending arrival of a multiply injured patient, the team should assemble in the resuscitation room. Members of the team can then be briefed to ensure that each member is aware of his or her role. Information should be obtained from ambulance control about the nature of the accident, number of casualties, type of injuries, conscious state, and estimated time of arrival.

It is essential that members of the trauma team are suitably dressed with protective gear. The minimum is: gloves, aprons, and eye protection. It is the responsibility of the team leader to ensure that these standards are maintained.

The size of the team will depend on local resources. Ideally there should be:

- a medical and nursing team leader
- an airway doctor and nurse
- two circulation doctors and two nurses
- a relatives' nurse
- a radiographer.

Once all the life-threatening emergencies of the patient have been identified and treated, surplus members of the team may stand down.

The principal role of the trauma team leader is to coordinate effectively a structured resuscitation of the trauma patient, to assimilate clinical findings, to direct investigations, and to liaise with specialists who have been consulted. They are also responsible for obtaining relevant prehospital information and the patient's past medical history. The medical team leader may also perform particular tasks, e.g. pericardiocentesis, depending on the skill of the team members.

The nursing team leader coordinates the nursing team members. He or she may also assume the role of recorder. This includes recording vital signs, quantity of fluid administered, urine output, procedures performed, and drugs administered.

The role of the airway doctor and nurse is to assess and secure a patent airway together with cervical spine immobilisation. The circulation group establishes vascular access, using two large-bore cannulae, and ensures that blood is sent for cross-matching, full blood count, urea, and electrolytes, and, blood glucose estimation. They will also establish external haemorrhage control, if required, and catheterise the patient if no contraindications exist.

## Primary survey

Primary survey consists of:

- **A**irway with cervical spine control
- **B**reathing and ventilation
- **C**irculation with haemorrhage control
- **D**isability – neurological status
- **E**xposure with environmental control.

The objectives here are to perform a rapid evaluation with simultaneous management of acute life-threatening injuries. The patient may have more than one acute life-threatening injury so the approach to the patient must be prioritised to treating the greatest threat to life first; this is often called the ABC approach. The emphasis is on the resolution of each problem as it is identified, before going on to the next stage. Continual assessment of response to treatment should be carried out, and any deterioration should prompt a rapid systematic re-evaluation

### Airway

A compromised airway is the quickest killer of the multiply injured patient. Evaluation should always be linked with manoeuvres to maintain cervical spine immobilisation. This becomes especially important in unconscious patients. Cervical spine immobilisation can initially be achieved by holding the head and neck in line manually. Then an appropriately sized semirigid cervical collar should be applied, with head blocks or sand bags secured to a spinal board. A dilemma arises in the combative patient; it is unsafe to immobilise the neck forcibly if the rest of the patient is moving about, as this increases the probability of doing further harm. In this situation one member of the team should hold the neck in line with the trunk as best as he or she can. The cause of irritability should then be identified (e.g. hypoxia) and appropriately corrected.

Talking to the patient yields valuable information. If the patient can respond coherently, with a normal voice, then the airway is patent and there is adequate perfusion and oxygenation of the brain. If there is no response, then the airway should be opened by the chin lift or jaw thrust manoeuvre, with care to maintain cervical spine immobilisation. This is often enough to relieve an obstructed airway which is most commonly secondary to the tongue falling backward against the pharynx. Airway opening can be maintained using either an oropharyngeal airway, if tolerated, or alternatively a nasopharyngeal airway. Any foreign material should be removed under direct vision either with a Magill's forceps or a rigid suction device.

All patients require high-flow oxygen. This is best achieved, in spontaneously breathing patients, with the use of a well-fitting oxygen mask with a reservoir bag (Hudson mask) at 15 l/min. In the unconscious patient with an absent gag reflex the risk of aspiration is high. Therefore, early consideration should be given to endotracheal intubation in order to protect the airway and administer high-flow oxygen.

Occasionally extreme facial injuries, glottic oedema, foreign body obstruction, fracture of the larynx, or severe oropharyngeal haemorrhage makes it impossible to intubate a patient. In this instance a cricothyroidotomy should be performed. A large-bore cannula is used to pierce the cricothyroid membrane. The cannula is connected to wall oxygen at 15 l/min with a Y-connector in the tubing enabling intermittent ventilation to be achieved by occluding the open port for 1 second and releasing it for 4 seconds. Owing to inefficiency of $CO_2$ clearance this technique is valuable for only 30–45 min. In an emergency, a surgical cricothyroidotomy is preferred to a tracheostomy, because it is associated with minimal haemorrhage and fewer complications. This is performed by making a transverse incision in the cricothyroid membrane and inserting either a small (5 or 6 mm) endotracheal or tracheostomy tube. Because of the potential damage to the cricoid cartilage, it is not recommended in children under the age of 12 years.

Once intubated the patient should be appropriately ventilated. However, it is important to recognise a potential tension pneumothorax with the combination of positive pressure ventilation and chest trauma. Hence it is often safer to perform a tube thoracotomy electively in a patient known to have fractured ribs when the decision has been taken to ventilate.

## Breathing

Breathing and ventilation may be adversely affected centrally, for example, hypoventilation associated with reduced level of consciousness, or peripherally from thoracic injuries. Chest injuries account for 25% of all trauma deaths and many could be prevented by prompt diagnosis and treatment. Less than 10% of blunt chest injuries and less than 30% of penetrating injuries require surgery. Most can be managed initially by experienced intensivists or emergency physicians.

There are six life-threatening chest injuries that should be identified and managed in the primary survey:

- airway obstruction
- tension pneumothorax
- open pneumothorax
- flail chest
- cardiac tamponade
- massive haemothorax.

In order to identify these injuries the chest and abdomen must be adequately exposed. The chest should be inspected for respiratory rate and effort, chest expansion, abrasions, open wounds, and penetrating trauma. The position of the trachea and the presence of surgical emphysema or fracture crepitus can be identified by palpation. Resonance to percussion and equality of air entry should also be established. In this way an open pneumothorax, tension pneumothorax, massive haemothorax, and flail chest can be diagnosed. In the conscious patient with a flail chest, paradoxical movement of the chest wall rarely exists, as splinting of the chest wall occurs secondary to pain.

A tension pneumothorax is a clinical diagnosis and is treated promptly with placement of a 12 gauge cannula in the second intercostal space in the midclavicular line on the affected side. This should yield a large hiss of air escaping from the chest, relieving the tension; a definitive tube thoracotomy should then be performed as soon as possible.

A massive haemothorax is defined as a haemothorax of >1500 ml or a continued loss >200 ml/h out of the chest drain. Although this may be due to bleeding from intercostal vessels, the pulmonary vessels at the hilum may have been damaged. Urgent referral to a cardiothoracic surgeon is indicated as the patient will probably require a thoracotomy.

An open pneumothorax causes ventilatory problems because an opening of more than two thirds the diameter of the trachea allows air preferentially to traverse the opening in the chest. The immediate life-saving manoeuvre in this situation is simply to cover the hole with an occlusive dressing sealed on three sides only, to avoid precipitating a secondary tension pneumo-thorax. A chest tube should be inserted on the same side but away from the site of the wound.

Cardiac tamponade is usually secondary to penetrating chest or abdominal trauma. The heart is within a fairly rigid fibrous pericardial sac, so the accumulation of only 15–20 ml fluid is enough to cause difficulty with diastolic filling. This leads to a reduction in cardiac output, ultimately resulting in cardiac arrest secondary to electromechanical dissociation. Cardiac tamponade should be suspected when there is a reduction of pulse pressure, muffled heart sounds, and elevation of the jugular venous pressure – known as Beck's triad. The presence of hypovolaemia may make elevation of the jugular venous pressure an unreliable sign. A true paradoxical sign is raised jugular venous pressure on inspiration – known as Kussmaul's sign. The immediate life-saving manoeuvre is a needle pericardiocentesis followed by definitive surgery (pericardiotomy). This is performed with a 16 gauge 15 cm over-the-needle cannula connected to a three-way stopcock and a 50 ml syringe. The patient must be connected to an ECG monitor. With an aseptic technique the skin is punctured 1 cm below and lateral to the xiphisternal junction, at an angle of 45° to the skin, the needle aimed towards the tip of the left scapula. As the needle is advanced, continual aspiration is carried out, and the ECG is observed for evidence of myocardial injury (ST wave changes, widening of the QRS complex). Aspiration of only 20 ml of blood can be life saving. In the case of a positive aspiration, the cannula should be secured in place, in order to allow for repeated aspiration while definitive surgery is organised.

### Circulation and haemorrhage control

Failure to recognise and correct occult haemorrhage after injury is the leading cause of preventable death in the United Kingdom. Common sites of occult haemorrhage are the abdomen, pelvis, and thorax.

The first objective in assessing the circulation is to identify clinical signs of shock and establish baseline circulatory parameters in order to evaluate response to resuscitative measures. Unfortunately, clinical examination is unreliable and there are no simple early indicators of shock. Hypovolaemia is associated with increased sympathetic activity leading to peripheral vasoconstriction. However, by the time this is evidenced by skin pallor and sweating, together with a tachycardia, tachypnoea, and narrowed pulse pressure, there has been at least a 20–30% blood loss. It is important to be aware of this in order that resuscitative efforts are proactive rather than reactive.

Two large-bore (12–14 gauge) intravenous cannulae should be sited preferably in the antecubital fossae. Peripheral venous cannulation is preferred to central access because it is associated with less complications, especially in inexperienced hands. Blood (20 ml) should be taken for cross-matching, full blood count, urea and electrolytes, blood sugar estimation, and creatinine. Toxicology and a pregnancy test are performed if indicated. The patient should be resuscitated with warmed intravenous fluid. A patient with >40% haemorrhage will be hypotensive and tachycardic, have an altered mental state, and require blood urgently. A full cross-match takes approximately 1 hour and type-specific blood 15 min to prepare. In these cases it is often more appropriate to use uncross-matched O-negative blood. Obvious external haemorrhage is initially controlled by the application of sustained pressure over the bleeding site. Tourniquets should be avoided because they exacerbate damage to the distal aspect of the limb, and if they are incorrectly applied they exacerbate distal oozing. Attempts to clamp arterial/venous bleeding should be avoided in the emergency setting because of the high risk of clamping associated nerves.

It is important to monitor response to treatment closely in order to identify continuing haemorrhage early. Failure to achieve haemodynamic stability after the first fluid bolus indicates the presence of uncontrolled haemorrhage which requires early surgical intervention.

Intrathoracic bleeding can be identified on erect or decubitus chest radiograph or through blood loss via the chest tube. Occult intra-abdominal haemorrhage is more difficult to detect. Diagnostic peritoneal lavage, computed tomography, and ultrasound are commonly used. Retroperitoneal haemorrhage is usually not detected by diagnostic peritoneal lavage. Ultrasound is gaining in popularity. Computed tomography may be inappropriate in the unstable patient.

Pelvic spring is now largely discontinued as a reliable test for pelvic fracture because excessive pelvic stressing can increase pelvic venous bleeding. Plain radiographs can fail to identify the presence of a posterior pelvic ring fracture. If suspected, this is best confirmed using computed tomography. Pelvic fractures can be associated with occult haemorrhage of >3 litres. The early application of external pelvic fixators reduces haemorrhage by up to 50%. Arterial bleeding can be controlled by directed embolization.

Haemorrhage associated with fractures can be reduced by 50% by early realignment and splinting. Open fractures are associated with twice the amount of haemorrhage. Open pelvic fractures in particular are associated with a very high mortality rate.

## Disability

The next imminent cause of death, after airway, breathing, and circulatory problems, is the presence of an expanding extradural haematoma. A rapid neurological assessment should therefore be carried out during the primary survey (AVPU mnemonic):
* **A**lert
* Responds to **V**oice
* Responds to **P**ain
* **U**nresponsive.

The conscious state can be rapidly and simply evaluated using this AVPU mnemonic. This characterises the patient's neurological status as alert, responding to voice or to pain, or as unresponsive. Pupillary responsiveness and equality should be evaluated together with any obvious motor lateralising signs.

## Exposure

It is now necessary to expose the patient completely. Particular attention should be given to the back and the perineum. Trauma impairs thermoregulatory control and therefore attention must be directed to ensuring that the patient is kept warm with blankets and overhead heaters. Resuscitation fluids should be warmed.

### Initial investigations

Portable radiographs showing the lateral cervical spine, chest, and pelvis are an important component of the primary survey. Response to resuscitation should be monitored by continually re-evaluating the patient's overall status, and specifically blood pressure, heart rate (ECG monitor), respiratory rate, temperature, $O_2$ saturation (pulse oximeter), and urine output. Blood will have been withdrawn for haemoglobin, packed cell volume, urea and electrolytes, blood sugar, and cross-match as indicated.

All trauma patients should have continual ECG, blood pressure, and oxygen saturation (pulse oximeter) monitoring. A nasogastric tube should be passed in order to relieve gastric dilatation which commonly accompanies injury. If there is a suspicion of a basal skull fracture, an orogastric tube is preferred. Urine output is monitored with a urethral catheter. A disrupted urethra, often associated with pelvic fractures, requires a suprapubic catheter.

## Secondary survey

The objectives of the secondary survey are to:

1. perform a detailed head-to-toe examination;
2. take a good medical history;
3. examine results;
4. develop management plan for definitive care.

The priorities now are to identify occult, potentially life-threatening injuries, together with injuries that may be either limb threatening or lead to future disability. A safe approach is to begin examination at the head and proceed down through each region of the body in order not to miss any area. The back is examined by log-rolling the patient.

### Head/scalp/face

The scalp is examined for evidence of underlying skull fractures and penetrating wounds. CSF otorrhoea or rhinorrhoea suggests the presence of a basal skull fracture. Facial bone fractures, whilst not of immediate concern, need to be identified for future management. Multiple fractures of the mandible can cause acute airway problems if the tongue falls backwards to occlude the airway. This can be corrected by putting a suture through the tip of the tongue and securing it to the cheek.

Early examination of the eyes is important. Contact lenses and foreign bodies should be removed to avoid permanent damage. Penetrating ocular trauma requires early identification. Even the most swollen eyes can be examined with an ocular speculum. This becomes especially important if an ocular compartment syndrome is present; this is identified by swelling associated with loss of visual acuity. Early decompression will prevent permanent loss of vision. This can be achieved by a lateral canthotomy and inferior cantholysis and must be performed within 80 minutes.

## Neck

The neck should be examined for evidence of elevated jugular venous pressure, tracheal position, obvious wounds, or penetrating trauma. The cervical spine can be palpated for tenderness, swelling, or deformity.

## Chest

There are six potentially life-threatening injuries that should be considered in the secondary survey of the chest:

- aortic disruption
- myocardial contusion
- pulmonary contusion
- traumatic diaphragmatic rupture
- tracheobronchial disruption
- oesophageal disruption.

The identification of these injuries is dependent on having a high index of suspicion. Aortic disruption must be considered in all patients who have sustained significant deceleration injuries. Radiological signs include a widened mediastinum, together with obliteration of the aortic knob on chest radiograph. In addition there may be an associated pleural cap, depression of the left main stem bronchus, or deviation of the oesophagus to the right (nasogastric tube). The diagnostic test of choice is an arch aortogram. Failure to identify and treat this injury is associated with a 30% mortality rate each day the patient is left untreated.

The presence of blunt chest injury or fractured sternum suggests the possibility of underlying myocardial contusion. The ECG may demonstrate changes suggestive of an infarct, new onset right bundle-branch block, or multiple ectopics. The investigation of choice for myocardial contusion is an echocardiogram.

Pulmonary contusion is the most common thoracic injury. As the contused lung is highly sensitive to under- or overhydration, patients who sustain significant pulmonary contusion will require invasive monitoring. Failure to maintain a normal $Pao_2$ despite oxygen therapy will require early ventilation.

A ruptured hemidiaphragm is more commonly seen on the left, as the right is relatively shielded by the liver. It is often missed initially if the chest radiograph is misinterpreted as showing an elevated hemidiaphragm or a distended gastric air bubble. The presence of a nasogastric tube curled up in the chest is diagnostic and eliminates the need for special contrast studies.

Tracheobronchial disruption usually presents as a large pneumothorax, which is associated with a continued large air leak from the chest tube. This requires early surgical repair.

Oesophageal disruption is usually secondary to penetrating trauma, but may also occur as a result of blunt injury to the epigastrium, causing expulsion of the gastric contents up into the chest; this results in a linear tear of the lower oesophagus. A ruptured oesophagus should be suspected in a patient who has gastric contents draining through the chest tube. It should also be suspected in a patient with a pneumomediastinum and in patients found to have a left-sided pneumothorax or haemothorax without overlying rib fractures. If it is left untreated, these patients have a very high mortality rate because of the development of malignant mediastinitis.

## Abdomen

Unrecognised abdominal injury remains a frequent cause of preventable death. Peritoneal signs may be masked by the coexistence of a head injury or intoxication. It may also be overshadowed by pain from extra-abdominal injuries. Approximately 20% of patients who have significant intra-abdominal haemorrhage will have an initially normal abdominal evaluation. Consequently re-evaluation is essential.

A diagnostic peritoneal lavage or computed tomography is indicated if abdominal examination is unreliable (head injury or intoxication), equivocal (fractured lower ribs or pelvis), or impractical (anticipated lengthy radiological studies or general anaesthesia).

## Pelvis and perineum

A fractured pelvis will already have been identified during the primary survey. Coexisting injury to the urethra is suspected from the presence of blood at the urethral meatus and a scrotal haematoma. A rectal examination may demonstrate a high-riding prostate secondary to urethral injury, or bony fragments penetrating the wall of the rectum. Priapism or a lax anal sphincter may be the first suggestion of spinal cord injury.

## Extremities

A detailed examination of the extremities can be carried out at this stage to assess:

- perfusion
- open wounds
- closed wounds: fractures and joint injuries
- neuromuscular function.

The early management priorities are to:

- restore limb alignment together with the application of splints;
- perform appropriate wound care;
- restore perfusion;
- relieve pain.

Appropriate wound care involves adequate cleansing of wounds, removal of foreign bodies, identification of underlying structural damage, and ensuring tetanus protection.

With regards to amputated parts, they should be cleaned well, wrapped in moist sterile gauze, and put in a sterile bag. This should then be placed in a bag of crushed ice and transferred with the patient. The intention is to cool not freeze the part. An amputated part is viable for only 4–6 h at room temperature, but up to 18 h if kept cool. Even if not salvageable for re-implantation, they may be useful for skin and bone grafting.

### Back

All trauma patients must be presumed to have spinal column injuries until proven otherwise. Therefore it is important to log-roll the patient to examine the back. During this manoeuvre, any debris can be removed from under the patient. The whole spinal column should be palpated for tenderness, swelling, or deformity, and a detailed neurological examination is performed. Isolated findings such as priapism or loss of anal tone may be the first warning of an unstable spinal column injury.

### Medical history

Coexistent medical conditions are much more prevalent and more important than had been previously recognised. Evaluation of the patient is incomplete without a detailed history. A useful mnemonic is AMPLE:

- **A**llergies
- **M**edications
- **P**ast medical history
- **L**ast meal
- **E**vents (at the scene and in hospital).

## Definitive care

During the course of assessment a management plan for definitive care needs to be decided upon. Patient outcome is directly related to the time from injury to delivery of definitive care. If the patient's needs exceed the facilities of the department, then referral to another centre will be necessary. It is the trauma team leader's responsibility to ensure that the patient is stable prior to transfer and that the necessary communication with the receiving physician has occurred early. In addition all documents and radiographs should accompany the patient, along with an experienced doctor with the necessary supplies of drugs, fluids, oxygen, and instruments to deal with emergencies en route.

## Trauma in pregnancy

The treatment priorities here are the same as in the non-pregnant state. Survival of the unborn baby is dependent on efficient resuscitation of the mother. Early involvement of an obstetrician and surgeon is important.

It is essential to have an appreciation of the anatomical and physiological changes of pregnancy that influence the response to trauma. There is a greater risk of aspiration owing to increased gastric stasis and oesophageal reflux during pregnancy. It is normal for pregnant women to hyperventilate and a $Pa_{CO_2}$ of 4 kPa (30 mm Hg) is normal. Hence a $Pa_{CO_2}$ of 5·3 kPa (40 mm Hg) in a pregnant woman signifies maternal and fetal acidosis. During pregnancy the blood volume increases by approximately 50% and cardiac output by 1·0–1·5 litres. With the development of hypovolaemia, blood is directed away from the uterus and there is consequent delay in the appearance of signs of blood loss.

If a pregnant woman is laid on her back the uterus will compress the vena cava and reduce venous return by up to 40% causing the "supine hypotension syndrome". This can be avoided by elevating the right hip and displacing the uterus manually over to the left side.

Once the uterus is out of the pelvis, the fetus becomes vulnerable to the effects of blunt trauma. Placental abruption is the most common cause of fetal death. It is important that the fetus is monitored with a cardiotacograph for at least 6 hours after admission. In rhesus-negative women it is also important to consider the possibility of isoimmunisation of the mother. As little as 0·01 ml of Rh-positive blood will sensitise 70% of Rh-negative patients; therefore Rh immunisation therapy needs to be considered.

## Paediatric trauma

There are a number of important differences that distinguish children from adults:

- The small size and close proximity of major organs result in an increased frequency of polysystem trauma.
- Incomplete calcification of the skeleton renders it more resilient, therefore there is an increased tendency to significant underlying organ damage without overlying fractures.
- Because the ratio of the child's body surface area to body volume is higher than in adults, heat is lost more rapidly. Hypothermia complicates the management of hypotension as it causes resistance to fluid resuscitation.

• Children compensate for hypovolaemia well and a fall in blood pressure occurs late and is a preterminal event.

## Conclusion

Trauma is an important clinical problem. In order to be effective in trauma care, the clinician needs a good understanding of the biomechanics of injury and how it relates to specific anatomical regions of the body. A knowledge of both the physiological and pathophysiological responses to trauma will help the team to provide optimum patient resuscitation. Teamwork is vital.

Tasks must be allocated prior to the patient arriving and must be executed simultaneously. This will reduce the time for the team to complete life-saving procedures.

Finally, the morbidity and mortality associated with injury will be reduced by more focused and effective prevention programmes, and by improving our knowledge of the pathophysiological responses to injury through basic scientific, clinical, and epidemiological research.

## Further reading

Advanced Life Support Group. *Advanced paediatric life support*, 2nd edn. London: *BMJ* Publishing Group, 1997.

Anderson ID, Woodford M, de Dombal FT, Irving M. Retrospective study of 1000 deaths from injury in England and Wales. *BMJ* 1988;**296**:1305–8.

Barton R (ed.). Trauma and its metabolic problems. *Br Med Bull* 1985;**41**(3).

Committee on Trauma of the American College of Surgeons. *ATLS Program*. Chicago: American College of Surgeons, 1989.

Driscoll P, Vincent C. Organising an efficient trauma team. *Injury* 1992;**23**:107–10.

Driscoll P, Vincent C. Variation in trauma resuscitation and its effects on patient outcome. *Injury* 1992;**23**:111–15.

Driscoll P, McMahon G. Trauma. In *Clinical surgery in general: Royal College of Surgeons course manual* (Kirk RM, Mansfield AO, Cochrane J, eds), 2nd edn. Edinburgh: Churchill & Livingston 1998: in press.

Driscoll P, Gwinnutt C, LeDuc Jimmerson C, Goodall O. *Trauma resuscitation: the team approach*. London: Macmillan Press Ltd, 1994.

Grundy D, Swain A. *ABC of spinal cord injury*, 2nd edn. London: BMA Publications, 1993.

Little RA, Kirkman E, Driscoll P, Hanson J, Mackway-Jones K. Preventable deaths after injury: Why are the traditional "vital" signs poor indicators of blood loss? *J Accid Emerg Med* 1995;**12**:1–4.

Skinner D, Driscoll P (eds). *ABC of major trauma*. London: BMJ Publishing Group, 1995.

Stoner H. Metabolism after trauma and in sepsis. *Circ Shock* 1986;**19**:75–87.

Yates DW. Airway patency in fatal accidents *BMJ* 1977;**ii**:1249–51.

Yates DW. Trauma in the elderly. In *1995 Yearbook in intensive care and emergency medicine* (Vincent JL, ed.). Berlin: Springer, 1995.

Yates DW. Trauma care in Europe 1995. In *Update in intensive care and emergency medicine 22: The integrated appproach to trauma care – the first 24 hours* (Goris RJA, Trentz O, eds), Berlin: Springer, 1995.

Yates DW, Woodford M, Hollis S. Preliminary analysis of the care of injured patients in 33 British hospitals: first report of the United Kingdom major trauma outcome study. *BMJ* 1992;**305**:737–40.

# 26: Mass casualty and major disaster planning

M V PRESCOTT and A D REDMOND

A major incident is "any emergency that requires the implementation of special arrangements by one or more of the emergency services, the NHS, or the local authority". For NHS purposes it can be defined as "any occurrence which presents a serious threat to the health of the community, disruption to the service, or causes such numbers or types of casualties as to require special arrangements to be implemented by hospitals, ambulance services, or health authorities".

Incidents may be "simple" with an intact infrastructure, or increasingly "complex" with overwhelming casualties, destruction of local resources, and breakdown of local command structures. The most complex disasters are those that are continuing and national, requiring an international response.

The ability of a hospital to cope will depend fundamentally upon the normal arrangements for responding to everyday, common emergencies. This response will not improve in a major incident. What is in daily use will form the basis of any "special" response.

In a major incident a hospital has two main areas of responsibility:

* *pre-hospital*: to provide a Site Medical Incident Officer, and a Mobile Medical Team;
* *hospital*: to manage patients admitted to the accident and emergency department.

## Major incident planning

The NHS Executive wishes health authorities in Britain to ensure that providers have adequate plans for a response in the event of a major incident. This planning process will involve taking into consideration a number of issues.

### Designated hospitals

The ambulance service will decide which hospitals become the main receiving hospitals for an incident at a particular site and which hospitals will act in support. Increasingly planning is occurring across districts, using more than one hospital to take casualties who will be despatched from the scene to various hospitals in the area. This distribution may be based on geography (fill up the nearest, then move to the next) or on clinical requirements (for example, head injuries sent to the hospital with neurosurgery, burn cases to a burns facility).

### The alert procedure

Notification of a major incident will come from the ambulance service. Exceptionally the hospital accident and emergency (A&E) department can declare a major incident if it is thought that the hospital is likely to be overwhelmed. This decision is passed to ambulance control.

Nationally agreed nomenclature is used (Box 26.1).

## Prehospital response

The site of a Major Incident may be contained or spread out, controllable or confused.

Three different services work there, each having a different command and control system: the police, the fire service, and the ambulance and medical services. Each has different responsibilities and duties:

- The *police* are in overall charge of the scene except in special circumstances when the military may assume command. They coordinate the overall activity of the emergency services at the site, maintain law and order, and investigate the cause of the incident.
- The *fire service* controls rescue and extraction, and contains hazards such as fire, chemicals, or radioactivity.
- The *ambulance and medical services* are concerned with saving and preserving life at the scene and subsequently at hospital. The ambulance service will provide communication facilities for NHS staff and establish

---

**Box 26.1** *Major incident messages*

- **Major incident – standby**
  This is used to notify a hospital of a threatened or impending event (for example, a bomb threat or an aircraft in difficulty).

- **Major incident declared – activate plan**
  This message triggers a full hospital response. The full activation is not always preceded by a warning standby.

- **Major incident cancelled**
  This is used to stand-down the response.

- **Major incident – casualty evacuation complete**
  All receiving hospitals should be notified by this message once all casualties have been removed from the site.

---

a Casualty Clearing Station on-site, treat patients, and transport patients from the scene.

Other agencies may become involved, particularly with a large or an environmental disaster. These include local authorities, industry, and various voluntary organisations.

Traditionally transport of casualties is by land vehicle, but increasingly helicopters and occasionally fixed-wing planes are used. Air transport may decrease the time to hospital and increase the distribution of cases.

## The Medical Incident Officer

The Medical Incident Officer (MIO) is the doctor in charge of the medical resources at the scene. The MIO will wear protective and identifying clothing. Most importantly this doctor must not become clinically involved with patients. The duties of the MIO are to:

- work closely with the Ambulance Incident Officer and liaise with the police and the Fire Incident Officers;
- assess the medical situation;
- establish site triage and with the ambulance incident officer control the distribution of patients to the receiving hospitals;
- direct and control doctors and nurses who attend the scene;
- control treatment of casualties at the scene;
- assess the requirement for additional medical resources and obtain them through the ambulance service;
- communicate with the receiving hospitals' control rooms.

## Mobile medical team

Ideally these teams should come from supporting hospitals, not the receiving hospital. The teams usually comprise one or two doctors and two to four nurses. They should:

- wear protective clothing which is warm, weatherproof, and reflectives and displays their status and identity;
- carry portable medical resuscitation equipment with which they are familiar;
- have available further equipment from the ambulance service;
- be trained in prehospital work and the hazards that could be encountered;
- on arrival, report to the Site Medical Officer and work under his or her direction;
- usually be based at the Casualty Clearing Station;
- be familiar with the assessment and treatment of injured and ill casualties;
- communicate through the Site Medical Incident Officer.

# Hospital response

## Principles

1. A hospital managing a Major Incident cannot function normally. Routine work must stop and resources must be channelled into the response.
2. The management of cases continues after the patients have been admitted. This will require special staffing arrangements on subsequent days, not just the day of the event.
3. Everyday routine emergency cases must also be managed as part of the incident (if it is not possible to divert them elsewhere). Priority of care must be established by taking into account all emergency cases – both from the incident and others.
4. Planning can be based only on the staff who will definitely be available, i.e. those on call. Anyone else who attends should be looked upon as a bonus, deployed immediately, or stood-by.

The responsibility of a hospital is to:

- call out sufficient staff;
- receive, triage, and treat the patients from the incident in the A&E department;
- receive, triage, and treat other emergencies (if not diverted);
- establish a coordination team and a hospital control room;
- make arrangements to admit and further treat patients from the incident;
- open up facilities for the patients (wards, theatres, additional ICU beds);
- liaise with surrounding hospitals to take any overflow;
- manage the patients' relatives;
- manage the media.

## The call-out procedure

Staff can be called in a variety of ways, with bleeps, telephones, tannoy, and "runners". Key staff and departments will be contacted by the hospital switchboard operators. The initial call-out will be to doctors on call in the hospital and to others, to establish control of the hospital. Other staff will be called to support this response. Each department must have a list of staff to call in, usually by telephone. Each member of the first group to be called is tasked to telephone another group who in turn can call more – the "cascade system". These calls should not be via the switchboard, but by direct-dial lines or ward pay-phones. Call-out takes time. Unnecessary calls to switchboard cause further delay. Staff must not 'phone in to recheck messages. Staff and departments will be busy. Media calls must be diverted to an information desk away from the clinical response.

## Identification

In the A&E department the gathering of many staff from various departments may lead to confusion. Others may intrude (for example, voyeurs and reporters). All staff must be clearly identified. Tabbards with roles and status clearly marked are best. For professional groups, such as doctors or nurses, these can be colour-coded.

## Control

A control room is established. This is usually separate from A&E. A senior doctor (usually the medical director), a senior manager (chief executive), and a senior nurse form a team to control the overall hospital response. Information and requests from the treatment areas are passed to this team who will also link with the police information centre.

## Documentation

With a sudden influx of cases there will not be time to register everyone on their arrival. However, it is still important that patients be treated immediately and records made. Hospitals must have a unique set of prenumbered records in special packs held in A&E for the early phase of the response. These packs should also have labels, pathology request forms, and property bags, all prenumbered to avoid confusion. It is important that doctors make notes on each case before moving on to the next – again to reduce confusion.

## Triage

Patients must be sorted into priorities for care. This process will occur at the scene, both for treatment and transport, in the A&E department, and further on into the hospital (theatre lists, intensive care). Triage is a dynamic, continuous process, and priorities will change. The patients' conditions may alter, and so will the required treatment. The aim is to "get the right patient, to the right place, at the right time, and to do the most for the most".

There are many systems of triage. Conventionally a four-point scale is used in the UK:

- *Priority 1*: patients needing immediate life-saving care.
- *Priority 2*: patients needing urgent care (within 6 h).
- *Priority 3*: patients whose care can be delayed.
- *Priority 4*: the dead.

On some occasions a fifth priority is required when the caseload overwhelms the medical resource available:

- *Priority 5*: expectant patients – where a decision is taken not to treat.

Conventionally, the different groups are identified on arrival at A&E and care provided in special areas of the department (for example, Priority 1 in resuscitation, Priority 3 in a clinic area). Triage will also have been carried out at the scene to a varying extent. For prehospital use there are several labels that indicate priority. The best allow the triage category to be changed without fresh documentation (an example is the cruciform card).

Triage is based on the "ABC", but beware of the silent casualty. Noisy patients can be very distracting but are unlikely to be as ill or injured as someone who is quiet. As circumstances change, be prepared to change triage categories.

## Special circumstances

Individual hospitals will have general plans appropriate to their facilities and available staff. However, these plans should also consider the response to special incidents such as multiple paediatric casualties, multiple burns, terrorism, or "medical" disasters such as food poisoning or chemical or radioactive contamination. Unambiguous arrangements must be established with relevant staff (for example, a senior paediatrician, a medical physicist, microbiology) and form part of the general plan. Medical disasters will not require a surgical response but multiple resuscitations will involve anaesthetists, A&E, and ICU staff.

### Burns

There are a limited number of burns units in the country. Burn injuries are therefore a good illustration of triage in the face of local hospital facilities.

An essential part of planning is the identification of a burns care specialist who will attend the receiving hospital to direct triage. Further organisation of care will be required at the receiving hospital. This should be under the direction of a plastic surgeon. These special arrangements may involve inviting specialist teams to work in the receiving hospital (for example, the Bradford stadium disaster) or the tertiary distribution of patients to other hospitals with plastic surgery on-site.

The best place of treatment is a triage decision. Most small partial thickness burns can be managed initially with the patient as an outpatient, either at the receiving hospital or by arrangement with a plastic surgical unit. Those requiring admission can be divided into those who will benefit from admission to a specialist burns centre (intermediate and major burns) and those with lethal injuries. There is little point in sending a severely burned patient to a specialist unit when death is inevitable. This will deny a potential survivor specialist care. Appropriate comfort care should be provided in the receiving hospital.

Burns cases may be complicated by airway burns and smoke inhalation which require early "ABC" assessment and intervention. In the absence of a significant skin burn these patients will need intensive care, but not always in a burns centre. The patients should be taken promptly to the receiving hospital where these triage decisions can be made. Burns cases require quantities of dressings over and above those available in a standard A&E department. Hospital supplies departments must, as part of the planning process, identify a regional source that will be readily available on the day. Fluid resuscitation should follow standard guidelines, for example, the use of Hartmann's solution according to the Parkland formula.

## Chemical, radioactive, and gas incidents

Injuries from gas escape may produce both inhalational injuries and poisoning. Victims are usually not a contamination risk to others. Their management follows the arrangements for a "medical" incident. However, the management of chemical and radioactive contamination and injury is complicated by the need to remove the contamination as well as provide medical care.

Contamination may be on the body surface – fluid spillage or particle/dust contact. Clothing may be contaminated and will continue to act as a source of chemicals until removed. Ingestion or inhalation of chemicals causes more complex problems of elimination and neutralisation. A major problem is monitoring of the substance and quantity involved and adequacy of elimination.

Some types of contamination may injure not only the patient but the people providing care as well, particularly in the case of radioactive spillage. Few hospitals have adequate arrangements to manage these cases. Most A&E departments provide only a simple domestic shower draining into the mains drainage system, yet many chemicals should not be released into mains drains. Washings should be kept for later safe disposal. Monitoring radioactive contamination is easy using the various emission counters available, but there are few available tests for monitoring chemical clearance. Washing with copious amounts of water is appropriate in most cases, except special circumstances such as those involving skin contamination with phosphorus.

Ideally, cases should be decontaminated at the scene before transportation to hospital. This involves establishing zones with access limited only to rescuers wearing protective clothing with airway protection. Decontamination will be performed in the "warm zone" and the patients passed through to a "clean zone" where medical care can start, inevitably after a delay. The establishment of decontamination on site is the responsibility of the fire service assisted by medical and ambulance staff.

Despite these principles (only "clean" patients being delivered to hospital), there may be cases of contaminated patients arriving at the A&E department, often unannounced. Every department must have a clear protocol for their management. This will include setting up a contaminated-to-clean pathway for patients. They should be isolated. Staff must wear protection, which may have to include airway protection. A decontamination unit will need to be used. This may be a portable shower/trolley arrangement where the washings are collected for later disposal, or a mobile unit provided by the fire or ambulance service. Exceptionally a few hospitals have a separate facility. Staff working in these areas are effectively lost to the rest of the department, and will have to be supervised when they remove contaminated protective clothing. They themselves may need to be decontaminated as they leave the contaminated zone. The basic principle is that the main areas in the A&E department must be kept clean.

Only certain hospitals are designated to manage radioactive contamination. These hospitals have a medical physics department. Ambulance authorities should take contaminated patients only to these hospitals. Hospital plans must involve a medical physicist who will establish decontamination areas and supervise and monitor decontamination.

In a large chemical incident there may well be patients who are injured as well as contamined and poisoned. Important decisions will have to be made as to the priority of care in these cases in order to protect and preserve both staff and patients. This is a situation where the principle of the "best for the most" must apply.

## Training and exercises

In the development of a response to a major incident, planning is only the first stage. For any plan to be effective it must be practised in order to familiarise all staff with their duties, and to revise the plan in the light of lessons learnt. Practice exercises can be staged:

- *Communications testing.* A switchboard callout of key staff involved should occur every few months. Staff can respond to the switchboard without leaving their normal duties, causing minimal disruption.
- *Table-top exercise.* Individual departments and the control room responses can be tested this way; scenes can be set and practised with models, either in real time or by taking responses at various times after the incident (e.g. 1 h, 6 h, 24 h).
- *Departmental exercise.* A single department can practise in real size and real time.
- *Full-scale practice.* A major exercise should be conducted at least every two years: the whole hospital can participate. Time has to be set aside and staff have to respond (seriously). Many valuable lessons can be learned, not least that of the real limitations to the response. The main organisational difficulty is arranging the practice in such a way that the routine business of the hospital can continue without disrupting contractual commitments.

319

- *On-site exercise.* The prehospital response is easier to practise for hospital staff because it involves less disruption to the hospital's normal function; linking a prehospital practice to a  full-scale hospital practice, however, can be extremely valuable.

# Major disasters

### The spectrum of disasters

Disasters may be natural or artificial and range in complexity from the most *simple* (a contained, single event such as a train crash, with an intact infrastructure), through increasing complexity (earthquakes, floods, famine), to the most *complex* situation of a war, where the cause of the disaster persists and remains a threat to all those involved, and there is disruption to social infrastructure, roads, clean water, waste disposal, power supplies, communications, law and order, and even government.

A complex disaster may involve population disruption and mass migration. This will require special public health measures to support the people who have moved as well as those left behind. The ability of a single country to cope diminishes as the scale of the disaster increases. Local medical services can become overwhelmed. The initial response in a major disaster is from remaining local facilities. A national response follows and often this will involve the military. International medical aid is required in more complex disasters but will inevitably arrive late.

For many doctors reports of a major disaster or complex medical emergency are compelling. Many would like to help but feel constrained for a number of reasons which include family responsibilities, being in a full-time job, and having no previous experience of this type of work. A doctor's sudden departure may interrupt their patients' treatment, place a burden on their colleagues, and disrupt waiting lists and outpatient clinics.

### Foreign disasters

The needs of those involved in a foreign disaster must be set against the needs of those already in a doctor's care and their current professional and personal commitments. If you are genuinely free to volunteer, only go if you have something to offer. You can ascertain this by contacting major government and voluntary relief organisations. If your skills are required, proceed only if the local authorities in the disaster area specifically request your presence. Otherwise you will only add to their problems rather than relieve. If you are invited, then again do only what is wanted and not what you like. If there is to be any effective coordination, it will come from the host country.

If you do not wish to become part of the disaster, be self-sufficient in food, water, clothing, shelter, and medicines. It is possible that "UNDAC"

(United Nations Disaster Assessment and Coordination Team) will be on site, and will have already established a control centre and liaison between the host government and foreign helpers. Make contact on arrival and take their advice.

## Further reading

Advanced Life Support Group *Major incident medical management and support – the practical approach.* London: BMJ Publishing Group, 1995.

Baskett PJ, Weller R. *Medicine for disasters.* Bristol: John Wright, 1987.

British Burn Association. *Burn injuries – management in major disasters.* BBA correspondence. June, 1996.

Daynes T. Redmond AD. *Chemical and radiation incidents. The Cambridge textbook of emergency medicine.* Cambridge: Cambridge University Press, 1996.

Department of Health. *Emergency planning in the NHS: Health Service arrangements for dealing with major incidents.* NHS Executive Good Practice Document. London: DoH, 1998.

Masellis M, Gunn SWA. *The management of mass burn casualties and fire disasters.* London: Kluwer Academic Publishers Group, 1992.

Redmond AD, Jones J. The Kurdish refugee crisis – what have we learned? *Arch Emerg Med* 1993;**10**:73–8.

Wallace WA, Rowles JM, Colton CL. *Management of disasters and their aftermath. London:* BMJ Publishing Group, 1994.

321

# 27: Metabolic and acid–base disturbances

M MANJI and J BION

The regulation of blood gas partial pressures and hydrogen ion concentration in body fluids is of prime importance for the normal functioning of physiological systems. This chapter describes acid–base and electrolyte disorders, together with relevant aspects of blood gas measurement and their disorders in critical illness.

## Blood gas analysis

Blood gas measurements should never be interpreted in isolation from clinical information: look at the patient first. Trainees often have difficulty with the interpretation of blood gas analyses, perhaps because of the large number of symbols and derived variables offered by the standard printout from a blood gas analyser. The following approach may be helpful.

- **Time and date.** Check that the analyser is correct – the data may be important for medicolegal reasons. Clip the original print-out in the case record.
- **Temperature** (patient, not environmental). The default value is 37°C. Gases are more soluble in solution at lower temperatures, and come out of solution when the sample is warmed. Thus, a sample from a hypothermic patient when measured at 37°C will overestimate the true partial pressures unless the analyser is instructed to "correct" the results for the patient's actual body temperature. This is important only at extremes.
- **pH or $H^+$.** Defines whether the patient is acidotic or alkalotic. The $Pa_{CO_2}$ and base deficit will clarify whether this is respiratory or metabolic in origin.
- **$Pa_{O_2}$ (or $Pv_{O_2}$).** The partial pressure of oxygen in arterial (or venous) blood. Many analysers are calibrated in système internationale (SI) units, so the results will be given in kPa. At normal barometric pressure (1 atmosphere), kPa and percentages are the same (100 kPa = 100%). $P_{O_2}$ measurement identifies hypoxaemia or hyperoxaemia, and requires a knowledge of the inspired oxygen concentration for interpretation. A low

$P$ao$_2$ usually means venous admixture, or "shunting": blood is getting into the arterial side of the circulation without being adequately oxygenated.

- **$P$aco$_2$ or ($P\nu$co$_2$).** An elevated $P$aco$_2$ identifies inadequate alveolar ventilation – a common cause would be chronic obstructive airway disease or respiratory depression from opioids. Hypercapnia acutely produces a respiratory acidosis. Hyperventilation reduces the $P$aco$_2$ but has little if any effect on $P$ao$_2$.
- **Base excess or deficit.** Calculates the metabolic contribution to acid–base disturbance, or metabolic compensation for respiratory acidosis or alkalosis.
- **$S$ao$_2$ or $S\bar{\nu}$o$_2$.** The percentage oxygen saturation. Remember that, because of the sigmoid relationship between haemoglobin oxygen saturation and partial pressure, saturations are well maintained until the $P$ao$_2$ reaches a critical value (around 7–8 kPa) after which the $S$ao$_2$ falls rapidly.
- **Haemoglobin ($0.3 \times$ haematocrit).** These values are estimates and are only accurate to within 1 g either way.
- **Other chemistry.** May include electrolytes, lactate, and glucose. Extreme values may occur if venous blood was taken from the "drip" arm because too much added heparin if a non-blood gas syringe was used, or the results may be genuine.

## Acid–base definitions and values

Acids and bases can be defined in a number of ways; the Brönsted–Lowry definition of an acid and base is used in clinical practice. An acid is a substance that releases hydrogen ions ($H^+$), whilst a base is a hydrogen ion acceptor. The relative affinity for losing or gaining hydrogen ions determines how strong the acid or base is. A strong acid readily and almost irreversibly gives up an $H^+$, whilst a strong base avidly binds $H^+$. The converse is true for a weak acid and base. Acids and bases usually exist in conjugate pairs, examples of which are given in Box 27.1. The dominant species is determined by prevailing conditions as the chemical reaction can proceed both ways.

---

**Box 27.1** *Conjugate pairs*

- Acid $\Leftrightarrow$ $H^+$ + Base
- $H_2CO_3$ $\Leftrightarrow$ $H^+$ + $HCO_3^-$
- $NH_4^+$ $\Leftrightarrow$ $H^+$ + $NH_3$
- $CH_3COOH$ $\Leftrightarrow$ $H^+$ + $CH_3COO^-$

---

---

**Box 27.2** *Normal acid–base values*

- pH $\quad = \quad 7\cdot4 \pm 0\cdot04$
- $H^+ \quad = \quad 4\cdot0 \pm 4\cdot0$ nmol/l
- $PaCO_2 \quad = \quad 5\cdot3$ kPa (40·0 mm Hg)
- $HCO_3^- \quad = \quad 24\cdot0 \pm 2\cdot0$ mmol/l

---

The hydrogen ion concentration $[H^+]$ in extracellular fluids averages 0.00000004 mol/l. Because chemists deal with a wide range of $[H^+]$, Sorenson in 1909 introduced pH, which expresses $[H^+]$ as the negative logarithm to the base 10 and reduces the extremes of the scale to manageable proportions. For example, an $[H^+]$ of 0·00000004 mol/l is more easily expressed as pH 7·4, $[H^+]$ of 0.00000016 mol/l as pH 6·8, or $[H^+]$ of 0.000000016 mol/l as pH 7·8. However, pH is non-linear, non-intuitive, and unnecessary for the range of values encountered in clinical practice. In 1962 Campbell[1] reintroduced arithmetic rather than logarithmic expression for $[H^+]$, and the term nanoequivalent was adopted (a unit equal to $10^{-9}$ equivalent, commonly known as a nanomole). The normal $[H^+]$ of blood and extracellular fluid is therefore 40 nmol/l, equivalent to pH 7·4. In this chapter we use pH as shorthand for "acid–base status", but refer to $[H^+]$ when discussing specific changes in acid or base measurements.

Box 27.2 shows the normal acid–base values.

## Disorders of acid–base balance

Disturbances of acid–base balance are common in intensive care, and reflect a wide range of disease states and therapeutic interventions. Acid–base status is usually determined by analysis of arterial blood pH and $PaCO_2$, but venous blood can be used as a substitute in many circumstances.

### Definitions and classification

Acidaemia or alkalaemia means that the blood $[H^+]$ exceeds or falls below the normal range of 36–44 nmol/l (pH 7·36–7·44). The terms acidosis and alkalosis refer to the disorders or physiological conditions that cause this to occur.

Disorders of acid–base balance are classified as respiratory or metabolic, compensated or uncompensated. A primary respiratory acidosis (or alkalosis) results when the $PaCO_2$ rises above (falls below) the normal range of 36–44 mm Hg or 4·8–5·8 kPa. By definition all other processes that alter arterial pH are metabolic in origin. Thus, four potential primary disturbances exist (Table 27.1) and each can be identified by examining the pH, $PaCO_2$, and bicarbonate concentration $[HCO_3^-]$.

Table 27.1 Compensatory mechanisms in acid-base disturbances

| Primary disorder | pH | $HCO_3^-$ | $P$aco$_2$ | Mode of compensation |
|---|---|---|---|---|
| *Metabolic* | | | | |
| Alkalosis | ↑ | ↑ | | Hypoventilation ↑ $P$aco$_2$ |
| Acidosis | ↓ | ↓ | | Hyperventilation ↓ $P$aco$_2$ |
| *Respiratory* | | | | |
| Alkalosis | ↑ | | ↓ | Renal elimination of $HCO_3^-$ |
| Acidosis | ↓ | | ↑ | Renal conservation of $HCO_3^-$ |

*Standard bicarbonate (SBC)*

This is the concentration of bicarbonate in plasma after fully oxygenated whole blood has been equilibrated in the blood gas analyser with carbon dioxide to achieve a $P$aco$_2$ of 40 mm Hg (5·3 kPa) at 37°C. The purpose of correcting the sample to a normal $P$aco$_2$ is to eliminate respiratory contributions to changes in pH.

*Base excess*

The base excess of whole blood is a measure of the metabolic component of acid–base disorders. It is the amount of acid or base (in mmol) required to return the pH of 1 litre of blood to the normal value at a $P$aco$_2$ of 40 mm Hg (5·3 kPa) at 37°C, and it relies upon the same principle of correcting the $P$aco$_2$ (or $P$vco$_2$) to normal in order to exclude respiratory contributions to pH shifts. It is calculated by multiplying the deviation in SBC by an empirical factor of 1·2 which accounts for the greater buffer content of the red blood cells compared to plasma. Its precision depends on the haemoglobin concentration. For this reason the acid-buffering capacity of blood is decreased in the presence of anaemia.

# Compensatory mechanisms and buffers

The physiological responses or adaptation to pH disturbances involves three phases of compensation:

1. Short-term chemical buffering capacity of the body.
2. Intermediate-term respiratory compensation.
3. Long-term renal metabolic compensation.

Buffers are weak acids and their conjugate salts, which bind reversibly with $H^+$ to neutralise them, reduce their free concentration and hence their effect on pH. The five main buffer systems in humans are:

- Bicarbonate: $H_2CO_3 \Leftrightarrow H^+ + HCO_3^-$
- Phosphate: $H_2PO_4^- \Leftrightarrow H^+ + HPO_4^{2-}$
- Haemoglobin: $HHb \Leftrightarrow H^+ + Hb^-$
- Proteins: $HProt \Leftrightarrow H^+ + Prot^-$
- Ammonia: $NH_4^+ \Leftrightarrow H^+ + NH_3$

Bicarbonate is the most important, providing 75–80% of the extracellular buffering capacity. The $HCO_3^-/H_2CO_3$ buffer system is in a state of dynamic balance with $Paco_2$, thus:

$$CO_2 + H_2O \Leftrightarrow H_2CO_3 \Leftrightarrow H^+ + HCO_3^-$$

The weak carbonic acid $H_2CO_3$ allows changes in pH to be accommodated by subsequent shifts in respiratory $CO_2$. The relationship between these three variables is given by the Henderson–Hasselbalch equation, where $K$ = dissociation constant, and $pK = -\log_{10}K$:

$$pH = pK + \log_{10}([\text{metabolic}]/[\text{respiratory}]).$$

Given a solubility coefficient for $CO_2$ of 0·03 mmol/l:

$$pH = pK + \log_{10}([HCO_3^-]/[0·03 \times Paco_2]).$$

$Paco_2$ and $[HCO_3^-]$ are regulated by alveolar ventilation and renal regeneration respectively. In this way the lungs and kidneys are the predominant control mechanisms for arterial pH.

Haemoglobin functions as a non-carbonic buffer in extracellular fluid because of its large quantity. Proteins are important intracellular buffers, but contribute less to extracellular buffering. Other compensatory mechanisms are of less importance in terms of direct buffering, but are essential for longer-term renal compensation (phosphate, ammonia).

## Acidosis

The $[H^+]$ must be controlled within a tight range because the body's enzyme systems are intolerant of extremes in pH. The effects of systemic acidosis include pulmonary hypertension, reduction in cardiac output, dysrhythmias, and hyperkalaemia. Direct myocardial and smooth muscle depression reduce cardiac contractility and peripheral vascular resistance, resulting in progressive hypotension and decreased organ perfusion. Both cardiac and smooth muscle become less responsive to catecholamines. Severe acidosis may also depress CNS function and cause coma. Progressive hyperkalaemia is seen as a result of compensatory $K^+$ efflux from cells attempting to maintain electrochemical neutrality by exchanging extracellular $H^+$ with intracellular $K^+$. Acidoses may be respiratory or metabolic, compensated, or uncompensated.

---

**Box 27.3** *Causes of respiratory acidosis and alkalosis*

*Respiratory acidosis*
- Alveolar hypoventilation
  - CNS depression
  - neuromuscular disorders
  - chest wall abnormalities
  - pleural abnormalities
  - airway obstruction
  - parenchyma lung disease
- Increased $CO_2$ production:
  - malignant hyperthermia
  - thyroid crisis
  - severe shivering
  - seizures

*Respiratory alkalosis*
- CNS stimulation/disease:
  - pain, anxiety, fever/infection
  - meningitis/encephalitis
  - trauma/tumour/haemorrhage
  - drug-induced, e.g. salicylate
- Pulmonary causes:
  - infection, pulmonary emboli
  - pulmonary oedema
  - high altitude/hypoxaemia
- Shock
- Iatrogenic – ventilator induced

---

## Acute respiratory acidosis

Respiratory acidosis is caused by an acute increase in $Paco_2$ with associated production of excess $H^+$ (Box 27.3). The $Paco_2$ represents a balance between production and excretion. Hypercapnia means inadequate alveolar ventilation for the body's needs, and may be a consequence of primary ventilatory failure (disease, drugs), excessive production (hyperthermia, excessive enteral nutrition), or failure to adjust the ventilator appropriately in mechanically ventilated patients. As with any blood gas disturbance, treatment involves identifying and correcting the cause, not merely treating the effect. Arterial hypoxaemia may also be present together with circulatory failure in hypercapnic patients, resulting in a combined respiratory and metabolic acidosis.

## Chronic respiratory acidosis

Renal compensation for respiratory acidosis is accomplished by retention of $HCO_3^-$, and takes several days to become effective. The blood gas sample demonstrates a normal or near-normal $H^+$, an elevated $Paco_2$, a positive base excess, and markedly elevated $HCO_3^-$. The compensatory metabolic alkalosis may impede weaning from ventilation, and can be aggravated by loop diuretics; acetazolamide may be helpful in this circumstance. The commonest cause is chronic obstructive pulmonary disease. In these patients acute-on-chronic hypercapnic acidosis may occur as a result of an intercurrent process such as infection, trauma, or surgery. Some patients become dependent on hypoxic drive for respiration, and the response to oxygen therapy should always be carefully monitored. However, more patients suffer from too little oxygen than too much, and the risks of oxygen-induced respiratory depression are often over-emphasised. The decision to provide mechanical ventilatory support for patients with chronic $CO_2$ retention is best made in discussion with the patient and family, and well before any acute event precipitates a crisis.

## Metabolic acidosis

Approximately 13 000–15 000 mmol of ("respiratory") carbonic acid and 260 mmol of ("metabolic") non-volatile acids are produced daily by normal cellular metabolism. The non-volatile acids include organic (lactic, hydroxybutyric, and free fatty acids) and inorganic (sulphuric and phosphoric acid) acids. The organic acids can be used by many tissues as a source of fuel under normal circumstances; for example, lactic acid is used by the kidneys, heart, and liver. Under normal circumstances the metabolic acid load is relatively small, but in diseases such as diabetic ketoacidosis this can increase markedly (up to 1000 mmol of hydroxybutyric acid/day).

Metabolic acidoses are characterised by a reduction in $[HCO_3^-]$. Calculation of the anion gap serves as a useful guide to the nature of the abnormality. The anion gap is defined as the difference between the major measured cations and the major measured anions:

$$\text{Anion gap} = ([Na^+] + [K^+]) - ([Cl^-] + [HCO_3^-]).$$

The number of cations and anions in plasma are the same because electroneutrality must be maintained. There is normally an anion gap of 12–18 mmol/l because of the negatively charged proteins, phosphate, lactate, and organic anions. Box 27.4 shows some of the causes of metabolic acidosis.

Treatment depends on the nature of the primary disorder. Any respiratory contribution to the acidosis must be corrected. The role of bicarbonate for correcting severe acidoses caused by excess acid generation or failure of clearance remains controversial. Resuscitation councils do not recommend it routinely in cardiopulmonary resuscitation, because $CO_2$ produced as a consequence of the reaction between $H^+$ and $HCO_3^-$ will diffuse rapidly into cells where it dissociates, producing $H^+$ and worsening the intracellular acidosis. The use of bicarbonate also increases the sodium load and, by artificially correcting the acidosis, may produce a false sense of security. Bicarbonate is evidently appropriate for those conditions associated with excess bicarbonate loss, such as small bowel or pancreatic fistulae, and certain forms of renal disease.

## Lactic acidosis

Elevated blood lactate and $H^+$ are a common cause of metabolic acidosis in critically ill patients. It should be suspected in the presence of an increased anion gap acidosis or a base deficit not explained by ketones or uraemia. Lactic acidosis is commonly caused by anaerobic respiration from

---

**Box 27.4** *Causes of metabolic acidosis*

*Increased anion gap metabolic acidosis*
- Overproduction of non-volatile acids
  - diabetic ketoacidosis
  - starvation
  - lactic acidosis type A, B1, B2, B3
  - rhabdomyolysis
- Exogenous/ingestion of acids
  - salicylates
  - methanol
  - ethylene glycol
  - paraldehyde
  - toluene
- Reduced excretion
  - acute renal failure
  - chronic renal failure

*Normal anion gap metabolic acidosis*
- Increased gastrointestinal $HCO_3^-$
  - biliary/pancreatic fistula
  - diarrhoea
  - ureterosigmoidostomy/ileal loop
  - ileostomy
  - anion exchange resins
- Increased renal losses
  - hypoaldosteronism
  - renal tubular acidosis
  - carbonic anhydrase inhibitors
- Total parental nutrition
- Addition of acid with chloride
  - ammonium chloride
  - lysine and arginine hydrochloride

---

hypoperfusion and tissue hypoxia. Lactic acid is an indirect product of anaerobic metabolism, which permits (inefficient) glycolysis to proceed despite the absence of oxygen, by removing pyruvic acid and $H^+$ from the system, the accumulation of which would otherwise block glycolysis and ATP production.

Aerobic metabolism is energy efficient:

$$Glucose + ADP + Pi + O_2 + H^+ \rightarrow 38 \text{ ATP molecules} + CO_2 + H_2O.$$

Anaerobic metabolism is not:

$$Glucose + ADP + Pi \rightarrow 2 \text{ ATP} + lactate + H_2O.$$

Once oxygen supply is restored, lactate is metabolised via the citrate cycle and the excess hydrogen ions are consumed in the production of further ATP. Aerobic metabolism can also result in $H^+$ accumulation and an acidosis if ATP utilisation is greater than ATP production, as may occur in extreme exercise or malignant hyperthermia.

The normal blood lactate concentration in an unstressed patient is $1 \cdot 0 \pm 0 \cdot 5$ mmol/l. An upper limit of 2 mmol/l can be considered "normal" in critically ill patients.[2] The more common causes are listed in Box 27.5.

Lactic acidosis is conventionally classified as type A and type B according to the presence or absence of clinical evidence of tissue hypoperfusion, but the distinction may be misleading. Type A lactic acidosis most commonly results from imbalance between tissue oxygen supply and use, and may be systemic or regional. Cardiogenic and hypovolaemic shock are examples of states in which systemic delivery of oxygen is inadequate. Impaired tissue

329

---

**Box 27.5** *Lactic acidosis*

*Type A – clinical evidence of tissue hypoxia*
- Hypoxia
- Shock (cardiogenic, septic, hypovolaemic)
- Ischaemia/regional hypoperfusion (mesenteric or limb ischaemia)
- Severe anaemia, carbon monoxide poisoning

*Type B – no clinical evidence of tissue hypoxia*
- B1 associated with underlying disease, e.g. liver disease, diabetes mellitus, malignancy, thiamine deficiency
- B2 associated with drugs/toxins, e.g. biguanides, ethanol, methanol, sorbitol, salicylates, adrenaline, ritodrine, salbutamol, cyanide, nitroprusside, isoniazid, propylene glycol
- B3 associated with inborn errors of metabolism, e.g. pyruvate dehydrogenase deficiency, pyruvate carboxylase deficiency, glucose-6-phosphate deficiency.

---

oxygen use occurs in sepsis and in cyanide poisoning. Decreased oxygen supply in carbon monoxide poisoning or severe anaemia can cause lactic acidosis.[3,4] Mesenteric ischaemia is an example of regional hypoperfusion causing lactic acidosis, as the gut is one of the main lactate-producing organs. Increased muscular work (status epilepticus) may result in increased production of lactate and hydrogen ions. Cocaine in combination with muscular activity may be implicated in lactic acidosis by stimulating glycogenolysis, glycolysis, and vasoconstriction. $\beta$ Agonist therapy (for example, in asthma, isoprenaline as an inotrope) can also provoke lactic acidosis,[5,6] by stimulating glycogenolysis and glycolysis.

A worsening lactic acidosis identifies patients at greater risk of developing multi-organ failure and a high mortality. In type A lactic acidosis, the blood lactate concentration may have prognostic value;[7] where this is caused by inadequate tissue oxygen supply, lactate may therefore be a useful index of severity and a guide to the adequacy of resuscitation.

## Alkalosis

As with acidoses, an alkalosis may be respiratory (hyperventilation) (see Box 27.3) or metabolic, compensated, or uncompensated. Regardless of the cause, there is an exchange of intracellular for extracellular $K^+$ resulting in hypokalaemia. This may decrease cardiac output, increase ventricular irritability, and even precipitate fibrillation if severe. Hypokalaemic alkalosis in the presence of digitalis is hazardous. An alkalosis increases the number of anionic binding sites for calcium on plasma proteins, thus decreasing ionised plasma calcium concentrations, which reduces myocardial performance and increases neuromuscular irritability. The $P_{50}$ of the oxygen dissociation curve is decreased as a result of leftward shift of the oxygen dissociation curve. Hypocapnic alkalosis produces short-term cerebral vasoconstriction, increases systemic vascular resistance, and may produce coronary vasospasm. Severe alkalaemia with compensatory hypoventilation may cause hypercapnia-induced CNS depression.

Metabolic alkaloses are defined as a primary increase in plasma $[HCO_3^-]$. The compensatory hypoventilation is usually ineffective. Metabolic alkaloses may be chloride sensitive (associated with NaCl deficiency and extracellular fluid depletion) and chloride resistant (due to enhanced mineralocorticoid activity). Causes are summarised in Box 27.6. The distinction between chloride-sensitive and chloride-resistant alkaloses is important because the former responds to volume expansion with physiological saline.

## Chloride-sensitive metabolic alkalosis

This is the most common form of metabolic alkalosis and is associated with chloride depletion, a low urine chloride concentration (usually < 20 mmol/l), and a decrease in serum chloride concentration, equivalent approximately to the increase in plasma $[HCO_3^-]$. Physiologically, maintenance of extracellular fluid volume is given priority over acid–base balance. Extracellular fluid depletion results in an increased quantity of cations ($Na^+$) reabsorbed and compensatory obligatory renal tubular loss of $H^+$. The net effect is excess $HCO_3^-$ reabsorption. Electroneutrality can also be maintained by excretion of $K^+$ ions. In addition hypokalaemia enhances the excretion of $H^+$. Indeed, severe hypokalaemia causes metabolic alkalosis.

The most common causes of this type of disorder are the administration of diuretics, and loss of gastric acid either by vomiting or by continuous nasogastric drainage. The gastric juice contains 25–100 mmol/l of $H^+$, 40–160 mmol/l of $Na^+$, approximately 15 mmol/l of $K^+$, and 200 mmol/l of chloride.

---

**Box 27.6** *Causes of metabolic alkalosis*

| *Chloride-sensitive (urine Cl⁻ <20 mmol/l)* | *Chloride-resistant (urine Cl⁻ >20 mmol/l)* |
|---|---|
| • Loss of gastric juice | • Hyperaldosteronism |
| • Diuretic therapy | • Cushing's syndrome |
| • Sweat losses | • Licorice ingestion |
| • Congenital chloridorrhea | • Bartter's syndrome |
| | • Oedema (secondary hyperaldosteronism) |

---

### Chloride-resistant metabolic acidosis

This is characterised by urinary chloride concentrations $>20$ mmol/l, and is usually a consequence of increased mineralocorticoid activity causing extracellular fluid expansion by $Na^+$ reabsorption. This is balanced by compensatory excretion of $K^+$ and $H^+$ resulting in a hypokalaemic alkalosis. Other causes include iatrogenic administration of citrate and acetate in blood and blood products, relative chloride deficiency in lactate-buffered fluid replacement for continuous renal replacement therapy, and high doses of sodium penicillin. The last acts as non-absorbable anions in the renal tubules, resulting in compensatory secretion of $H^+$ and $K^+$ to maintain electrochemical neutrality.

# Electrolyte balance

Fluid distribution within the body is determined by electrolyte and protein distribution. Osmolality and volume control are two independent but complementary systems controlling the composition of the extracellular fluid. Electrolyte imbalance is common in critically ill patients and reflects altered metabolic status.

## Sodium

Sodium is the major extracellular cation in the body. $Na^+$ requirements vary with age. Infants born at 32 weeks' gestation require 3 mmol/kg per day whilst normal adults require approximately 1 mmol/kg per day. Regulation of $[Na^+]$ is achieved by the renal and endocrine systems. The kidney conserves $Na^+$ given the two very different stimuli of hypovolaemia and hyponatraemia. Aldosterone and atrial natriuretic peptide are the main hormones responsible for $Na^+$ conservation and excretion respectively. Antidiuretic hormone does not directly regulate $Na^+$, but controls water balance by affecting its absorption in the renal collecting ducts. Thus $Na^+$ balance is influenced mainly by intake and renal regulation of excretion, whilst plasma $[Na^+]$ is maintained mainly by changes in water content.

### Hyponatraemia

Hyponatraemia (serum $Na^+ < 135$ mmol/l) is a common electrolyte disorder in critically ill patients and may occur in the setting of normal, elevated, or low serum osmolality. True hyponatraemia must be distinguished from pseudohyponatraemia, which occurs with a normal serum osmolality and results from severe hyperlipidaemia (for example, primary lipidaemia, diabetic ketosis, nephrotic syndrome) or elevated serum proteins. This is because the measured concentration is expressed in terms of plasma volume, that is, millimoles per litre of whole plasma and not plasma water. This problem has largely been overcome by the use of ion-specific electrodes.

Hyponatraemia in the presence of an elevated serum osmolality may result from high concentrations of impermeable solutes such as glucose, mannitol, or toxins such as ethylene glycol, which replace $Na^+$ as the osmotically active solute. Hyponatraemia in association with a reduced plasma osmolality is the most common type of sodium disorder. Before determining the cause and initiating treatment, clinical examination of the patient should determine whether the hyponatraemia is associated with a low, high, or normal total body water. Box 27.7 shows some of the causes.

Severe acute hyponatraemia (serum $Na^+$ < 120 mmol/l) is associated with significant morbidity and mortality.[8] It may present as muscular weakness and cramps, lethargy, disorientation, coma, seizures, and even cerebral oedema, with uncal and tonsillar herniation and neuronal death. Chronic hyponatraemia must not be corrected rapidly, as doing so is associated with cerebral dehydration and bleeding, demyelination, and the syndrome of central pontine myelinolysis which has a high morbidity and mortality. The rate of correction of acute hyponatraemia should aim for an increase in serum $Na^+$ of no more than 1 mmol/l per h, and half this rate (12 mmol/l per day) for chronic hyponatraemia. The method by which this is achieved depends on the cause, but will involve either $Na^+$ administration or water restriction in conjunction with treatment of the underlying cause.

*Hypernatraemia*

Hypernatraemia (plasma $Na^+$ > 150 mmol/l) indicates that the body fluids are hypertonic, and that it is a consequence of either $Na^+$ overload or water loss. ADH secretion and thirst are powerful preventive mechanisms; the latter is not available to most acutely ill patients. Initial fluid losses are from the extracellular compartment, followed by progressive reduction in total body water. The common factor in all hypernatraemic states is intracellular dehydration from extracellular hyperosmolality. The clinical features of hypernatraemia affect first the central nervous system[9] (changes in mental status, weakness, seizures, focal deficits, and cerebral haemorrhage), followed by cardiovascular and renal dysfunction. The cells of the central nervous system tend to adapt to chronic hypernatraemia by accumulating increased intracellular solute, and rapid correction may result in cerebral intracellular oedema and further cerebral injury.

Assessment of the patient's extracellular fluid status and circulating volume must be made before correcting hypernatraemia. Hypovolaemic hypernatraemia occurs as a result of renal water losses such as diabetes insipidus, osmotic diuretics, adrenal failure, or non-renal water losses, such as diarrhoea or excess sweating. Oedema in the presence of hypernatraemia

**Box 27.7** *Hyponatraemia in association with hypo-osmolality[a]*

*Low*
- Renal losses (urine sodium > 20 mmol/l)
  - diuretics
  - hypoadrenalism
  - salt-losing nephropathy
  - renal tubular disease
- Extrarenal losses (urine sodium <15 mmol/l)
  - gastrointestinal
  - third space
  - skin (burns)
  - dietary insufficiency

*High*
- Urine sodium < 20 mmol/l
  - CHF
  - cirrhosis
  - nephrotic
- Urine sodium >30 mmol/l
  - renal failure

*Normal*
- SIADH (urine sodium >30 mmol/litre)
- Excess intravenous therapy
  - water intoxication
- Drugs
- Hypothyroidism
- Renal failure
- Glucocorticoid deficiency

[a] Assessment of total body water. CHF, congestive heart failure; SIADH, syndrome of inappropriate secretion of ADH.

indicates $Na^+$ and water overload and is either iatrogenic in origin or due to mineralocorticoid excess.

## Potassium

Potassium is the main intracellular cation, and 98% of total body $K^+$ is intracellular. Plasma levels are a poor guide to total body $K^+$. Its intracellular to extracellular ratio is the principal determinant of transmembrane potentials in conducting tissue such as nerves and muscle. The Nernst equation describes the potential difference (PD) across the membrane:

$$PD = -61 \log (\text{intracellular } K^+ / \text{extracellular } K^+).$$

Thus, relatively small changes in extracellular potassium have considerable influence on membrane electrical stability, as manifest by cardiac dysrhythmias such as atrial fibrillation in the presence of hypokalaemia.

The kidney is the primary regulator of $K^+$, although less efficient in this respect than for $Na^+$. Endocrine control involves insulin, adrenaline ($\beta_2$-receptor mediated), and aldosterone. Acid–base balance is also important in determining the relation between plasma and cellular potassium, as $H^+$ will exchange for $K^+$ as described above: an alkalosis may be either the cause or the effect of hypokalaemia.

### Hypokalaemia

Hypokalaemia is present when the plasma concentration is $< 3.5$ mmol/l. As an estimate during chronic deficiency, a 1 mmol/l reduction corresponds to approximately a 200 mmol deficit in total body $K^+$. Hypokalaemia may be renal or non-renal in origin. The former includes diuretic administration, alkalosis, aldosterone secretion, and nephrotoxic renal tubular damage. The commonest "non-renal" cause of hypokalaemia is that associated with loss of gastric fluid (vomiting, drainage) in which the predominant effect is loss of chloride with secondary inhibition of renal reabsorption of $K^+$.

Acute hypokalaemia tends to produce more serious effects than chronic. Clinical features include cardiac dysrhythmias, impaired catecholamine pressor responses, digoxin sensitivity, muscle weakness, and impaired weaning from mechanical ventilation. Gastric paresis and ileus may occur in critically ill patients. Severe potassium deficiency may cause rhabdomyolysis.

The amount required to correct the deficit can be difficult to predict because it is mainly an intracellular ion; saturation can occur rapidly, and the effect of supplementation should be checked at regular intervals. $K^+$ supplements may be given enterally if there is no urgency, or intravenously by peripheral vein in a concentration of $\leq 60$ mmol/l in 8 hours. More rapid correction using concentrated solutions requires central venous administration (never give concentrated $K^+$ into a peripheral vein), using controlled rate infusion devices in a monitored environment with skilled staff, not unmonitored in an ordinary ward. Spironolactone may be useful for primary or secondary hyperaldosteronism.

*Hyperkalaemia*

Hyperkalaemia is defined as $>5\cdot5$ mmol/l. Pseudohyperkalaemia may occur from haemolysis in the sample tube, or if blood has been taken from the "drip arm". Renal insufficiency is a common cause of hyperkalaemia in hospital. In critically ill patients, acidosis, increased catabolism, tissue necrosis, and rhabdomyolysis can cause hyperkalaemia in the presence of preserved renal function. Pharmacological causes include non-steroidal anti-inflammatory drugs, angiotensin-converting enzyme inhibitors, and potassium-sparing diuretics.

Clinical effects of hyperkalaemia involve predominantly the cardiovascular and neuromuscular systems. ECG changes include peaked T waves progressing to prolonged QRS complexes and ventricular fibrillation, aggravated by acidosis, hypocalcaemia, hyponatraemia, and hypermagnesaemia. Neuromuscular features include ascending muscular weakness, flaccid quadriplegia, and respiratory paralysis.

A rising serum $K^+$ requires urgent treatment. The membrane effects can be reversed in an emergency by depressing the membrane threshold potential with calcium. Insulin with glucose, bicarbonate, and $\beta_2$ agonists can also reduce serum levels by promoting intracellular uptake. Increased $K^+$ excretion requires diuretics, potassium-binding resins, or dialysis.

## Chloride

Chloride is the body's principal anion and the most abundant in extracellular fluid. A knowledge of $[Cl^-]$ is required for calculation of the anion gap. The kidneys are mainly responsible for regulation of $Cl^-$, which acts as the main counteranion for $Na^+$ (80%), $K^+$, and $H^+$, or exchanges for $HCO_3^-$. $Cl^-$ depletion is associated with a metabolic alkalosis and hypokalaemia, correction of which requires $Cl^-$ repletion. The mechanism is related to failure of $Na^+$ reabsorption in the proximal renal tubule because of the lack of the $Cl^-$ anion, with exchange for $K^+$ and $H^+$ in the distal tubule where $Na^+$ does not need a counteranion for reabsorption. Common causes for hypochloraemia in critically ill patients include plasma dilution (mannitol), gastrointestinal tract losses, loop diuretics, and hypokalaemia, and secondary to chronic respiratory acidosis. Hyperchloraemia may accompany a respiratory alkalosis, intravascular volume depletion, and metabolic acidosis.

## Calcium

Calcium is essential for maintaining normal cellular function. It is required for excitation–contraction coupling, enzyme activation, hormone and neurotransmitter secretion, cell division, blood coagulation, membrane stability, and bone structure. In addition it is the most important component of the second messenger systems linking extracellular receptor activation to intracellular events. Failure to maintain intracellular free calcium at low levels during ischaemia and sepsis leads to cellular damage and death. It is regulated by parathyroid hormone, calcitonin, and the active form of vitamin D.

Only half of plasma calcium is both unbound and ionised (1·2 mmol/l), and therefore physiologically active, and it is ionised calcium that should be measured. Moderate to severe hypocalcaemia results in hypotension, dysrhythmias, heart failure, digitalis insensitivity, and QT prolongation. Neuromuscular effects include respiratory muscle failure, bronchospasm, tetany, and paraesthesia, and psychiatric manifestations such as irritability, confusion, and psychoses. Acute hypocalcaemia may complicate inadvertent or intentional parathyroidectomy. Hypercalcaemia usually occurs in renal failure, but may also follow immobilisation, calcium administration, and various hormonal disorders. Clinical manifestations include cardiovascular instability, weakness and lethargy, seizures and coma, gastrointestinal symptoms, dehydration, polyuria, and (when a primary event) renal failure. Treatment involves identification of the cause, fluids and diuretics if renal function is satisfactory, corticosteroids (most effective for tumour-related hypercalcaemia), and calcitonin.

## Magnesium

Magnesium is the second most common intracellular cation and the fourth most abundant cation in the body. Magnesium is a cofactor for numerous enzymatic processes, in particular glycolysis and adenosine triphosphatase. It is used therapeutically as an anticonvulsant, and a prophylactic in eclampsia.

Magnesium homeostasis is primarily determined by the kidneys. Hypomagnesaemia results from gastrointestinal or renal losses, or malnutrition. Clinical features are related to increased neuromuscular irritability and include weakness, respiratory insufficiency, tremors, tetany, and seizures. Cardiovascular effects include digitalis sensitivity, QT interval prolongation, dysrhythmias, vasospasm, and angina pectoris. Hypocalcaemia, hypokalaemia, and hypophosphataemia may accompany hypomagnesaemia and contribute to the clinical features.

Hypermagnesaemia occurs in renal insufficiency, adrenal insufficiency, hypothyroidism, and lithium intoxication. Clinical features are seen at levels greater than 2·5 mmol/l and include neuromuscular blockade, weakness and paralysis, depressed mentation, lethargy, and respiratory depression or failure. Cardiovascular effects include ECG changes (PR–QRS–ST prolongation), bradycardia, heart block, hypotension, and vasodilatation, and eventually cardiac arrest. Intravenous calcium is an effective but transient emergency treatment of severe hypermagnesaemia, and must be followed by enhanced magnesium removal (physiological saline, loop diuretics, or dialysis).

## Phosphate

Phosphate is the major intracellular anion, and it is essential for metabolic activities that include synthesis of cell membrane phospholipids, the phosphonucleotides involved in protein synthesis, and the body's energy storage molecule adenosine triphosphate (ATP). Like magnesium and phosphate it exists in three forms: ionised, chelated, and bound; only the ionised form is physiologically active and regulated. Severe hypophosphataemia is associated with widespread organ dysfunction. This includes muscle weakness and respiratory failure, cardiomyopathy, hepatic dysfunction, metabolic acidosis, immune dysfunction, haemolysis and impaired platelet function, and impaired oxygen dissociation from haemoglobin. Hypophosphataemia should be actively excluded in ill patients, particularly alcoholics, and those with muscle weakness causing ventilator dependence. The clinical effects of hyperphosphataemia are mainly due to the accompanying renal failure or hypocalcaemia from calcium precipitation.

## Zinc and selenium

Zinc has been identified as a constituent of many enzymes. Its deficiency has a marked effect on nucleic acid metabolism, preventing protein and amino acid synthesis. Zinc deficiency impairs growth, cellular immunity, wound healing, and plasma protein regeneration. Selenium forms an integral part of the enzyme glutathione peroxidase which, together with superoxide dismutase, controls the levels of superoxide and peroxide in cells. Without this antioxidant defence, lipid peroxidation of fatty acids would continue unchecked. Selenium and vitamin E are interrelated in their actions. Patients receiving long-term parenteral nutrition should receive zinc and selenium supplementation.

1 Campbell EJM. RI pH. *Lancet* 1962;**i**:681.
2 Mizock BA. Lactic acidosis. *Diseases a Month* 1989;**35**:241–300.
3 Buehler JH, Berns AS, Webster JR, *et al*. Lactic acidosis from carboxyhaemoglobin after smoke inhalation. *Ann Intern Med* 1975;**82**:803–5.
4 Geerken RG, Gibbons RB. Lactic acidosis associated with iron deficiency anaemia. *JAMA* 1972;**22**:292–3.
5 Assadi FK. Therapy of acute bronchospasm: complicated by lactic acidosis and hypokalaemia. *Clin Pediatr* 1989;**28**:258–60.

6 Bracken GL, Johnston SS, German MJ, *et al.* Lactic acidosis associated with the therapy of acute bronchospasm. *N Engl J Med* 1985;**313**:890–1.
7 Vitek V, Cowley RA. Blood lactate in the prognosis of various forms of shock. *Ann Surg* 1971;**173**:308–13.
8 Sterns RH. The management of hyponatremic emergencies. *Crit Care Clin* 1991;7:127.
9 Arieff AI. Central nervous system manifestations of disordered sodium metabolism. *Clin Endocrinol Metab* 1984;**13**:269.

# 28:  Disorders of thermoregulation

A P H STEELE and J H COAKLEY

## Accidental hypothermia

### Definition

Hypothermia is defined as the presence of a body core temperature <35°C. It usually occurs in patients who are vulnerable to the cold because of pre-existing disease or drug overdose. However, it may arise in fit people following exposure to extreme environments, for example, after mountain accidents.[1] In Britain, in winter, about 3% of elderly patients admitted to hospital have a core temperature <35°C.

### Clinical features

The physiological changes in hypothermia are conveniently considered in two stages. The shivering phase, most prominent between 30 and 35°C, is marked by a dramatic increase in oxygen consumption. As core temperature falls to <30°C, thermoregulation is inhibited, shivering stops, and the direct physiological effects of low temperature predominate.[2]

*Metabolic changes*

The large increase in metabolic rate brought about by shivering ceases as core temperature falls. By 28°C, basal metabolic rate is 50% of normal. Blood glucose levels are usually modestly raised as part of the stress response, although in patients with prolonged hypothermia or starvation, levels may be low.

*Acid–base physiology*

Hypothermic patients are prone to metabolic acidosis as a result of increased lactic acid production in vasoconstricted tissues and reduced hepatic capacity for lactate clearance. In the early stages there may be respiratory alkalosis; however, as the temperature decreases below 30°C, respiratory acidosis is usual.

340

Interpretation of blood gases and pH is complicated by several factors.[3,4] At low temperature the partial pressure of gases in solution is decreased and there is an increase in pH from a change in the dissociation constant of the haemoglobin buffer. This means that the readings from a blood gas machine that warms samples to 37°C will underestimate the pH and overestimate the $P_{CO_2}$ and $P_{O_2}$ of a patient with a lower core temperature. The most common practice is to use these uncorrected values to guide clinical management. Temperature therefore leads to a relative alkalosis but probably provides the best internal environment for enzyme function and cell metabolism.

*Cardiovascular system*

Shivering is accompanied by an increase in cardiac output. As core temperature approaches 30°C there is progressive cardiac depression with decreased heart rate and stroke volume. Hypovolaemia arises secondary to a marked diuresis. Despite these changes blood pressure is initially maintained by increases in systemic vascular resistance. Below 25°C, however, hypotension is common. Conduction and rhythm abnormalities of the heart occur with decreasing temperature. Sinus bradycardia may progress through first-degree heart block, associated with prolonged QRS complexes and QT intervals, to complete heart block. The characteristic J wave of the ECG is seen at below 33°C. Atrial fibrillation is common below 33°C, and below 28°C there is a high risk of ventricular fibrillation.

*Central nervous system*

Conscious level begins gradually to decrease at around 33°C until below 27°C patients lose consciousness completely. Cerebral metabolic rate for oxygen falls, once shivering has stopped, by about 50% for each 10°C fall in temperature. This largely explains why the brain tolerates hypothermia well, despite a progressive decrease in cerebral blood flow to 20% of normal at 20°C.

*Renal system*

In mild hypothermia cold diuresis is probably mediated by peripheral vasoconstriction causing stimulation of volume receptors in the central vessels. However, as core temperature falls, decreased renal tubular activity and direct suppression of ADH release maintain the diuresis in the face of hypovolaemia and decreases in renal blood flow and glomerular filtration rate of ≥75%.

*Respiratory system*

The early increase in minute volume changes to a decrease as the shivering phase subsides. At 25°C respiratory rate may be only three or four per minute, and anatomical dead space is increased by 50%.

341

*Gastrointestinal system*

Ileus, hepatic dysfunction, and pancreatitis are all common.

*Haematological system*

With severe hypothermia, platelet and white cell counts fall. There is a rise in haematocrit secondary to the haemoconcentration brought about by cold diuresis. Both disseminated intravascular coagulation and deep venous thrombosis have been described in hypothermic patients.

## Presentation and diagnosis

The diagnosis in a deeply hypothermic patient with a clear history of exposure may be obvious. However, less severe cases are easily and frequently missed. All patients with risk factors (Box 28.1), who appear cool, should have a deep body temperature measured with a low reading thermometer. Core temperature may conveniently be measured with a rectal or oesophageal probe. Infrared aural thermometers, which are becoming more widely available, give accurate temperature readings and are non-invasive.

## Immediate treatment

All patients should have immediate assessment of their airway, ventilation, and circulation. Wet clothing should be removed and replaced with blankets. Patients should be nursed horizontally to avoid the risk of postural hypotension.

## Resuscitation

There have been many reports of survival, often with no neurological abnormality, in hypothermic adults who have suffered cardiac arrest. It is

---

**Box 28.1** *Risk factors for hypothermia*

*Environmental*
- Cold water immersion
- Avalanche
- High wind speeds
- Inadequate or wet clothing

*Patient factors*
- Extremes of age
- Malnutrition
- Male sex

*Disease*
- Myocardial infarction
- Hypothyroidism
- Trauma
- Diabetic coma
- Spinal cord transection
- Erythroderma

*Drugs*
- Alcohol
- Opioids
- Benzodiazepines
- Phenothiazines
- Carbon monoxide

---

generally accepted that hypothermic patients should not be pronounced dead until they have been re-warmed to 35°C. Exceptions to this rule are the patient with unsurvivable injuries, a rectal temperature less than ambient temperature, or an airway blocked by ice or snow.[5]

There is no reason to avoid tracheal intubation in the patient with respiratory failure, as the risk of inducing ventricular fibrillation is small in comparison with the advantages of controlled ventilation and airway protection.

Defibrillation should be used sparingly or even delayed until core temperature is 30°C. Below this temperature there is a reduced chance of success and a risk of myocardial damage. Similar caution should be applied to the use of antiarrhythmic drugs and cardiac pacing at low temperature.

## General measures

Apart from steady warming, the management of hypothermia includes monitoring cardiac rhythm and haemodynamic status with the treatment of complications as they occur. The patient with mild hypothermia may be managed with a peripheral venous line, non-invasive blood pressure measurement, ECG monitor, and urinary catheter. Deep hypothermia requires full invasive monitoring in an intensive care unit (ICU). All patients should have arterial blood gas and routine haematology and biochemistry measurement, including serum amylase. A 12-lead ECG will detect myocardial ischaemia and allow accurate diagnosis of cardiac arrhythmias.

There is no proven benefit from resuscitation with any particular fluid, but Hartmann's solution should be avoided because clearance of the lactate may be reduced by the hypothermic liver. Inotropic support may be necessary, but it makes sense to accept a lower mean arterial pressure than in the normothermic patient. Metabolic acidosis usually corrects with warming alone and bicarbonate administration is not recommended. There is no conclusive evidence to support the use of prophylactic antibiotic therapy.

## Warming

In the absence of randomised controlled trials, there remains considerable uncertainty about the best method of warming hypothermic patients.[4,5] However, the broad aims of treatment should be to start warming at the earliest opportunity, to support the circulation as necessary, and to raise the core temperature by no more than 2°C per hour. Faster rates of warming are likely to provoke cardiovascular instability and are only advisable for patients in cardiac arrest or on cardiopulmonary bypass. All patients should receive warmed humidified oxygen and warmed intravenous fluids in addition to the chosen warming method.

*Passive external warming*

Wrapping the patient in blankets has the advantages of simplicity and freedom from direct complications. However, average rates of warming are only about 0·5°C/h. Passive warming is therefore suitable only for patients who are cardiovascularly stable with a core temperature of more than 32°C. Even in these patients, if core temperature rises by less than 0.5°C/h, then active warming should be considered.

*Active external warming*

There have been several concerns about this method of warming. It has been associated with "cold after-drop" – a fall in core temperature after initiation of treatment. Immersion in warm water, one of the previously favoured methods of active external warming, clearly makes monitoring and therapeutic intervention difficult. Finally, methods involving direct contact between the skin and a heat source can cause burns.

Nevertheless, active external warming is effective and, provided warming is concentrated on the trunk and careful attention is paid to fluid replacement, the risks are small.

Forced hot air warming systems designed for perioperative use have recently been used in accidental hypothermia.[6] The method is convenient, non-invasive, and in one small series of patients there were no complications from cardiac arrhythmia or cold after-drop. This may prove to be the best method of warming even deeply hypothermic patients who have a perfusing cardiac rhythm.

*Active internal warming*

Providing heat directly to the body core is more rational than external warming and avoids the potential risk of cold after-drop. However, it often requires expensive equipment and is necessarily more invasive than other methods.

*Intracorporeal methods*

Box 28.2 shows the methods that have been used successfully. Colonic, bladder, and gastric lavage are of limited efficiency, and gastric lavage also requires tracheal intubation. Peritoneal lavage is effective, relatively simple, and may have particular benefit in some patients with drug overdose. However, it is not risk free and has been associated with fatal infarction of abdominal organs in a 27-year-old patient. Closed pleural lavage has been less widely used but offers the advantage of allowing more rapid warming of the heart rather than other less vital organs. Closed-circuit oesophageal tubes share this benefit without the potential to compromise respiratory function. Radiowave regional hyperthermia (originally developed for treatment of solid tumours) has been used successfully to warm hypothermic dogs. It is potentially the least invasive method of warming the body core preferentially.

**Box 28.2** *Methods of warming*

*Surface warming*
- Forced hot air system
- Radiant heater
- Electric blanket
- Water filled mattress
- Warm water immersion

*Core warming*
- Intracorporeal
  - humidified warm air
  - peritoneal lavage
  - colonic or stomach lavage
  - oesophageal warming tube
  - radiowave energy
  - mediastinal lavage
  - pleural cavity lavage
- Extracorporeal
  - cardiopulmonary bypass
  - arteriovenous or venovenous circuit
  - haemodialysis or haemofiltration

*Extracorporeal methods*

Haemodialysis and arteriovenous or venovenous warming circuits allow rapid increases in core temperature. They are more readily available than cardiopulmonary bypass (CPB) and may be the best methods for patients with a non-perfusing rhythm when CPB is unavailable.

Cardiopulmonary bypass has the advantages of ensuring tissue oxygenation while allowing increases in core temperature >12°C/h.[7] It is the method of choice for warming patients in cardiac arrest, who have a survival rate of about 50% with the method. CPB should also be considered in patients with core temperature <25°C because of the increased risk of ventricular fibrillation on warming. The main problems with CPB are its restricted availability and the need for anticoagulation. A heparin-coated bypass circuit which avoids the latter problem has been used successfully to treat a 13-year-old child with severe trauma. It may be advisable to continue cardiopulmonary resuscitation (CPR) during femoral–femoral bypass to reduce ventricular dilatation in the fibrillating heart.

**Late complications**

Although recovery from hypothermia may be rapid and complete, a number of late complications are well described (Box 28.3). These may largely be explained by the combined effects of direct immunosuppression and severely impaired tissue oxygenation.

---

**Box 28.3** *Late complications of hypothermia*

*Pulmonary*
- Pneumonia
- Adult respiratory distress syndrome

*Cardiac*
- Myocardial infarction

*Haematological*
- Thrombocytopenia
- Disseminated intravascular coagulation
- Venous thromboembolism

*Neurological*
- Seizures
- Cerebrovascular accident

*Gastrointestinal*
- Pancreatitis
- Ileus

*Metabolic*
- Hypophosphataemia
- Temporary adrenal insufficiency

*Renal*
- Myoglobinuria
- Acute tubular necrosis

*Musculoskeletal*
- Frostbite
- Compartment syndrome

---

## Summary

1. Hypothermia usually occurs in association with an underlying medical condition or drug overdose.
2. A core temperature should be taken with a low reading thermometer in all patients who have been found collapsed in the cold.
3. With few exceptions CPR should not be terminated until the core temperature is 35°C.
4. All patients should receive warm humidified oxygen and warm intravenous fluids.
5. Patients with temperatures >32°C may be warmed passively.
6. Patients who have a non-perfusing cardiac rhythm should be warmed on CPB if available.
7. There is no consensus about the best method of warming other patient groups.

However, for all patients, treatment should start promptly and close attention should be paid to fluid resuscitation.

# Hyperthermia

## Definition

Hyperthermia is defined as the presence of a body core temperature of >37°C; severe hyperthermia (or heat stroke) is defined as a core temperature of ≥40·5°C sustained for over one hour. Like hypothermia, it may be associated with environmental exposure or drug toxicity, but may also follow severe exertion. Mild hyperthermia encompasses heat cramps or heat exhaustion, and severe hyperthermia the more extreme cases of heat stroke, malignant hyperthermia, and neuroleptic malignant syndrome.[8]

## Clinical features

Heat cramps usually occur in muscles after exercise, and are due to a combination of water and sodium loss, often exacerbated by replacing lost fluid but not salt. Heat exhaustion is characterised by systemic symptoms such as headache, malaise, dizziness, nausea, and vomiting. It may be distinguished from heat stroke by a core temperature of <39°C and by the absence of confusion. It is important to recognise that, at presentation, the core temperature may have started to fall, and thus the patient with altered mental state and a marginal temperature should be assumed to have heat stroke. The latter is divided into classic heat stroke occurring in high ambient temperatures in those with compromised homeostatic mechanisms, and exertional heat stroke, which typically affects a younger population following either severe exertion or drug ingestion. Drugs may also cause hyperthermia without concomitant exertion.

Classic heat stroke is of slower onset, and often not associated with sweating in contrast to exertional heat stroke. Like hypothermia, hyperthermia is a multisystem disorder, the latter characterised by excess heat production, failure of dissipation, or both. The causes of hyperthermia are summarised in Box 28.4. Most cases in the United Kingdom follow strenuous exertion[9] or drug abuse.[10] Elsewhere, high ambient temperature may be more important.[11]

Drugs implicated in hyperthermia include amphetamines and derivatives, cocaine, lysergic acid diethylamide, mescaline, and phencylidine. Anticholinergic drugs such as tricyclic antidepressants and antihistamines, and those increasing metabolic rate such as salicylates may also cause elevation of core temperature.[12]

### Acid–base physiology

Metabolic acidosis is common, as are production of lactic acid from over-exertion, muscle rigidity, convulsions, or circulatory insufficiency. A respiratory acidosis may also occur.

---

**Box 28.4** *Causes of hyperthermia*

*Increased heat production*
- Increased muscular activity
  - exercise
  - seizures
  - agitation
  - rigidity
- Uncoupling of oxidative phosphorylation
- Stimulation of hepatic metabolism
- Alterations in brain chemistry

*Reduced heat dissipation*
- Behavioural dysfunction
- High ambient temperature and humidity
- Pre-existing disease
- Drug-related

*Specific syndromes*
- Malignant hyperthermia
- Neuroleptic malignant syndrome

---

*Cardiovascular system*

The physiological response to hyperthermia is to maximise heat dissipation by elevation of cardiac output combined with peripheral vasodilatation. The combination of sweating and transudation of fluid into interstitial and intracellular spaces produces a relative hypovolaemia.

Fluid resuscitation should be cautious, since as the body cools volume may be redistributed from the periphery to the core. Cardiac failure may occur, with a low cardiac output and normal or high peripheral vascular resistance. Myocardial contractility decreases when body temperature is >40°C.

*Central nervous system*

Neurological symptoms and signs usually resolve following prompt treatment; however, long-term complications may occur and include cerebellar ataxia, paresis, and personality changes. This is more likely in prolonged hyperthermia and is associated with cardiovascular failure. Petechial haemorrhages and oedema in the brain have been observed *post mortem* in children who have died of hyperthermia.

*Renal*

Renal failure is a well-recognised complication of severe hyperthermia. The causes of acute renal failure are complex but direct thermal injury coupled with hypovolaemia and hypotension are major factors. Myoglobin and haemoglobin release into the circulation, following rhabdomyolysis and haemolysis, exacerbate the adverse effects on the kidney.

*Respiratory system*

Pulmonary oedema may occur from congestive cardiac failure or acute lung injury following severe hyperthermia. The underlying mechanism is probably direct thermal injury to pulmonary vascular endothelium compounded by myocardial dysfunction. Additionally the return of large fluid volumes to the central circulation, as vasoconstriction occurs following cooling and overexuberant intravenous fluid therapy, may lead to pulmonary oedema.

*Gastrointestinal*

Liver injury in severe hyperthermia is almost universal and is reflected in biochemical abnormalities of liver function and clinically obvious jaundice in severe cases. The damage is due to a combination of direct thermal injury, circulatory failure, and hypoxia. Liver failure may compound coagulopathy produced directly by the heat injury.

*Haematological system*

Disseminated intravascular coagulation (DIC) is a common and serious complication of hyperthermia, the presence of which increases mortality. The consequent severe haemorrhage is the usual mode of death.

Clotting factors are probably denatured by the heat and the clotting cascade is activated via vascular endothelial damage resulting in DIC.

*Muscle*

Muscle damage and rhabdomyolysis are commonly seen in severe hyperthermia, particularly that associated with drug abuse and exercise. Muscles swell and become painful, serum muscle enzymes, such as creatine kinase, become grossly elevated, and myoglobinuria occurs. Rhabdomyolysis rapidly impairs renal function and, if not treated aggressively with intravenous fluids and alkali, leads to acute renal failure.

## Presentation and differential diagnosis

The most important differential diagnosis in a hyperthermic patient with altered mental function is meningitis. If signs of meningeal irritation are present and the history unclear, appropriate antibiotic treatment should commence immediately in addition to cooling measures. Later lumbar puncture if necessary preceded by CT scan may clarify the diagnosis.

Hyperthermia may be present in generalised sepsis, which may also be associated with altered mentation. It is important to ask about any recent history of foreign travel, in particular seeking evidence of malaria or other tropical fevers.

Numerous agents may be responsible for toxic hyperthermia and a history of drug intake should be elicited. It is essential to consider this if muscular rigidity is present.

Prolonged status epilepticus or other disorders of increased muscle tone such as abrupt discontinuation of antiparkinsonian treatment, or some psychoses, may occasionally present as hyperthermia.

Rarely neurological conditions involving the pons or hypothalamus or endocrine emergencies such as thyrotoxicosis or phaeochromocytoma may present with severe hyperthermia and altered mental state.

## Immediate treatment

Simple measures may suffice to prevent serious complications; the patient should be removed promptly from the heat stress. Clothing should be removed and cooling instituted by whatever means available. The subject should be sprayed or splashed with water and fanned to encourage cooling by evaporation. Alternatively, exposing the subject to a draught by keeping doors or windows open may be of help.

If available, ice packs should be applied to the neck, axillae, and groin. Oxygen should be given together with a peripheral intravenous infusion of crystalloid. Immediate transfer to hospital should be arranged, after assessment of airway, breathing, and circulation, and support of those functions given if necessary.

## Resuscitation

### General measures

Aggressive cooling measures should be instituted immediately once the diagnosis is suspected.

Immersion in iced baths has been advocated, but may produce peripheral vasoconstriction, thus interfering with heat exchange and diminishing the capacity for heat loss. The difficulties of managing a critically ill patient submerged in a bath make this method impractical, as in hypothermia.

Evaporation of water consumes seven times as much heat as melting the same quantity of ice and thus the most effective methods for cooling use evaporation combined with convection. Splashing or sponging the patient with tepid water and combining this with a continuous current of air may be useful.

The most effective method[13] involves spraying the naked subject with lukewarm atomised water (at 15°C) whilst warm air (at 40–45°C) is blown over the body with the skin temperature kept > 30°C to maintain cutaneous vasodilatation.

Other methods of cooling are of only minor significance; cold humidified oxygen and cold intravenous fluids contribute little to heat loss, but iced gastric lavage has been used and, as a simple procedure, may be used in combination with the above measures.

If cooling methods have failed to reduce core temperature to < 40°C after 30 minutes, then additional methods, such as iced peritoneal lavage, may be useful. This is achieved by instilling 2 litres of iced physiological saline via open peritoneal lavage and draining after 30 minutes.

Cardiopulmonary bypass provides the most rapid technique for cooling concomitant with maintenance of oxygen delivery to tissues, but is only of use if instituted early and is likely to be of use only for cases of malignant hyperthermia occurring in the anaesthetic room. Dantrolene is usually cheaper and safer (see below)!

Antipyretics such as aspirin and paracetamol have little place in the treatment of severe hyperthermia but other specific therapies may be indicated according to the aetiology of the condition.

## Specific therapies

Dantrolene, a hydantoin derivative, inhibits the release of calcium from the sarcolemma of skeletal muscle as well as having muscle relaxant properties. It prevents muscle contraction and thus reduces heat production.

Dantrolene may rapidly reverse the clinical features of malignant hyperthermia and is also effective prophylactically in malignant hyperthermia-susceptible patients when given prior to anaesthesia.

It has been suggested that dantrolene may be effective in neuroleptic malignant syndrome, exercise-induced hyperthermia, and drug-induced hyperthermia. Whilst dantrolene may have a role in neuroleptic malignant syndrome, a large randomised double-blind trial in Mecca suggests that it is of no benefit in non-drug-induced hyperthermia.[11] Although dantrolene has been advocated for use in severe hyperthermia secondary to amphetamine sulphate (and its derivatives such as Ecstasy and Eve), there is as yet little evidence to support any additional benefit over and above that provided by cooling measures and other supportive therapy, and its use as yet cannot be recommended.[10]

Specific therapy to redress neurotransmitter imbalance has been successful in neuroleptic malignant syndrome with the use of bromocriptine, amantidine, and levodopa. These agents lead to increased dopaminergic activity although, as they have always been used in combination with other therapies, clear evidence of their efficacy (as with dantrolene and drug-induced hyperthermia) is lacking.

## Supportive measures

Even after successful resuscitation and stabilisation, further emergency department and ICU management of a severely hyperthermic patient can be difficult and challenging.

Tracheal intubation and mechanical ventilation may be necessary in an unconscious patient to avoid hypoxia and hypercapnia. Agitation increases heat production, and sedation with benzodiazepines may be indicated.

351

Neuromuscular blocking agents reduce muscular activity (and thus heat production), although they may not reduce the muscular rigidity seen after drug toxicity.

Pulmonary oedema from cardiac failure or adult respiratory distress syndrome may require a prolonged period of mechanical ventilation. Hypotension is common and, although it may partially resolve with aggressive cooling, intravenous fluid therapy is almost always necessary to restore circulating volume. Colloids should be administered, and their use guided with central venous pressure monitoring. Fluid therapy should be cautious to avoid volume overload and pulmonary oedema. If hypotension or congestive cardiac failure is refractory, then a pulmonary artery flotation catheter should be used to guide fluid replacement and the cautious use of inotropes. $\alpha$-Agonists such as noradrenaline and ephedrine should be avoided if possible as they cause peripheral vasoconstriction and impair heat loss.

Seizures are common, often manifesting during cooling, and animal studies have shown that prevention of seizures reduces mortality in cases of amphetamine and cocaine toxicity.

Rhabdomyolysis is a common problem particularly with sympatho-mimetic toxicity (for example, amphetamine sulphate, Ecstasy, and Eve), and may also occur in exercise-induced hyperthermia. Patients should be well hydrated to maintain a high urine output (100 ml/h)[8] and mannitol or frusemide may be indicated.

In cases of severe rhabdomyolysis and hyperpyrexia, early use of haemofiltration should be considered to provide rapid cooling, remove toxins (including myoglobin and potassium), and correct acidosis. Hyperkalaemia may be severe, and treatment with dextrose and insulin may be required urgently until haemodynamics have effected normokalaemia. Disseminated intravascular coagulation is a common complication of severe hyperthermia and indicates a poor prognosis. If bleeding occurs, treatment should proceed with blood products.

Liver injury following severe hyperthermia is almost universal and treatment should be supportive. Hypoglycaemia must not be missed and is treated with intravenous glucose.

## Conclusions

1. Rapid institution of cooling and basic resuscitation are essential for the treatment of severe hyperthermia.
2. The accident and emergency department should have a treatment protocol readily available.
3. Attempts to cool patients should not provoke peripheral vasoconstriction.

4. The intensive care team should be involved from an early stage and, in severe cases, the use of cardiopulmonary bypass and early haemofiltration should be considered.

1 Ledingham IM, Mone JG. Treatment of accidental hypothermia: a prospective clinical study. *BMJ* 1980;**280**:1102–5.
2 Cantineau JP, Regnier B. Accidental hypothermia. In *Care of the critically ill patient* (Tinker J, Zapol WM, eds), 2nd edn. London: Springer-Verlag, 1992:1091–114.
3 Stoneham MD, Squires SJ. Prolonged resuscitation in acute deep hypothermia. *Anaesthesia* 1992;**47**:784–8.
4 Danzl DF, Pozos RS. Accidental hypothermia. *N Engl J Med* 1995;**331**:1756–60.
5 Larach MG. Accidental hypothermia. *Lancet* 1995;**345**:493–8.
6 Chevalier P. Accidental hypothermia. *Lancet* 1995;**345**:1048–9.
7 Vretenar DF, Urschel JD, Parrot MD, Unruh HW. Cardiopulmonary bypass resuscitation for accidental hypothermia. *Ann Thorac Surg* 1994;**58**:895–8.
8 Tek D, Olshaker JS. Heat illness. *Emerg Med Clin North Am* 1992;**10**:299–310.
9 Whitworth JAG, Wolfman MJ. Fatal heatstroke in long distance runner. *BMJ* 1983; **287**:948.
10 Watson JD, Ferguson C, Hinds CJ, Skinner R, Coakley JH. Exertional heat stroke induced by amphetamine analogues. *Anaesthesia* 1993;**48**:1057–60.
11 Bouchama A, Cafege A, Devol EB, Labdi O, El–Assil K, Serjaj M. Ineffectiveness of dantrolene sodium in the treatment of heatstroke. *Crit Care Med* 1991;**19**:176–80.
12 Ali MT, Coakley JH. Hyperthermia. In *Cambridge textbook of emergency medicine* (Skinner D, Peyton R, Robertson C, Swain A, Worlock P, eds). Cambridge: Cambridge University Press, 1995.
13 Weiner JS, Khogali M. A physiological body-cooling unit for treatment of heatstroke. *Lancet* 1980;**ii**:507–9.

# 29: Poisoning

K-L KONG and R E FERNER

Acute self-poisoning accounts for about 100 000 admissions to hospital in the United Kingdom each year. Most patients are women, and most are between the ages of 20 and 35 years. Accidental exposure to poisons is rare in adults and, although common in children, harm rarely results. Most self-poisoning is by drugs, of which the commonest are paracetamol, benzodiazepines, and antidepressants. The prognosis is good in those patients who reach the hospital alive: less than 1% will die. Some of the indications for intensive care or high dependency care following acute poisoning are listed in Box 29.1. Supportive care is generally much more important than treatment with specific antidotes. There are exceptions, most particularly paracetamol poisoning, where prompt antidotal treatment can be life-saving. Procedures such as gastric lavage or administration of ipecacuanha can lead to unpleasant and occasionally fatal complications. As the mortality rate in hospital is low, elimination procedures should be reserved for those patients who are most likely to benefit from them, that is, those who present soon after ingesting large amounts of potentially very toxic drugs. This chapter discusses the generalities of diagnosis, management, and supportive care, and also deals with some of the most common specific agents.

## Diagnosis

The history is important and, if the patient is unconscious or uncooperative, additional information may be obtained from parents, spouses/partners, friends, or rescuers. Circumstantial evidence is important in establishing a diagnosis, particularly in unconscious patients and in children. A search may yield empty drug containers, tablets, capsules, or other diagnostic clues. Drug overdose should always be considered in the unconscious patient. Other causes of coma must also be excluded. Whenever possible, the history should include the following:

- nature of the poison;
- route and time of exposure;
- amount and strength of the poison;
- use of other prescription, over-the-counter, or illegal drugs;
- previous psychiatric disorders and self-poisoning episodes;
- evidence of complicating illnesses, such as liver or renal disease, which might impair the patient's ability to handle poisons.

---

**Box 29.1** *Criteria for admission to the intensive care/high dependency unit following acute poisoning*

*CNS depression or excitation*
- Unconsciousness with no response to verbal stimuli
- Uncontrolled seizures

*Respiratory insufficiency*
- Need for tracheal intubation
- Pulmonary aspiration
- $Paco_2$ >45 mm Hg (6·0 kPa) and rising

*Cardiovascular instability*
- Inadequate perfusion pressure (e.g. systolic arterial pressure of <80 mm Hg/10 kPa)

*Rhythm disturbances*
- Cardiac arrhythmias
- Sinus tachycardia >125 beats/min with tricyclic overdose
- Second- or third-degree atrioventricular block
- QRS > 0·12 s (>0·1 s with tricyclic overdose)

*Metabolic disturbances requiring urgent correction*
- Metabolic acidosis or alkalosis
- Hyper- or hypokalaemia

*Need for therapeutic drug monitoring and/or specific treatment*
- Intravenous *N*-acetylcysteine for paracetamol overdose, for example

*Other major organ system failure*
- Hepatic or renal, for example

*Uncontrolled hyperthermia or severe hypothermia*

---

Commonly, a mixture of drugs will have been ingested, often including alcohol and a benzodiazepine. Some poisoning syndromes have been described and their recognition may aid early diagnosis and appropriate treatment (Table 29.1).

## Assessment, resuscitation, and continuing supportive therapy

The initial physical examination should assess vital functions to prioritise treatment and to recognise poisoning syndromes, so that those patients most at risk of developing serious complications may be treated appropriately and specific treatment instituted at an early stage. It is important to appreciate that patients who have taken toxic doses of poisons such as paracetamol may not present with any physical signs initially.

### Airway and ventilation

Food, vomitus, and dentures should be cleared from the airway. An unconscious patient should be nursed in the left lateral position with the head down to reduce the risk of pulmonary aspiration. Comatose patients without an adequate gag reflex and those (few) requiring gastric lavage will need endotracheal intubation to secure and protect the airway. Respiratory function must be assessed at frequent intervals by clinical observation of ventilatory adequacy and rate, and by arterial blood gas analyses. All unconscious patients should receive supplementary oxygen, and mechanical ventilation will be required in those with ventilatory failure.

Opioids, sedatives–hypnotics, and salicylates can produce non-cardiogenic pulmonary oedema. The addition of positive end–expiratory pressure in these patients on mechanical ventilation is beneficial. Patients who develop the adult respiratory distress syndrome with persistent hypoxaemia despite 100% inspired oxygen and optimal ventilatory support should be considered for extracorporeal membrane oxygenation.

### Circulation

The blood pressure, pulse rate, peripheral perfusion, and urine output should be assessed and recorded. Continuous ECG monitoring is particularly important in patients who are poisoned by agents with an arrhythmogenic potential, such as tricyclic antidepressants. Hypotension severe enough to need treatment usually responds to an increase in the intravascular volume.

*Table 29.1 Common poisoning syndromes*

| Poisoning syndrome | Clinical features | Likely poisons |
|---|---|---|
| Narcotic syndrome | Coma, miosis, ventilatory depression | Opioid analgesics |
| Sedative–hypnotic syndrome | Coma, hypotonia, hyporeflexia, hypotension | Barbiturates, benzodiazepines, ethanol |
| Anticholinergic syndrome | Hypertension, tachycardia, mydriasis, dry mouth, hypertonia, hyperreflexia, extensor plantar responses, coma, convulsions, ventilatory depression | Tricyclic antidepressants |
| Cholinergic syndrome | Increased salivary, lacrimal and bronchial secretions, sweating, bradycardia, abdominal cramps, diarrhoea, miosis, muscle fasciculations, seizures | Organophosphate insecticides, nerve gases, anticholinesterases |
| Salicylism | Tinnitus, deafness, nausea, vomiting, hyperventilation, sweating, vasodilatation, tachycardia | Aspirin |

## Conscious level and neurological signs

Assessment of the patient's conscious level should be repeated at regular intervals to follow progress and may also indicate the need for further interventions. Convulsions are commonly observed in poisoning and may be related to convulsant activity of the drugs, or they may be secondary to cerebral hypoxia or hypoglycaemia. When correction of hypoxia, hypoglycaemia, and acidosis fails to terminate the convulsions, parenteral diazepam should be used to treat them. Occasionally, they can be controlled only with an infusion of thiopentone. Refractory situations may require muscle paralysis and mechanical ventilation.

## Body temperature

Salicylates, stimulants such as Ecstasy, and drugs with anticholinergic properties may produce hyperthermia by interfering with metabolism and reducing perspiration. Often, observation and a low environmental temperature will suffice. Patients with dangerously elevated body temperature ($>39°C$) will require active cooling measures such as tepid sponging and cold saline gastric lavage, and dantrolene may be needed.

Overdoses of tricyclic antidepressants, alcohol, opioids, barbiturates, and other sedatives may produce hypothermia from disturbance of central mechanisms, vasodilatation, and prolonged exposure. Careful and gradual rewarming with humidified gases, space blankets, and warmed infusion fluids is the usual treatment. ECG monitoring is essential since arrhythmias may occur during rewarming.

## Metabolic complications

Metabolic acidosis is a common complication of severe poisoning and may arise indirectly as a consequence of poor tissue perfusion and hypoxia, or may be due to specific toxic effects such as those following the ingestion of salicylates, alcohols, ethylene glycol, or phenformin. An elevated osmolar gap in the presence of metabolic acidosis is suggestive of poisoning with methanol or ethylene glycol. Treatment of metabolic acidosis should be directed at the cause, such as the restoration of an adequate perfusion pressure and the correction of hypoxia, as the use of compensatory hyperventilation and sodium bicarbonate has inherent limitations.

## Psychiatric and social assessment

All adult patients admitted with acute poisoning should be referred for psychiatric and, if necessary, social assessment.

## Non-toxicological investigations[1-3]

Standard haematological and biochemical investigations, and blood gas analyses are sometimes helpful in managing poisoned patients and may also provide clues to the diagnosis.

- *Blood sugar.* Hypoglycaemia is usually due to overdosage with insulin, oral hypoglycaemics, ethanol, or salicylates. It may also occur following paracetamol-induced liver failure.
- *Electrolytes.* Hypokalaemia is commonly seen in poisoning with theophyllines and $\beta_2$ agonists. Hyperkalaemia is caused by poisons that cause acute renal failure, haemolysis, or rhabdomyolysis, or which inhibit the membrane $Na^+/K^+$ pump such as digoxin. Measurement of serum electrolytes also allows calculation of the anion gap. An elevated anion gap in conjunction with a low serum bicarbonate is suggestive of poisoning with salicylates, methanol, or ethylene glycol.
- *Urea and creatinine.* These are useful baseline measurements since many drugs are dependent on normal renal function for elimination, and some drugs cause renal failure.
- *Liver function tests.* These are useful baseline investigations, particularly important in suspected paracetamol overdose, when the plasma liver enzymes' activity can be massively elevated and the prothrombin time prolonged.
- *Osmolality.* An elevated osmolar gap suggests poisoning with methanol or ethylene glycol.
- *Arterial blood gas analysis.* This is essential, in severely ill patients, for determining acid–base status and oxygenation, and as a guide to severity of poisoning, particularly with paracetamol.
- *Urinalysis.* Haemoglobinuria occurs in haemolysis, and myoglobinuria in rhabdomyolysis.
- *Chest radiograph.* Pulmonary aspiration is common in severely poisoned patients, especially if gastric lavage has been performed with an unprotected airway. Pulmonary oedema may occur in overdosage with opioids or salicylates.
- *ECG.* Many agents cause myocardial irritability, tachycardia, or conduction disturbances. Characteristic ECG changes are seen in overdosing with tricyclic antidepressants, cardiac glycosides, or potassium salts.

## Role of the toxicology laboratory

In general, toxicological investigations should be requested only if they are likely to aid diagnosis or influence the management of the patient. These requests are rarely an emergency except in patients who may have taken paracetamol, where urgent measurements are crucial. There is no simple test that would detect all of the drugs and other poisons that might have been ingested by a patient. A wide variety of substances could be involved and patients may also have ingested "cocktails" of substances with or without alcohol. If laboratory screening is considered necessary, this must be discussed in advance with the laboratory staff to ensure optimum patient care.

---

**Box 29.2**  *Useful indications for toxicological investigations*

- Assessment of the severity of poisoning (quantitative analyses)
- Where a diagnosis of poisoning is uncertain, particularly in children
- In the differential diagnosis of coma
- Where administration of an antidote depends on the rapid identification of a poison and its concentration in blood
- To predict complications and plan for subsequent management
- To monitor the efficacy of an active elimination technique or antidote

---

Box 29.2 summarises some of the useful indications for toxicological investigations. A toxicological screen is usually carried out on specimens of urine (30 ml for qualitative tests) and blood (10 ml for qualitative and quantitative tests). Most district general hospitals will have the facilities to screen for paracetamol, salicylate, and ethanol overdosage. Screening for some other common drugs such as phenytoin, digoxin, carbamazepine, and lithium may also be available locally. Hospitals with co-oximeters will also be able to determine carbon monoxide saturations. For more comprehensive screening and for more unusual qualitative and quantitative tests (such as poisoning with herbicides), referral to a regional laboratory is necessary. Box 29.3 lists the centres of the United Kingdom Poisons Information Service. These centres should be contacted for further poisons information, clinical advice, and local availability of specialist tests.

---

**Box 29.3**  *The United Kingdom Poisons Information Service – list of centres*

- *Belfast.* Poisons Information Centre, Royal Victoria Infirmary, Grosvenor Road, Belfast BT12 6BB. Tel: 01232 240503.
- *Birmingham.* West Midlands Poisons Unit, City Hospital, Dudley Road, Birmingham B18 7QH. Tel: 0121 5075588.
- *Cardiff.* Welsh National Poisons Unit, Ward West 5, Llandough Hospital NHS Trust, Cardiff CF64 2XX. Tel: 01222 709901.
- *Edinburgh.* Scottish Poisons Information Bureau, The Royal Infirmary, Lauriston Place, Edinburgh EH3 9YW. Tel: 0131 5362300.
- *Leeds.* Leeds Poisons Information Service, Pharmacy Department, The General Infirmary, Great George Street, Leeds LS1 3EX. Tel: 0113 2340715.
- *London.* Medical Toxicology Unit, Avonley Road, London SE14 5ER. Tel: 0171 6359191.
- *Newcastle:* Northern and Yorkshire Regional Drug and Therapeutics Centre, Wolfson Unit, Claremont Place, Newcastle upon Tyne NE1 4LP. Tel: 0191 2325131.

---

# Reducing drug absorption

## Decontamination

Measures that help to reduce the amount of poison absorbed systemically from the skin, eyes, and mucous membranes may prevent the development or reduce the seriousness of poisoning. Certain agents, such as organophosphate and carbamate insecticides, are readily absorbed through the intact skin. Liberal body washes with water can be life-saving.

## Induced emesis

Although syrup of ipecacuanha 6% is an effective emetic in children, there is little evidence that its use prevents significant absorption of poison. Clinical studies have found no benefit from ipecac-induced emesis.[4,5] The technique is also associated with significant adverse effects: aspiration pneumonitis, Mallory–Weiss tear of the oesophagus, intracranial haemorrhage, and ipecac poisoning. Inducing emesis cannot be recommended.

## Gastric lavage

The current view is that gastric lavage has a very limited role.[5] Gastric emptying studies in experimental animals have shown no impressive drug recovery, particularly if lavage was delayed for an hour. Volunteer studies also provide no support for the use of gastric lavage. Gastric lavage should be considered only in patients who have ingested a life-threatening amount of poison within an hour previously. It should not be performed in a patient with an unprotected airway. Other important contraindications to its use include:

- poisoning with corrosives, caustics, and acids because oesophageal or gastric perforation may occur;
- poisoning with petroleum derivatives or hydrocarbons, because inhalation causes intense pneumonitis;
- patients who are at risk of haemorrhage or perforation due to pathology or recent surgery.

Gastric lavage may result in significant morbidity secondary to laryngospasm, pulmonary aspiration, and cardiac arrhythmias.

## Activated charcoal

Activated charcoal has now replaced induced emesis and gastric lavage as first-line treatment for acute poisoning. Activated charcoal is a fine, black powder produced by burning organic materials and treating the residue with chemicals or steam to increase surface area and remove impurities. Oral activated charcoal is not absorbed through the gastrointestinal tract but is very absorbent of most drugs and poisons. However, it is not useful for the treatment of poisoning with ethanol, methanol, ethylene glycol, strong acids or alkalis, iron, or lithium.[6] It is probably ineffective more than 1–2 hours after ingestion.

## Enhancing elimination

Methods of enhancing elimination of poisons, such as repeated dose oral activated charcoal, diuresis with ion trapping, dialysis, and haemoperfusion (Table 29.2) are all potentially dangerous, and should be used only when they will clearly be of benefit to the patient.

Table 29.2 Enhancing the elimination of poisons

| Techniques used | Agents for which technique may be helpful |
| --- | --- |
| Repeated dose oral activated charcoal | Aminophylline, theophylline, amitriptyline, nortriptyline, carbamazepine, phenytoin, dapsone, phenobarbitone, quinine, paracetamol, salicylates |
| Diuresis with ion trapping | Salicylates |
| Dialysis | Salicylates, methanol, ethylene glycol, lithium, metformin |
| Haemoperfusion | Theophylline, barbiturates, phenytoin, carbamazepine |

### Repeated dose oral activated charcoal

Repeated dose oral activated charcoal removes poisons by three distinct mechanisms:

- Drug that is still in the gut can be adsorbed before systemic absorption can occur. This particularly applies to slow-release preparations, such as theophylline, and to drugs that are absorbed slowly because they decrease gut motility.
- Charcoal adsorbs drugs secreted in bile, thereby preventing enterohepatic recirculation.
- Activated charcoal can trap any drug that diffuses from the circulation into the gut lumen. After absorption, a drug will re-enter the gut by passive diffusion, provided that the concentration there is lower than that in the blood. Adsorption of drug by charcoal in the gut lumen ensures that this concentration gradient is maintained.

The efficacy of charcoal depends on the dose ratio of charcoal to drug; the higher this ratio the more efficacious the elimination of poison.[7] For maximum efficacy therefore charcoal should be given at a rate that keeps the small intestine filled. It is administered orally or by nasogastric tube. The initial dose in an adult is 50 g of oral activated charcoal as a slurry in 400 ml of water; in a child this is 1 g in 10 ml/kg bodyweight. Half the initial dose (25 g in 200 ml water in an adult) should be given every two hours until the patient is asymptomatic, or the plasma level of poison has fallen below the toxic range, or charcoal fills the gut, as evidenced by charcoal black stool. Oral activated charcoal has some disadvantages. It is a black and unpalatable slurry, commonly inducing vomiting in the conscious patient. There is a danger of aspiration pneumonia, and severe constipation may lead to intestinal obstruction.

## Diuresis with ion trapping

Drugs cross biomembranes most readily when unionised and remain in aqueous solution most readily when ionised. If a drug is excreted in the urine, reabsorption can be prevented by ensuring that it remains ionised. For a drug that is acidic, the concentration of ionised drug increases as the pH increases. Urinary alkalinisation will increase the proportion of ionised drug and reduce reabsorption. The converse is true for a basic drug.

Whilst these techniques were widely used in the past, acid diuresis is now largely of historical interest. Alkaline diuresis is still used for treating poisoning with carbamate insecticides and sometimes aspirin. It can be induced by infusing sodium bicarbonate solution or giving sodium bicarbonate orally to a target urinary pH > 7·5, although this is difficult to achieve in practice. The technique requires careful biochemical and haemodynamic monitoring because hypokalaemia, hypernatraemia, and pulmonary or cerebral oedema can result.

## Dialysis

The efficacy of the technique depends on the permeability of the dialysis membrane to the drug, the concentration gradient, and the proportion of the drug that is in the circulating blood volume. It is of no practical value for drugs that have large volumes of distribution such as the tricyclic antidepressants. Only free drug is dialysable, so drugs that are highly protein bound cannot be efficiently removed. Haemodialysis is more effective than peritoneal dialysis, but is less widely available, takes longer to set up, and is more expensive.

## Haemoperfusion

In haemoperfusion, blood is pumped down a column containing the adsorbent from which it is separated by a biocompatible membrane. The poison is retained by the adsorbent: activated charcoal is the most popular choice. The major indication for haemoperfusion at present is severe theophylline overdosage in a critically ill patient in whom conventional therapy with repeated dose oral activated charcoal is impossible.

# Specific poisoning agents

## Paracetamol[8]

Paracetamol is the commonest cause of hospital admission with potentially serious poisoning in Britain, but fortunately antidotal treatment in the early stages can prevent serious damage. It tends to be less common in other countries. Paracetamol does not itself cause damage, but in overdosage it is metabolised to a toxic metabolite, $N$-acetyl-$p$-benzoquinoneimine (NABQI or NAPQI). NABQI binds preferentially to sulphydryl (-SH) groups, initially in hepatic glutathione and then in cellular proteins, which are damaged. Hepatic and renal failure ensue. They can be prevented by giving $N$-acetylcysteine, which acts as a source of -SH groups. Methionine, given orally, can also be effective, but there is the danger that a seriously poisoned patient will vomit it. Patients who become sufficiently ill to require intensive care will usually have received antidotal treatment too late, or not at all.

### Clinical features

One of the cruelties of paracetamol poisoning is that early symptoms can be few or absent, even in cases that will end fatally. Nausea is common; vomiting should be taken as a sign of potentially serious overdosage, not an indication that there is little drug left in the body. After a day or so, severely poisoned patients may develop right upper quadrant abdominal pain, and over the next one or two days there can be oliguria, loin pain, and the gradual onset of jaundice, and then frank renal failure and hepatic encephalopathy. Rarely, patients can develop renal failure without hepatic failure. Death is due to hepatic encephalopathy, and usually ensues when the patient develops intractable cerebral oedema or cardiac instability.

### Management

$N$-Acetylcysteine is uniformly successful in preventing serious liver damage in patients with potentially severe poisoning, provided that it is given within eight hours of ingestion. It is beneficial up to 24 hours after ingestion, and also in those patients who have actually developed encephalopathy. Previous concerns that the drug would worsen encephalopathy have proved groundless.

The decision to treat rests on the history of paracetamol ingestion, the time from ingestion to intervention, and the value of the serum paracetamol concentration measured four hours or more after ingestion. Concentrations measured earlier than four hours after ingestion are uninterpretable, because absorption may not be complete. After 16 hours, it is possible for paracetamol concentrations to be below the limit of detection of the assay, even in patients who have been severely poisoned. In between these times,

363

a graph of paracetamol concentration against time from ingestion will guide treatment.[1,8]

Because of delays in establishing the concentration, and because the efficacy of the antidote wanes with time from about eight hours after ingestion, it is sensible to start antidotal treatment in all patients who present more than six hours after taking potentially toxic doses of paracetamol. In those whose plasma paracetamol concentrations are subsequently found to be "below the line" on the graph, treatment can be stopped. In those patients who are especially susceptible to the toxic effects of paracetamol (that is, those on enzyme-inducing drugs such as carbamazepine or phenobarbitone), those who chronically abuse alcohol, and those who are malnourished as a consequence of AIDS or other illness, treatment should be given at a paracetamol concentration half that which would indicate treatment in previously fit patients.

Patients who present > 16 hours from ingestion are those most likely to develop serious toxicity, although this can be excluded if 24 hours or more have elapsed from ingestion and there is no paracetamol in the blood, and serum creatinine concentration and prothrombin time are normal. All other patients should be treated as though they were at risk of serious renal or hepatic damage, and given N-acetylcysteine. Urinary metabolites of paracetamol are excreted for several days after overdosage, and so can be used to make the diagnosis even in patients who present in hepatic failure.

*Management of patients with severe paracetamol poisoning*

N-Acetylcysteine infusion reduces the chances of serious liver damage in the first 24 hours, and improves the prognosis in encephalopathic patients.[9] The infusion should be continued until there is evidence of recovery. Lactulose, and if necessary magnesium sulphate enemas, can be given. A prolonged prothrombin time will be followed by hypoglycaemia; frequent blood glucose estimations must be made, and hypoglycaemia corrected with intravenous glucose. Fluid management is often difficult, because dehydration can cause oliguria, but excessive fluid replacement in a patient developing hepatic encephalopathy will aggravate cerebral oedema. Serum sodium must be monitored; hypo- or hypernatraemia must be avoided. The development of a metabolic acidosis is a serious adverse prognostic factor, but in itself rarely requires correction. Because of the prognostic value of the prothrombin time, it should not be corrected with fresh frozen plasma unless there is active bleeding. Vitamin K has no beneficial effect.

Patients whose prothrombin times are rising rapidly or are very prolonged (> 180 s) and those with hypotension and a severe metabolic acidosis are likely to die. It is best to discuss the management of these patients with a specialist liver unit before they become encephalopathic. Delay in referral virtually guarantees subsequent death, as transplantation offers the only chance of survival. Encephalopathy develops rapidly, with progressive cerebral oedema and brain-stem herniation. Interhospital transfer must be conducted by an experienced anaesthetist or intensivist with full resuscitation equipment and adequate assistance. Patients should be transferred unintubated only if they have no evidence of encephalopathy, and if the medical attendant is prepared to intubate in the ambulance. Sedative drugs must not be given to unintubated patients. Mannitol 0·5 g/kg i.v. may be given to patients with grade IV encephalopathy if there is pupillary dilatation. Adequate mechanical (not manual) ventilation with satisfactory $CO_2$ clearance must be confirmed before departure.

## Tricyclic antidepressant drugs

Patients with depression are, *a priori*, at greater risk of attempting suicide than others, and so there is a disproportionate number of poisonings with antidepressant drugs. Tricyclic antidepressants are frequently taken and potentially lethal. All produce similar signs of anticholinergic action, convulsion, and cardiotoxicity.

*Clinical features*

Patients who are seriously poisoned often are, or become, deeply unconscious, and the combination of coma, tachycardia, and dilated pupils is characteristic. Early death is usually due to cardiac arrhythmia, and this can be precipitated by washing drug into the duodenum during gastric lavage. Intractable cardiogenic shock ("stone heart") can also occur. Convulsions and hypotension will be seen in many cases of moderate or severe poisoning.

Confusion and agitation are common, especially during recovery from coma. The ECG is a very useful index of the severity of poisoning. Sinus tachycardia, prolongation of the corrected Q-T interval, broadening of the QRS complexes, and then ventricular arrhythmias indicate poisoning of increasing severity. Blood or urine tricyclic concentrations can help to establish the diagnosis, but are not useful in determining management.

*Management*

Unconscious patients require endotracheal intubation if the gag reflex is absent, and if mechanical ventilation is necessary. If the ECG shows broad QRS complexes or there is a tachyarrhythmia, then the treatment is to infuse 50 mmol of sodium bicarbonate over 15–20 min (even if there is no acidosis), and to ensure that $Pao_2$ and electrolytes are normal. Standard antiarrhythmic drugs used for treating arrhythmia associated with ischaemia are contraindicated and can make matters worse. If life-threatening arrhythmias demand immediate treatment or fail to respond to bicarbonate infusion, then defibrillation or overpacing is necessary. Young patients with no pre-existing heart disease who sustain cardiac arrests can survive several hours of cardiopulmonary resuscitation. Fits or myoclonic jerks are often brief, and require no specific treatment. However, fits lasting long enough to cause hypoxia can be treated with intravenous diazepam. In patients who are stable, and in whom the airway is protected, it is sensible to wash out the stomach and then give activated charcoal orally or by nasogastric tube. Repeated doses enhance the elimination of amitriptyline,[10] and probably other tricyclics,[11] but have not been shown to produce clinical benefit. Even the most seriously poisoned patients usually recover consciousness within one or two days.

## Salicylates

Although poisoning with aspirin, methylsalicylate (oil of wintergreen), or other salicylates is now relatively uncommon in the UK, it remains common in other countries. The management of serious poisoning remains difficult.

### Clinical features

Salicylates act in several ways: there is stimulation of the respiratory centre, with consequent hyperventilation and respiratory alkalosis; cellular metabolism is disrupted, so that metabolic acidosis, hypoglycaemia, and hyperpyrexia occur; and gastric irritation leads to vomiting and dehydration, with haematemesis occasionally. Non-cardiogenic pulmonary oedema is an unexplained feature of severe overdosage. Tinnitus occurs in most patients with moderate or severe poisoning, and is therefore an important clinical feature. Central nervous system effects, such as excitement or unconsciousness, are rare in adults.

### Management

Patients with a normal venous bicarbonate and anion gap are unlikely to have salicylate poisoning sufficient to require treatment. However, in patients with abnormalities of blood chemistry who may have taken an overdose, arterial blood gases and plasma salicylate concentration should be measured. Patients with symptoms are likely to have salicylate concentrations >300 mg/l. Serious poisoning is indicated by the clinical state of the patient, the degree of acid–base disturbance, and a plasma salicylate concentration that is usually >700 mg/l.

Elimination of drug can probably be enhanced by repeated doses of oral activated charcoal,[12] and it is reasonable to administer this to all symptomatic patients until the symptoms have resolved. Urinary alkalinisation is an alternative or additional treatment. Glucose should be given to prevent or treat hypoglycaemia, and potassium to correct hypokalaemia if present. In seriously poisoned patients, the safest and surest method of removing salicylate, counteracting the acid–base disturbances, and avoiding pulmonary oedema is to institute haemodialysis.[13]

## Digoxin

Digoxin has a low therapeutic index, and so chronic iatrogenic poisoning is relatively common, but acute overdosage is rare. The drug is renally excreted, so intoxication can follow a deterioration in renal function. It acts at the membrane $Na^+/K^+$ ATPase pump, and this means that hypokalaemia enhances the toxicity, and that severe toxicity with paralysis of the pump is indicated by hyperkalaemia.

### Clinical features

The classic features of intoxication include anorexia, nausea, diarrhoea, visual disturbances, and cardiac arrhythmia. The ECG can show any arrhythmia, although first-, second-, or third-degree heart block with bradycardia is characteristic if the patient has been in sinus rhythm. Bigeminy is common, and other ventricular arrhythmias are important. Urea and electrolyte concentrations should be measured, and arterial blood gas analyses can be useful.

### Management

The serum potassium concentration is likely to be elevated in patients with severe poisoning, and should be treated, if >6 mmol/l, with intravenous insulin and glucose. Bradycardia can respond to atropine, but electrical pacing may be necessary. Malignant arrhythmias that cause hypotension are a reason for antidotal treatment with specific Fab fragments of goat antidigoxin antibodies. They may also respond to intravenous phenytoin or to amiodarone administered via a central venous catheter. If there is clinical or biochemical evidence of severe poisoning, digoxin concentrations should, if possible, be measured urgently, because the dose of Fab antidote is best calculated from it. The concentration does not, however, help much in the assessment of poisoning, since time from overdosage, and the acuteness or chronicity of intoxication, greatly influence the tissue effects of a given serum concentration. If a digoxin concentration cannot be measured at once, or at all, then the dosage can be calculated on the basis of the amount of digoxin ingested and the weight of the patient. The expense of the antidote means that it is best reserved for patients with serious arrhythmias or severe hyperkalaemia.

## Theophylline and aminophylline

These drugs are still used to treat asthma, and are often available in slow-release form. Intoxication can arise from therapeutic misadventure, for example, when the metabolism of theophylline is inhibited by concomitant prescription of erythromycin or ciprofloxacin, or from deliberate overdosage.

*Clinical features*

These include nausea, vomiting (sometimes with haematemesis), sinus tachycardia and tachyarrhythmias, restlessness, convulsion, coma, rhabdomyolysis, metabolic acidosis, hypoglycaemia, and hypokalaemia. Patients die either as a result of the convulsion or as a consequence of cardiac effects. Seizures, ventricular tachycardia, and hypotension are markers of severe poisoning when theophylline concentrations are usually > 50 mg/l.

*Management*

Correction of acidosis, hypokalaemia, and hypoglycaemia is important. In moderately severe poisoning in patients who are not asthmatic, a β blocker can help to alleviate tachycardia and restore normokalaemia. Convulsions can be treated with parenteral diazepam. Most patients have severe vomiting that may respond to parenteral haloperidol, but, when this is unsuccessful, ondansetron can be useful. When the patient has stopped vomiting and the airway is secure, repeated doses of activated charcoal by nasogastric tube will enhance the elimination of theophylline from the blood,[14] and reduce the absorption of slow-release preparations from the gut. In seriously poisoned patients, who cannot be treated with oral activated charcoal, charcoal haemoperfusion is a very effective method of reducing theophylline concentrations.[15]

# Conclusion

Acute poisoning is a common medical emergency. In general, supportive care is the mainstay of treatment, although specific antidotal treatment can be life-saving, as in paracetamol poisoning. In severely poisoned patients, it is often necessary to seek expert advice on their clinical management, and to enlist the help of the toxicology laboratory (see Boxes 29.1, 29.2, and 29.3).

1 Proudfoot AT. *Acute poisoning. Diagnosis and management*, 2nd edn. Oxford: Butterworth Heinemann, 1993.
2 Ellenhorn MJ, Schonwald S, Ordog G, Wasserberger J (eds). *Ellenhorn's medical toxicology*, 2nd edn. Baltimore: Williams & Wilkins, 1997.
3 Olson KR (ed.). *Poisoning and drug overdose*, 2nd edn. Norwalk, CT: Appleton & Lange, 1994.
4 Underhill TJ, Greene MK, Dove AF. A comparison of the efficacy of gastric lavage, ipecacuanha and activated charcoal in the emergency management of paracetamol overdose. *Arch Emerg Med* 1990;7:148–54.
5 Saetta JP, Quinton DN. Residual gastric content after gastric lavage and ipecacuanha-induced emesis in self–poisoned patients: an endoscopic study. *J R Soc Med* 1991;84:35–8.
6 Neuvonen PJ, Olkkola KT. Oral activated charcoal in the treatment of intoxications, role of single and repeated doses. *Med Toxicol* 1988;3:33–58.
7 Olkkola KT. Effect of charcoal–drug ratio on antidotal efficacy of oral activated charcoal in man. *Br J Clin Pharmacol* 1985;19:767–73.

8 Ferner RE. Paracetamol poisoning – an update. *Prescribers J* 1993;**33**:45–50.

9 Keays R, Harrison PM, Wendon JA, *et al.* Intravenous acetylcysteine in paracetamol induced fulminant hepatic failure: a controlled trial. *BMJ* 1991;**303**:1026–9.

10 Hedges JR, Otten EJ, Schroeder TJ, Tasset JJ. Correlation of initial amitriptyline concentration reduction with activated charcoal therapy in overdose patients. *Am J Emerg Med* 1987;**5**:48–51.

11 Crome P, Dawling S, Braithwaite RA, Masters J, Walker R. Effect of activated charcoal on absorption of nortriptyline. *Lancet* 1977;**ii**:1203–5.

12 Hillman RJ, Prescott LF. Treatment of salicylate poisoning with repeated oral charcoal. *BMJ* 1985;**291**:1472.

13 Jacobsen D, Wiik–Larsen E, Bredesen JE. Haemodialysis or haemoperfusion in severe salicylate poisoning? *Human Toxicol* 1988;**7**:161–3.

14 Shannon M, Amitai Y, Lovejoy FH. Multiple dose activated charcoal for theophylline poisoning in young infants. *Pediatrics* 1987;**80**:368–70.

15 Heath A, Knudsen K. Rate of extracorporeal drug removal in theophylline poisoning: a review. *Med Toxicol* 1987;**2**:294–308.

# 30: Obstetric critical illness

B N J WALTERS

Managing medical problems during pregnancy requires knowledge of the changes in anatomy and physiology induced by the gravid state. This is particularly important in intensive care, where so much emphasis is placed on achieving normal physiological values, as the normal ranges may be very different in pregnancy. For example, restoring a pregnant patient's cardiac output to her non-pregnant norm may result in underperfusion, as cardiac output increases 30–50% by mid-pregnancy to support the uterus and its occupant. Table 30.1 summarises a number of measurements likely to be used in the intensive care unit (ICU) that are altered by pregnancy. A complete discussion of these and many other changes may be found in Hytten and Chamberlain.[1] It should also be remembered that many drugs used in intensive care cross the placenta, and may affect the fetus.[2]

## Clinical implications of haemodynamic, respiratory, and other physiological changes during pregnancy

### Osmoregulation

Very soon after conception, even before the first missed period, major alterations occur in osmoregulation and volume regulation. The osmotic threshold for antidiuretic hormone (ADH) release is reduced by about 10 mosmol/kg. At the same time plasma osmolality falls to a mean of about 278 mosmol/kg (from 288 mosmol/kg non-pregnant) because of a reduction in plasma sodium and accompanying anions. Thus, at a plasma osmolality that would stimulate diuresis and inhibit thirst in the non-pregnant state, the gravid woman drinks, produces ADH, and behaves as though volume depleted, while plasma volume is steadily rising.

### Plasma volume and cardiac output

Plasma volume expansion follows generalised vasodilatation, a dominant feature of pregnant haemodynamics. Oestrogen, nitric oxide, prostacyclin, and other autacoids that relax vascular smooth muscle all contribute to this phenomenon. The renal response is to retain fluid early in pregnancy to correct this relative hypovolaemia. Cardiac output at rest is increased 40% by mid-pregnancy, even more with twins, and more also with exercise or uterine contraction. Average pulse rate rises in pregnancy by about

Table 30.1 Normal reference values for pregnancy

| References | Non-pregnant | Late pregnancy |
|---|---|---|
| *Haemodynamics* | | |
| Cardiac output (l/min) | 4·5±0·4 | 6·2±1·0 |
| CVP (mm Hg) | 4± | 4±3 |
| PCWP (mm Hg | 6±2 | 8±2 |
| PA pressure (mm Hg) | 9–16 | 9–16 |
| SVR dyne·s/cm$^5$ | 1400–1900 | 950–1300 |
| | | |
| *Respiratory* | | |
| Arterial pH | 7·35–7·40 | 7·40–7·44 |
| Arterial $Po_2$ (kPa)[a] | 12–12·6 (90–95) | 13–14 (98–105) |
| Arterial $Pco_2$ (kPa)[a] | 4·7–5·3 (35–40) | 3·7–4·3 (28–32) |
| Tidal volume (ml) | 470–610 | 660–760 |
| Functional residual capacity (ml) | 2800 | 2300 |
| | | |
| *Biochemistry* | | |
| Albumin (g/l) | 33–36 | 27–32 |
| AST (units/l) | 10–40 | 10–40 |
| Calcium (total) (mEq/l) | 2·2–2·7 | 2·15–2·45 |
| Creatinine ( mol/l) | 55–95 | 45–82 |
| Osmolality (molsm/kg) | 289 | 280 |
| Sodium (mEq/l) | 139±4 | 136±3 |
| Urea (mmol/l) | 3·4–5·2 | 3·1–3·9 |
| Colloid osmotic pressure (mm Hg) | 25±2 | 22±1·5 |
| | | |
| *Haematology* | | |
| Hb (g/l) | 125–155 | 110–130 |
| WCC (×10$^9$/l) | 4·5–11 | 5·5–16·5 |
| Platelet count (×10$^9$/l) | 150 | 130–350 |

[a] Values in parenthesis are mm Hg.
AST, aspartate aminotransferase; CVP, central venous pressure; PA, pulmonary artery; PCWP, pulmonary capillary wedge pressure; SVR, systemic vascular resistance.

15 beats/min and cardiac output from 4·5 to about 6 l/min. Stroke volume therefore rises by little more than 10%.

## Pulmonary function

Thoracic anatomy changes in pregnancy, with a 4 cm elevation in the diaphragm and 30° increase in the subcostal angle, both occurring before the gravid uterus even approaches the umbilicus. Thus on radiograph the cardiac apex is displaced up and outwards. Figure 30.1 displays alterations in lung volumes. Vital capacity is not consistently changed, but a 30–40% increase in tidal volume ($V_T$) is observed, encroaching upon expiratory reserve volume (decreased about 25%). As residual volume is also compressed (by the diaphragm), the functional residual capacity falls by 10–20%. All of these recordings have been made in the upright position, under experimental conditions, and the changes could well be greater in the

371

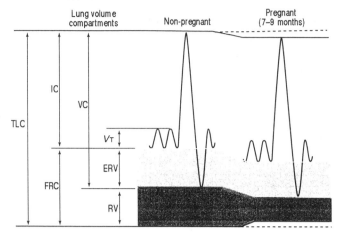

Fig 30.1    Alterations in components of lung volume in late pregnancy.

Abbreviations:  TLC = total lung capacity;
VC = vital capacity;
IC = inspiratory capacity;
RV = residual volume;
FRC = functional residual capacity;
ERV = expiratory reserve volume;
$V_T$ = tidal volume.

supine postion. Respiratory rate varies little. $V_T$ rises considerably as gestation proceeds, mostly secondary to central stimulation of respiration by progesterone and perhaps oestrogen, hence the "physiological hyperventilation" of pregnancy with minute ventilation increasing 50% or more.

## Arterial gas tensions and pH

The hyperventilation of pregnancy occurs early, and results in a fall in arterial $P_{CO_2}$ at rest to about 4 kPa (30 mm Hg). In compensation for this respiratory alkalosis, renal bicarbonate excretion is enhanced resulting in a fall of plasma bicarbonate, accompanied by sodium, and osmolality as detailed above. $O_2$ consumption is increased by 30–40 ml/min (about 15%) which approximately matches the increased requirements of fetus, placenta, and maternal tissues. The mother may therefore become hypoxaemic rapidly during short periods of apnoea, for example, during endotracheal intubation. Fetal haemoglobin has a higher $O_2$ affinity than that of the mother, and is present in a much higher concentration (160–180 g/l). Placental flow is the primary determinant of fetal oxygenation, but the fetus is also protected from short periods of maternal hypoxaemia because its haemoglobin $O_2$ dissociation curve is shifted to the left whilst that of the mother is shifted to the right.

### Blood pressure and systemic vascular resistance

Systolic blood pressure falls only slightly, but the diastolic decrement is 10–20 mm Hg by 20 weeks, lowering mean blood pressure appreciably. Given the increase in cardiac output described above, this implies a reduction in systemic vascular resistance (SVR) to around 980 dyn·s/cm⁵ in early pregnancy, rising later to 1300. These figures have been obtained from healthy pregnant women with the use of pulmonary artery catheters[3] (with ethics committee approval!) and the safer non-invasive Doppler ultrasound.[4]

### Aortocaval compression

It is essential that the "supine hypotensive syndrome" of pregnancy is not forgotten in the ICU. Particularly in late pregnancy, a profound fall in blood pressure may occur in the supine position from compression of the vena cava and obstruction to venous return by the gravid uterus. The aorta may also be compressed, impairing uterine blood flow. For this reason all pregnant patients (at least from 16 weeks onwards) must be nursed with lateral tilt using a wedge under one hip.

### Colloid osmotic pressure

Pregnancy increases susceptibility to pulmonary oedema for several reasons. Serum albumin declines markedly in normal pregnancy, and even more so in critical illness. The fall in plasma colloid osmotic pressure (COP) is partly counteracted by lower interstitial COP, but aggravated by capillary hydrostatic pressure which rises. Thus, the net balance of forces favours fluid movement from the circulation, and reduces the safety margin for pulmonary oedema. The endothelial dysfunction of critical illness contributes further to this, and pulmonary oedema will therefore occur at a lower pulmonary capillary wedge pressure (PCWP) than might have been expected. Intravenous crystalloid solutions will produce a greater decline in COP than colloids, and fluid resuscitation must therefore be handled with great care, particularly 3–12 hours post partum, in order to balance the competing demands of maximising oxygen supply and minimising pulmonary oedema. Tissue and lung oedema may take many days to resolve.

## Cardiopulmonary resuscitation (CPR)

The physiological changes of pregnancy described above must be taken into account in the conduct of CPR. Recommendations have been formulated into a policy document.[5] A wedge or manual traction should always be used to displace the uterus during CPR. Perimortem caesarean delivery may be necessary. This emotionally disturbing procedure must be considered very early during CPR as the time available to save the infant's life is short. It is also possible that the mother's chances of survival may be increased after delivery by improving venous return when the uterus is emptied.

# Severe pre-eclampsia and eclampsia

Severe pre-eclamptic toxaemia (PET) results from pathological derangements that begin in early pregnancy,[6] followed by a long preclinical asymptomatic stage. At the time of presentation, the disorder involves multiple organ systems (Box 30.1).

## Pathogenesis

The primary defect is thought to be vascular endothelial damage caused by humoral factors activating platelets and neutrophils, and an imbalance between prostacyclin and thromboxane. Loss of normal endothelial vasoregulation causes vasoconstriction and hypertension. In the utero-placental vascular bed (almost certainly the initial site of vascular disturbance in PET) there is occlusion of arteries supplying the placenta. This results in placental ischaemia and/or infarction,[6] resulting in fetal growth retardation or death. The incidence of placental abruption is increased. Increased vascular permeability results in proteinuria and the nephrotic syndrome, vasogenic oedema, and pulmonary oedema. Colloid oncotic pressure is low, with transfer of osmotically active substances into the extravascular space.[7] Contact activation with intravascular thrombin deposition together with vasospasm leads to ischaemic damage to the

---

**Box 30.1** *Complications of severe pre-eclampsia*

*Neurological*
- Eclampsia
- Cerebral haemorrhage
- Cortical blindness
- Cerebral oedema
- Cerebral infarct
- Cortical venous thrombosis

*Ocular*
- Retinal detachment
- Serous retinopathy

*Renal*
- Renal failure
- Nephrotic syndrome

*Cardiovascular*
- Pulmonary oedema

*Hepatic*
- Hepatic haemorrhage
- Focal liver infarction
- Liver rupture

*Haematological*
- Thrombocytopenia
- Haemolysis
- Coagulopathy

*Fetus/placenta*
- Fetal growth retardation
- Placental abruption
- Placental infarction

---

maternal liver and brain. Correction of hypovolaemia is complicated by the accelerated disappearance of even high-molecular-weight colloids from the circulation.[7]

## Clinical features

The presentation of PET varies depending on the main organ system involved. The likelihood of secondary PET (for example, with underlying hypertension, renal disease, lupus) is greater in multiparous women. Hypertension and proteinuria are the most common presenting features. In severe PET, thrombocytopenia may be profound and may worsen for some days after delivery. Other coagulation abnormalities are usually not severe unless there has been major haemorrhage or liver involvement. With placental abruption there may be disseminated intravascular coagulation. Fibrinogen levels are increased in most cases. Liver involvement is suggested by a severe, often nocturnal pain in the epigastrium or subcostal region, accompanied by elevated liver enzymes, often only the transaminases. Bilirubin may be elevated and will be pronounced if there is haemolysis (**H**) (a microangiopathic feature of severe PET) which often accompanies the liver abnormalities (**E**levated **L**iver enzymes) and thrombocytopenia (**L**ow **P**latelets), hence the acronym of the "HELLP" syndrome as a mnemonic to describe this presentation of atypical severe PET. Anaemia indicates either haemolysis, or intrahepatic or retroplacental haemorrhage. Intrahepatic haemorrhage is potentially lethal and better visualised by CT or MRI rather than by ultrasound.

## Therapy

Delivery is the only definitive treatment for PET, and recovery usually starts at this point. However, the pathological processes remain active and potentially life-threatening for 24–72 hours post partum. The intrinsic self-limiting nature of PET distinguishes it from most disorders seen in a general ICU. By implication, therefore, therapeutic and investigational manoeuvres must be supportive and corrective, and iatrogenic complications are all the more regrettable. The main requirements after delivery are control of hypertension, prevention of eclampsia, and avoidance of excessive fluid administration, while awaiting resolution. Before delivery, fetal monitoring is absolutely essential.

### Blood pressure control

Blood pressure must be controlled to prevent eclampsia and cerebral haemorrhage, which account for 30–40% of deaths from the condition, and to reduce the risk of heart failure. Treatment thresholds should be individualised: a patient whose non-gravid blood pressure is 90/50 mm Hg may be at serious risk with a systolic blood pressure of 150–160 mm Hg in PET. In general, systolic pressures of 170 mm Hg systolic or 110 mm Hg diastolic by standard sphygmomanometry require prompt treatment. Once a fit has occurred the threshold for further seizures is lowered, and they may recur unpredictably with no direct relationship to blood pressure. Acute pressure reduction may be achieved orally with nifedipine or parenterally using hydralazine, diazoxide, or labetalol. Nitroprusside or nitrates should be used only in an ICU with invasive monitoring. Once control is achieved, maintenance relies upon slower-acting oral agents such as methyldopa, labetalol, or atenolol, to any of which oral hydralazine may be added. These are all of confirmed safety for the fetus.

## Fluid therapy and invasive haemodynamic monitoring

Although haemodynamics may vary in severe PET,[8] the most common finding is a greatly increased SVR, often combined with hyperdynamic ventricular function, a low to normal central venous pressure (CVP) and normal pulmonary vascular resistance, and a low COP. Whilst these observations are of great interest, most women can be treated without invasive haemodynamic monitoring and the American College of Obstetrics and Gynecology has stated that benefits in excess of the risks of pulmonary artery catheterisation have yet to be demonstrated. Although invasive monitoring does have a limited place in certain circumstances (see below), minimally invasive techniques such as oesophageal Doppler flow analysis may provide a better substitute.

Although there are no controlled trials, careful plasma volume expansion using colloids is recommended on the basis that sudden falls in maternal blood pressure may compromise placental and renal perfusion, plasma volume is reduced in PET, and vasodilator therapy will expose this volume deficit. Accurate control of fluid management and cardiovascular function is difficult in the absence of invasive monitoring, which should probably be considered in the presence of pulmonary oedema, major haemorrhage, or renal failure complicating severe PET. It has also been recommended for the management of oliguria in PET,[9] but is usually unnecessary; oliguria often occurs post partum, is almost invariably short-lived, and probably reflects intrarenal vasospasm, not renal failure. Frusemide may increase hourly urine output but there is no evidence that it alters the prognosis. Mannitol may worsen pulmonary or cerebral oedema by traversing damaged endothelium. The benefits of low-dose dopamine for pre-eclamptic oliguria have not been subject to objective study. Perhaps 1% of patients with severe oliguria will develop acute tubular necrosis and may require a limited period of dialysis. All of these in our experience have recovered full renal function within four weeks. There is no evidence that invasive monitoring would prevent renal failure in these patients.

## Eclampsia

Eclampsia (fitting) is often preceded by less dramatic neurological disturbances, such as migrainous auras, twitching, dysphasia, or altered mental state. The fits may be focal or generalised, are usually brief, but may proceed to status eclampticus. Mortality rate increases with the number of seizures. Cerebral haemorrhage is a major cause of death in PET and eclampsia, and results from severe hypertension and endothelial damage. CT or MRI may be helpful if there is persisting neurological deficit or coma, or doubt about the diagnosis. Control of hypertension is the most critical factor in preventing cerebral haemorrhage, but prevention of eclampsia may require magnesium sulphate ($MgSO_4$) as well.

### Prevention and treatment of eclampsia

Does control of hypertension alone, without prophylactic anticonvulsants, prevent eclampsia? A large retrospective study in South Africa[10] showed that the risk of eclampsia in 996 parturients receiving hypotensive drugs was 0·5%; prophylactic $MgSO_4$ did not reduce the risk of seizures. In another study of more than 2000 women with hypertension in labour,[11] $MgSO_4$ significantly reduced the seizure rate compared with phenytoin; however, the overall incidence was <1%, and only 4% of the total population received antihypertensive treatment. At present, prophylaxis against eclampsia with $MgSO_4$ should be given to selected patients, but must be preceded by blood pressure control.

Eclamptic fitting is a medical emergency and must be controlled without delay. Airway patency and arterial oxygenation must be preserved; if in doubt, intubate and ventilate. Aortocaval compression must be avoided. $MgSO_4$ is given as a loading dose of 4 g intravenously over 5–20 min followed by an infusion at 1 g/h for 24 hours as prophylaxis against further fits. Maternal toxicity may include respiratory depression, muscular paralysis, cardiac arrest, and potentiation of neuromuscular blocking drugs during anaesthesia, but these are uncommon and can be easily reversed using calcium gluconate. Close monitoring of serum levels is mandatory particularly in patients with oliguria. A large multinational controlled trial of treatment *after* eclampsia showed magnesium sulphate to be superior to both phenytoin and diazepam in preventing further fits.[12] There was a non-significant reduction in maternal mortality. Benzodiazepines may be required for uncontrolled fitting, but will sedate both mother and baby. In status eclampticus, endotracheal intubation and mechanical ventilation are mandatory; a barbiturate infusion may be necessary.

*Postpartum phase*

Vigilance must be maintained for up to 72 hours: 30–50% of eclamptic seizures and 40–60% of deaths occur after delivery. Blood pressure may worsen on days 3–5, with a small associated risk of late postpartum eclampsia. The platelet count may fall for up to four days and haemolysis may appear after delivery. However, in the great majority of cases, recovery is complete. Late complications should prompt consideration of alternative diagnoses. The efficacy of plasma exchange is not known.

# Amniotic fluid embolism

Amniotic fluid embolism (AFE) usually presents as a catastrophic deterioration in haemodynamics and coagulation; many patients die within 30 minutes. The classic description of an older multiparous woman in tumultuous labour with a large fetus accounts for < 30% of cases, and many have been recorded in unexpected circumstances such as termination of early pregnancy, amniocentesis, uncomplicated pregnancy, closed abdominal trauma, and, more commonly, during caesarean section. AFE is responsible for 5–15% of all maternal deaths. As death occurs in 40–85% of recognized cases, the incidence of AFE may be as high as 1:10 000 deliveries. AFE most frequently presents during labour (70%) or caesarean section after delivery of the infant (19%) with 11% occurring after vaginal delivery.[13] Maternal mortality in this series was 61%, most within five hours, and only 7 of the 46 cases survived neurologically intact; 80% of the babies survived of whom only half were neurologically normal.

## Pathophysiology

The syndrome of AFE resembles septic and anaphylactic shock, suggesting that it is an excessive maternal host response to foreign fetal material, including squamous and other cells.[13] It is important to realise that amniotic fluid components are seen in blood from normal pregnant women. It is the response that is deleterious, not the mere presence of fetal material. Amniotic fluid has considerable thromboplastic activity and stimulates intravascular coagulation with rapid consumption of clotting factors; the resulting coagulopathy may become uncontrollable.

Haemodynamic studies are uncommon, performed late, and in contrast to animal research[14] show only mild or modest elevation of pulmonary artery (PA) pressures but significant left ventricular dysfunction, suggesting[13] that left heart failure is the dominant disturbance, at least in those who survive long enough to enter an ICU and undergo haemodynamic monitoring. Of the 14 adequately documented cases reported by 1993, pulmonary capillary wedge pressure exceeded the mean for normal pregnancy by at least three standard deviations in 85%.[14] In half, wedge pressure exceeded 17 mm Hg, and clinical pulmonary oedema is detailed in many reports.

In animal models, infusion of amniotic fluid causes major acute increases in both systemic and pulmonary vascular resistance. This is followed initially by hypoxaemia, acidosis, and perhaps coronary artery spasm, and then by pulmonary capillary damage and left ventricular failure. Most women reach the ICU during the second phase, by which time pulmonary capillary hyperpermeability and high hydrostatic pressures have both contributed to pulmonary oedema and acute respiratory distress syndrome (ARDS).

## Clinical features

The differential diagnosis includes pulmonary thromboembolism, air embolism, septic shock, aspiration pneumonia, placental abruption, and myocardial infarction, and gives some idea of the frightening clinical presentation of heart failure, cyanosis, seizures, shock, and massive haemorrhage that marks the fully developed syndrome. The initial symptoms are most commonly sudden dyspnoea or seizure and vascular collapse with profound cyanosis. In women undergoing electronic fetal monitoring, the initial sign may be fetal distress. The syndrome may present with widespread bleeding but in general this follows cardio-respiratory collapse. Disseminated intravascular coagulation (DIC) is common, and uncontrollable vaginal haemorrhage may complicate failure of uterine contraction after delivery. Intra-abdominal bleeding may occur after caesarean section.

## Diagnosis

As mentioned above, although characteristic embolic material (fetal squames surrounded by maternal neutrophils) can be identified in blood drawn from a wedged PA catheter, these findings have been noted in women without AFE syndrome. The diagnosis is therefore made on clinical grounds.

## Treatment

The immediate priorities for resuscitation are to stop haemorrhage, improve oxygenation, and correct cardiac failure. As large volumes of fluid may be required, and the pulmonary capillary permeability and ventricular dysfunction predispose to oedema, haemodynamic monitoring by PA catheter will be needed. Close liaison with the obstetrician is essential as uterine atony and torrential bleeding may require intramyometrial prosta-glandin, packing, or angiographic embolisation. Platelets, fresh frozen plasma, and fresh blood should be used. There is no evidence supporting the use of heparin to block the thrombotic element of DIC in AFE.

# Acute fatty liver of pregnancy (AFLP)

This is a rare maternal disorder (incidence approximately 1:10 000 pregnancies),[15] characterised pathologically by the presence of microvesicular steatosis in hepatocytes similar to that seen in Reye's syndrome in children and in hepatic tetracycline toxicity. Before 1980, 50–70% of reported cases were fatal, but the mortality rate has now fallen to around 25% presumably because of earlier diagnosis, reporting of milder cases, or improvements in management. The cause of AFLP is not known. Tetracycline is no longer implicated. AFLP occurred in one mother of infants with an acyl-fatty acid oxidation defect, but the lack of recurrence in subsequent pregnancies[15] argues against an underlying maternal metabolic disease. In survivors the liver returns to normal within weeks of delivery.

## Clinical features

The presenting feature in most cases is persistent vomiting in the third trimester of pregnancy. This is usually accompanied by tiredness and malaise for days or weeks followed by jaundice with drowsiness or confusion. A frequent symptom is polydipsia which may be extreme, with pseudodiabetes insipidus. Upper abdominal pain is present in many cases, but severe pain is suggestive of pre-eclamptic liver disease.[15] On presentation severe cases are jaundiced with a deteriorating conscious state leading to hepatic encephalopathy.[15] This is accompanied by renal failure, acidosis, coagulation failure, and occasionally pancreatitis. Gastrointestinal haemorrhage is common and hypoglycaemia may be profound.

## Diagnosis

Acute fatty liver of pregnancy may appear very similar to pre-eclamptic liver disease as described above ("HELLP" variant). Further confusion arises as hypertension and proteinuria are present in about 40% of cases.[16] If these features are severe, however, PET is more likely. Acute viral hepatitis may be similar and viral serology should always be ordered urgently, but the rise in transaminases is usually more severe in hepatitis than in AFLP, and other laboratory and clinical features are different. Accurate diagnosis requires liver biopsy, but coagulopathy usually precludes its performance. Moreover, unless an alternative diagnosis can be made quickly and with certainty, early delivery of the baby is essential for the survival of both mother and child, and waiting for biopsy confirmation usually cannot be justified. Liver function tests show combined hepatocellular and obstructive changes, with modest increases in aspartate transaminase (AST) and alkaline phosphatase, a more marked increase in bilirubin, and a reduction in albumin and blood glucose. The prothrombin time is prolonged, and hyperuricaemia is marked. The blood film may show leukaemoid or leukoerythroblastic change,[16] and thrombocytopenia.

## Management

Delivery of the baby is essential for maternal and fetal survival. Resolution of this disease before delivery has never been reported. Thus most cases will arrive at the ICU post partum. Delivery does not, however, guarantee survival, and many of the reported deaths have occurred in the puerperium. Even so, the prognosis is good where diagnosis and delivery are prompt.

Management is the same as for any form of fulminant hepatic failure. Parenteral glucose should be given to correct hypoglycaemia and to reduce protein catabolism and subsequent nitrogenous waste. Oral lactulose and neomycin may be used to reduce enterobacterial production of ammonia, together with a low protein diet in patients able to take enteral nutrition. Coagulopathy should be corrected with vitamin K, platelets, and fresh frozen plasma. Blood transfusion may be needed. The coagulopathy may preclude the use of epidural anaesthesia, and opioids may worsen encephalopathy; general anaesthesia and alfentanil for analgesia should be used for caesarean section in the sick patient. Standard measures should be employed to prevent infection and stress ulceration. Urgent liver transplantation should be considered in the presence of progressive liver failure.

# Pulmonary oedema due to tocolytic therapy

Preterm delivery contributes substantially to perinatal morbidity, mortality, and long-term handicap. The drugs used to prevent preterm labour (tocolytic agents) at one time included magnesium sulphate and alcohol, but these have largely been replaced by the $\beta_2^-$ sympathomimetic amines which have frequently been observed to cause pulmonary oedema.[17]

## $\beta_2$ Stimulation

Agents such as salbutamol, ritodrine, and terbutaline given by intravenous infusion relax vascular, bronchial, and uterine smooth muscle. The desired tocolytic effect is therefore accompanied by vasodilatation and an increase in cardiac output which is also a consequence of $\beta_2$-receptor-mediated tachycardia and stimulation of cardiac $\beta_1$-receptors. Myocardial oxygen consumption increases. $\beta$ Agonists also stimulate glucagon secretion resulting in glycogenolysis, hyperglycaemia, and enhanced production of ketone bodies, but significant acidosis is unusual. A transmembrane shift of potassium into cells occurs, sometimes resulting in hypokalaemia.

Arginine vasopressin (ADH) release is stimulated, which increases water reabsorption, with consequent haemodilution.

## Cardiorespiratory risk factors

Infection is a common precipitant of preterm labour (30%) and chorioamnionitis, pyelonephritis, etc., may contribute to pulmonary oedema by capillary membrane injury during the systemic inflammatory response. Multiple gestation is present in 10–15% of cases of preterm labour and, in twin pregnancy, blood volume is 50–60% above non-pregnant levels. The intravenous volume load that may be given by infusing $\beta$ stimulants may contribute to pulmonary oedema. Haemorrhage is a recognised complication of preterm labour, and transfusion may add to the intravascular volume load. Furthermore, labour alone accounts for an increase in cardiac output of 30–50%. The chronotropic, inotropic, volume-expanding, and possibly ischaemic effects on the heart of $\beta_2$ agonists contribute an additional burden to an already stressed system.

## Clinical features

Pulmonary oedema presents as dyspnoea, orthopnoea, and cough in a woman treated for preterm labour for a period usually in excess of 18 hours. Chest pain is reported by up to 20% and evidence of myocardial ischaemia may be found. Sinus tachycardia is universal, in part because it is standard obstetric practice to use an infusion rate that produces a maternal heart rate of about 120/min. Ventricular and supraventricular extrasystoles are likely. The tachycardia is particularly dangerous for women with stenotic valve disease such as mitral stenosis, in which condition $\beta$ agonists are contraindicated. Published haemodynamic measurements are few. Echocardiography was normal where reported, and elevated wedge pressure was found only in a minority, suggesting pulmonary endothelial dysfunction as a contributing factor. However, the evidence suggests that the dominant disorder is myocardial fatigue resulting from prolonged tachycardia, fluid overload, and excessive myocardial work when the heart is already operating near its limits.

## Treatment

Intravenous fluid and $\beta$ agonists should be stopped immediately. The patient should be sat upright and adequate supplemental oxygen must be given, together with morphine or equivalent opioid in small doses to relieve distress. Diuretics will usually result in considerable clearance of retained fluid. Continuous positive airway pressure (CPAP) by facemask may be helpful in more severe cases to maintain adequate oxygenation. Intubation and ventilatory support are rarely needed. Infection as a contributing cause must be excluded by blood culture and other microbiological samples as indicated.

# Other causes of acute lung injury in pregnancy

In addition to the conditions described above, there are two other significant disease processes in pregnancy that may cause acute lung injury: infection and acid aspiration.

## Infection

Pyelonephritis and chorioamnionitis causing a systemic inflammatory response in late pregnancy are often associated with acute lung injury. In 15 patients with acute pyelonephritis, respiratory distress, hypoxaemia, and pulmonary infiltrates developed a mean of 30 hours after admission.[18] In some cases the respiratory pathology and severe pyrexia overshadow urinary tract symptoms leading to an erroneous diagnosis of pneumonia. Thrombocytopenia, evidence of DIC, haemolysis and renal dysfunction are common. *Escherichia coli* or *Klebsiella* spp. are often grown from blood cultures and urine. In one study[19] pulmonary injury was more likely to complicate pyelonephritis if pulse rate was >110 beats/min and temperature >39·4°C. Gestational age was >20 weeks in these patients; tocolytic agents had been used in many and, although there was evidence of fluid overload, the pulmonary capillary wedge pressure was not elevated. The differential diagnosis includes intrauterine infection, intrauterine death, and pneumonia, all of which must be positively excluded in women with fever and signs of pulmonary injury.

## Acid aspiration

In 1946 Mendelson described the syndrome of aspiration pneumonitis following inhalation of gastric contents during obstetric anaesthesia administered via a facemask and spontaneous respiration.[20] The few deaths that occurred were a consequence of asphyxia from airway obstruction by undigested food. Avoidable maternal deaths from aspiration continue to be recorded, but the syndrome now carries a higher mortality rate, and it is assumed that this is because it is gastric acid or bile rather than food that is inhaled, and positive pressure ventilation through a cuffed endotracheal tube may facilitate wider dispersion of material through the lungs. All pregnant women, not just those nearing term, are at increased risk both at induction of and recovery from anaesthesia. Measures to prevent its occurrence include adequate provision of experienced and properly assisted anaesthetists, cricoid pressure at induction, non-particulate antacids (sodium citrate), and $H_2$-receptor antagonists.

# Conclusion

Critical illness in pregnancy is of particular importance not only because of the diseases unique to the gravid state but also because two individuals are involved. Close liaison between obstetrician and intensivist is essential so that correct management decisions are made for mother and baby during the antenatal period, for the timing and mode of delivery, and post partum to anticipate and prevent puerperal complications. Care of the fetus includes maintenance of placental blood flow and oxygenation, and care of the mother requires knowledge of the altered physiology of pregnancy. Emotional stress is considerable for the patient and her relatives, who will need full support. In the majority of cases, obstetric critical illness is reversible, and the woman will recover completely given physiological stabilisation, avoidance of iatrogenic complications, and resolution of the disease process, which often requires delivery of the infant.

1 Hytten F, Chamberlain G. *Clinical physiology in obstetrics*, 2nd edn. Oxford: Blackwell Scientific Publications, 1991.
2 Clark SL, Cotton DB, Hawkins GD, Phelan JP. *Critical care obstetrics*, 2nd edn. Boston: Blackwell Scientific Publications, 1991.
3 Clark SL, Cotton DB, Lee W, *et al*. Central haemodynamic assessment of normal term pregnancy. *Am J Obstet Gynecol* 1989;**161**:1439–42.
4 Easterling TR, Benedetti TJ, Schmucker BC, Carlson KL. Antihypertensive therapy in pregnancy directed by noninvasive haemodynamic monitoring. *Am J Perinatol* 1989; **6**:86–9.
5 Barth WH. Special resuscitation situations:pregnancy. *JAMA* 1992;**268**:2249–50.
6 Roberts JM, Redman CW. Pre–eclampsia: more than pregnancy-induced hypertension. *Lancet* 1993;**341**:1447–51.
7 Oian P, Maltau JM, Noddeland H, Fadnes HO. Transcapillary fluid balance in pre-eclampsia. *Br J Obstet Gynaecol* 1986;**93**:235–9.
8 Macphail S. Haemodynamics of hypertensive pregnancy. *Contemp Rev Obstet Gynaecol* 1992;**4**:116–20.
9 Clark SL, Cotton DB. Clinical indications for pulmonary artery catheterization in the patient with severe preeclampsia. *Am J Obstet Gynecol* 1988;**158**:453–9.
10 Odendaal JH, Hall D. Is magnesium sulphate really necessary to prevent eclampsia in patients with severe pre-eclampsia? *Abstracts of the International Congress of the International Society for the Study of Hypertension in Pregnancy*, Sydney, 1994.
11 Lucas MJ, Leveno KJ, Cunningham FG. A comparison of magnesium sulphate with phenytoin for the prevention of eclampsia. *N Engl J Med* 1995;**333**:201–5.
12 The Eclampsia Trial Collaborative Group. Which anticonvulsant for women with eclampsia? Evidence from the Collaborative Eclampsia Trial. *Lancet* 1995;**345**:1455–63.
13 Clark SL, Hankins GD, Dudley DA, *et al*. Amniotic fluid embolism: Analysis of the national registry. *Am J Obstet Gynecol* 1995;**172**:1158–69.
14 Hankins GD, Snyder RR, Clark SL, *et al*. Acute haemodynamic and respiratory effects of amniotic fluid embolism in the pregnant goat model. *Am J Obstet Gynecol* 1993;**160**:1113–30.
15 Purdie JM, Walters BNJ. Acute fatty liver of pregnancy: clinical features and diagnosis. *Aust N Z J Obstet Gynaecol* 1988;**28**:62–7.
16 Burroughs AK, Seong NH, Dojcinow DM, *et al*. Idiopathic acute fatty liver of pregnancy in 12 patients. *Q J Med* 1982;**51**:481–96.
17 Benedetti TJ. Life–threatening complications of betamimetic therapy for preterm labour inhibition. *Clin Perinatol* 1986;**13**:843–52.
18 Cunningham FG, Lucas MJ, Hankins GD. Pulmonary injury complicating antepartum pyelonephritis. *Am J Obstet Gynecol* 1987;**156**:797–807.

19 Towers CV, Kaminskas CM, Garite TJ, *et al.* Pulmonary injury associated with antepartum pyelonephritis: can patients at risk be identified? *Am J Obstet Gynecol* 1991;**164**:974–80.
20 Mendelson CL. The aspiration of stomach contents into lungs during obstetric anesthesia. *Am J Obstet Gynecol* 1946;**52**:191–205.

# 31: The critically ill child

M A STOKES and G A PEARSON

A child with life-threatening illness presents particular challenges for intensive care staff and services. Recognition of this has led to the development of paediatric intensive care as a separate speciality, with measurable improvements in morbidity and mortality. Good paediatric intensive care units distinguish themselves by doing simple things well rather than the number of innovative therapies that they have to offer. The aim is to offer a high standard of care to all admissions and not just to a small group of the sickest patients. Imbalance between the demand for and provision of specialist services, however, means that the care of critically ill children is shared among neonatal, paediatric, and adult intensive care units, depending on local arrangements. Consequently, clinical staff may either be involved in all aspects of recognition and treatment of critical illness in a child, or be responsible for stabilisation before transfer to a tertiary paediatric intensive care unit (PICU). This chapter aims to emphasise some key aspects of paediatric intensive care, to offer practical advice, and to highlight pitfalls for the unwary.

To put this topic in context, a specialist PICU admits a wide range of patients (Figure 31.1). The case mix includes neonates with major anatomical or physiological abnormalities, children with life-threatening infectious illness, and traumatic injuries to children of all ages. The age distribution is heavily skewed, however, such that 50% of admissions are children under 20 months of age (Figure 31.2). This finding is unsurprising because 70% of childhood deaths occur within the first year. As children grow older congenital abnormalities become less significant as a cause of death and other causes, such as trauma and malignancy, become more common (Tables 31.1 and 31.2). There is also a seasonal variation in admissions, trauma being more common in summer and respiratory infection in winter. Furthermore, some surgical specialties have a consistent rate of bed use, usually of short duration.

## Essential childhood pathophysiology and anatomy

Early childhood is characterised by physiological adaptation and growth. Physiological immaturity affects how critical illness presents and is managed, whilst some changes in body proportions (for example, airway anatomy) have important clinical and practical consequences. The key

386

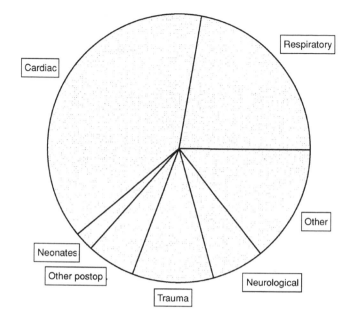

Fig 31.1 Typical case mix of a general PICU. Cases categorised by principal reason for admission.

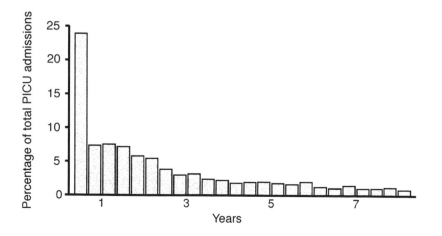

Fig 31.2 Frequency distribution of age of PICU admissions, abbreviated at eight years.

387

Table 31.1 Number of deaths in childhood by age group

| Age group | Number of deaths |
|-----------|------------------|
| 0–28 days | 2955 |
| 4–52 weeks | 1584 |
| 1–4 years | 874 |
| 5–14 years | 1037 |

Table 31.2 Common causes of death in childhood by age groupp

| Cause of death | 4–52 weeks No. (%) | 1–4 years No. (%) | 15–14 years No. (%) |
|----------------|--------------------|--------------------|---------------------|
| SIDS | 434 (27) | 22 (2.5) | 0 (0) |
| Congenital abnormality | 370 (23) | 163 (19) | 99 (10) |
| Infection | 77 (5) | 61 (7) | 32 (3) |
| Trauma | 83 (5) | 212 (24) | 370 (36) |
| Neoplasms | 20 (1) | 118 (13.5) | 229 (22) |
| Endocrine/immune | 45 (3) | 29 (3) | 47 (4·5) |

England and Wales, 1992, Office of Population Cencuses and Surveys (OPCS)
SIDS, sudden infant death syndrome.

aspects are the child's size and body composition, and the balance between oxygen delivery and demand.

**Thermoregulation**

Small children have a high surface area to mass ratio and the head accounts for a greater proportion of the surface area. Heat is lost readily, particularly by radiation, and control of this is the first step in nursing care.

If cold, a newborn baby tries to conserve heat through cutaneous vasoconstriction and by increasing heat production. Vasoconstriction has limited effect because there is little insulating subcutaneous fat. Neonates produce more heat by a generalised increase in metabolic activity, chiefly combustion of fatty acids and glucose. This non-shivering thermogenesis is stimulated by noradrenaline and occurs in several sites including a limited depot of brown adipose tissue, which is rich in mitochondria, blood vessels, and sympathetic innervation. Brown fat disappears later in infancy, by which time there is more subcutaneous fat.

The clinical significance of thermogenesis (and fever) is that oxygen consumption is greatly increased. Lowering the environmental temperature from 34 to 24°C increases a neonate's oxygen consumption by as much as 50%. Active measures to conserve heat are therefore necessary, and include a higher ambient temperature, radiant heaters, warmed intravenous fluids, and humidified inspiratory gases.

Table 31.3  Total body water

| Age | Total body water (% weight) |
| --- | --- |
| 0–1 month | 75 |
| 1–12 months | 70 |
| 1–12 years | 65 |

Table 31.4  Total fluid requirements

| Age | Water requirements (ml/kg per h) |
| --- | --- |
| 0–1 year | 5·0 |
| 1–3 years | 4·0 |
| 3–6 years | 3·0 |
| 7-14 years | 2·5 |
| Adult | 2·0 |

## Fluid and electrolyte balance

Children need a higher intake of fluid and electrolytes per kilogram of body weight than adults to compensate for proportionately higher insensible water losses, high metabolic rates, and limited ability to concentrate urine, all of which are more exaggerated in babies. Normal fluid requirements are given in Tables 31.3 and 31.4. Nutritional demands for growth are high, and liver glycogen stores are limited such that starvation is poorly tolerated. Enteral feeding is preferable, where possible, but parenteral supplementation may be necessary (Table 31.5).

Young children with immature renal tubular function, however, are also less able to excrete a water load and may produce high levels of antidiuretic hormone (ADH) during many illnesses. In practice, it is important to recognise the effects of water balance on serum electrolytes and to distinguish compartment shifts from fluctuations in the total body electrolyte content. Hyponatraemia, for example, may be dilutional (overhydration), or may reflect genuine sodium depletion. Similarly, serum potassium concentrations should be interpreted in the context of blood pH before any inference is made about total body potassium.

Oedema is common in ventilated children and a modest degree of dehydration is often beneficial, such as during ventilatory weaning. Fluid input is usually restricted to 50% of normal maintenance requirements in the acute phase of a critical illness, and liberalised as the child recovers. Circulatory volume is assessed and replaced separately. Oedema, however, may also reflect overhydration, high ADH levels, renal failure, or impaired venous return. More severe fluid restriction and/or diuretic therapy may then be needed. Hypoalbuminaemia and the ominous oedema of capillary

Table 31.5 Approximate requirements for parenteral nutrition in children

| Weight (kg) | Total fluid (ml/kg per day) day | Amino acids (g/kg per day) day | | | Dextrose (g/kg per day) day | | | Fat (Intralipid) (g/kg per day) | | | | Total calories needed/day |
|---|---|---|---|---|---|---|---|---|---|---|---|---|
| | | 1 | 2 | 3+ | 1 | 2 | 3+ | 1 | 2 | 3 | 4+ | |
| Neonates | 100 | 1·5 | 2·0 | 2·0 | 10 | 10–15 | 15–20 | 1·0 | 2·0 | 3·0 | 3·0 | 100/kg |
| <10 | 100 | 1·5 | 2·0 | 2·0 | 10 | 10 | 15–20 | 1·0 | 2·0 | 3·0 | 3·0 | 100/kg |
| 10–15 | 90 | 1·0 | 1·5 | 2·0 | 5 | 10 | 15 | 1·0 | 2·0 | 3·0 | 3·0 | 1000+(50/kg over 10 kg) |
| 15–20 | 80 | 1·0 | 1·5 | 2·0 | 5 | 10 | 10–15 | 1·0 | 2·0 | 2·0 | 3·0 | 1000+(50/kg over 10 kg) |
| 20–30 | 65 | 1·0 | 1·0 | 1–2 | 5 | 10 | 10–15 | 1·0 | 1·5 | 2·0 | 2·5 | 1500+(20/kg over 20 kg) |
| >30 | 50 | 1·0 | 1·0 | 1–2 | 5 | 5–10 | 10 | 1·0 | 1·5 | 1·5 | 2·0 | 1500+(20/kg over 20 kg) |

leak are more likely to be associated with intravascular volume depletion, and require the opposite approach. Dehydration is best recognised by weight loss although sometimes this can be confirmed only after rehydration.

### Respiratory function and failure

The important anatomical features of the child's airway are summarised in Box 31.1 and Figures 31.3 and 31.4. Oedema, from whatever cause, disproportionately reduces the cross-sectional area and greatly increases the resistance to air flow. Other important points are that an infant's ribcage is cartilaginous rather than bony, and its elasticity gives the chest wall a tendency to collapse. Lung compliance is low because there is little elastic tissue, and the ratio of closing volume to functional residual capacity (CV:FRC) is high. The neonate's ribs are aligned horizontally so that there is less movement in the anteroposterior direction during respiration. Breathing is primarily diaphragmatic and can be seriously impaired by abdominal distension, whether caused by pathology, air swallowing, or overzealous bag and mask ventilation. Small infants compensate for further increases in the CV:FRC ratio by grunting during expiration to give positive end-expiratory pressure. With increasing age, the ratio CV:FRC improves, the intercostal muscles contribute more to breathing, and the number of alveoli increases, reaching adult values by eight years of age. Respiratory variables such as tidal volume, dead space, vital capacity, functional residual capacity, and specific compliance are related to body weight. However, because the metabolic rate in neonates and infants is much higher than in older children and adults, respiratory rate (and therefore alveolar ventilation) is higher. This high level of alveolar ventilation makes

---

**Box 31.1** *Anatomical differences between a small infant's and the older child's or adult's airway*

- *Head*: relatively large with prominent occiput
- *Neck*: short
- *Tongue*: relatively large, fills the oral cavity
- *Larynx*: narrower, shorter and funnel shaped; situated more cephalad (C3–4) than in the adult (C4–5) with an anterior inclination
- *Epiglottis*: narrower, $\omega$-shaped epiglottis, angled away from the vertical axis of the trachea
- *Vocal cords*: angled compared with adult
- *Subglottis*: narrowest at the cricoid ring rather than at the vocal cords as in the adult

---

FRC a less effective buffer between inspired gases and the pulmonary circulation. Therefore, any interruption of ventilation very quickly leads to hypoxaemia.

Reduced muscle tone (due to residual anaesthetics, muscle relaxants, fatigue, etc.) causes a reduction of tidal volume and FRC, exacerbating the tendency to hypoxaemia. There is subsequent closure of the small airways, reduced compliance, decreased alveolar minute ventilation, and lung collapse. An infant breathing spontaneously partially compensates for this by breathing faster, but the combination of fatigue, increased physiological deadspace, and possible drug-induced depression of the ventilatory response to carbon dioxide makes it unlikely that normal alveolar minute ventilation is restored. Young infants are even more likely to tire because the diaphragm and intercostal muscles contain a lower percentage of type 1 (slow twitch, high oxidative) muscle fibres during the first few months of life.

Early intervention is important. The clinical picture of respiratory failure is that of a pale, quiet child, breathing quickly and using accessory muscles. Intercostal and subcostal recession are early signs of distress in babies but in children over five years they indicate severe distress. When arrest is

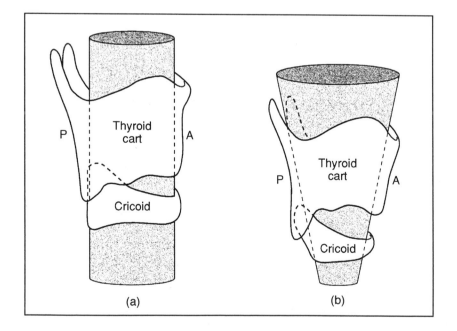

(a)   (b)

Fig 31.3 Diagram of adult (a) and infant (b) larynx. The adult larynx is cylindrical, with the narrowest part at the vocal cords; the infant larynx is tapered, with the narrowest part at the cricoid cartilage.

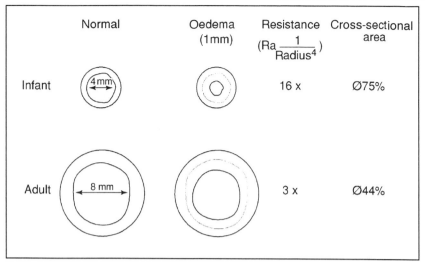

Fig 31.4 Schematic representation of effect of 1 mm oedema on airway cross-sectional area and resistance.

imminent the child becomes flaccid, and respiratory effort dwindles as consciousness is lost.

## Cardiovascular function and failure

The circulatory changes at birth are best considered by reviewing the effects on ventricular performance. As pulmonary vascular resistance falls and pulmonary blood flow increases, left ventricular preload starts to rise. With the separation of the systemic circulation from its low pressure placental sump, systemic vascular resistance and afterload rise correspondingly steeply.

Neonates have a small inotropic reserve that increases with age as some adaptation to these loading conditions occurs. The sudden increases in contractile indices at birth are probably related to surges in circulating catecholamines and thyroid hormone. The neonatal heart has a limited ability to alter cardiac output in response to changes in preload and afterload. Volume loading will increase stroke volume but only over a limited range, whereas overfilling results in a marked reduction in stroke volume. Similarly, increases in afterload significantly reduce cardiac output, whereas output can be preserved, but not greatly enhanced, when afterload falls. Neonatal cardiac output is also very sensitive to changes in heart rate, probably because of a reduced ventricular compliance, there being fewer contractile units (sarcomeres) in the neonatal myocardium. Hence, increases in heart rate in the newborn achieve little, whereas decreases in heart rate produce disproportionately large reductions in cardiac output. In

393

Table 31.6 Normal cardiovascular variables

| Age | Weight (kg) | Mean BP (95% range) | Mean heart rate (95% range) |
|---|---|---|---|
| Term | 3·5 | 40–60 | 95–145 |
| 3 months | 6·0 | 45–75 | 110–175 |
| 6 months | 7·5 | 50–90 | 110–175 |
| 1 year | 10·0 | 50–100 | 105–170 |
| 3 years | 14·0 | 50–100 | 80–140 |
| 7 years | 22·0 | 60–90 | 70–120 |
| 10 years | 30·0 | 60–90 | 60–110 |
| 14 years | 50·0 | 65–95 | 60–100 |

infancy and childhood the myocardium gradually adapts to its new loading conditions and becomes more responsive to $\beta$-adrenergic stimulation. Table 31.6 gives normal values of blood pressure and heart rate at various ages.

Heart failure is a term best avoided in children. Failure of the heart does occur with cardiomyopathy or myocarditis, but most children with physical signs that would represent "heart failure" in an adult are exhibiting a systemic to pulmonary or left to right (L–R) shunt. It is better to consider the effects of pressure and/or volume overload on each ventricle and to determine the causes and effects of the changes in loading conditions. Consider, for example, an infant who collapses as the result of a large ventricular septal defect. There may be little or no murmur because high flow through a large hole produces little turbulence. There are no symptoms for several weeks until pulmonary vascular resistance has completed its normal physiological decline. The presenting symptoms of pulmonary oedema and ventricular volume overload occur at a time when the cardiac output is positively athletic. Indeed the calorie requirement required to sustain this activity will be one component of the infant's failure to thrive.

Isolated L–R shunts are quantified by the ratio of net pulmonary to systemic flow whereas anatomical or physiological right to left (R–L) shunts cause cyanosis. Calculation of the shunt fraction in such circumstances can help to identify congenital heart defects but an accurate morphological (ultrasound) diagnosis is essential.

## Renal function and failure

Glomerular filtration rate (GFR) at term is 2–4 ml/min but is much reduced in the premature infant (0.7 ml/min before 34 weeks' gestation). After 34 weeks' gestation, the glomeruli mature at the same rate as those of a term infant. GFR increases in infancy and is complete at 5–6 months of age. Maturation of the tubules lags slightly behind, reaching adult values at about 8–9 months of age. Thus in early infancy the kidneys are relatively inefficient, excreting large volumes of low quality filtrate. Urinary losses of sodium and potassium are higher than in the adult and one expects urine production of at least 1–2 ml/kg per h in small children. Peak renal performance is reached at about 2–3 years, after which it decreases at a rate of 2·5% per year. Acute renal failure (ARF) is not as ominous a diagnosis in children as it is in adults, but prevention is still preferable. If treatment is prompt and appropriate, ARF is usually reversible. Nutrition plays an important role in this as catabolism leads to more rapid hyperkalaemia, uraemia, and hyperphosphataemia.

Renal failure owing to primary renal disease or postrenal obstruction are unusual reasons for PICU admission. ARF in children is usually secondary to prerenal insults and recovery rates slow markedly with age. Postoperative cardiac surgical patients constitute as many as 50% of cases, and sepsis and trauma comprise most of the remainder. As a general principle, dialysis is started early because fluid maldistribution and low cardiac output respond poorly to fluid restriction. Abdominal distension from the "dwell" of peritoneal dialysate can impair organ perfusion or compromise ventilation. The solution is to restrict cycle volumes or adopt a continuous "cross-flow" technique.

## Brain injury

Brain injury accounts for a large proportion of the deaths following trauma in children. The skull bones of an infant are thin and the sutures are not fused. Although this renders the vault more delicate than that of the older child, it fortuitously allows some expansion when intracranial pressure or volume changes. As the sutures close and the bony vault thickens with age, children are still susceptible to head trauma because of their size and the comparative weakness of neck musculature. Other acquired encephalopathies (hypoxic ischaemic, infective, metabolic) are also common in paediatric intensive care practice.

Management is aggressive, in expectation of a good recovery. Where raised intracranial pressure is anticipated, elective sedation, muscle paralysis, and artificial ventilation are mandatory. Body temperature is continuously monitored, and muscle paralysis is necessary if surface cooling to reduce oxygen demands is to be effective. The use of elective paralysis necessitates a continual search for signs of seizure activity and should not prevent an aggressive approach to seizure control. Rises in intracranial pressure from diffuse cerebral swelling or oedema can be anticipated but not reliably controlled without direct measurement of the intracranial pressure. Disturbance of cerebrovascular autoregulation makes cerebral perfusion pressure the critical determinant of cerebral blood flow in brain injury. Cerebral oxygen demand, intracranial pressure, and cerebral blood volume can be decreased by barbiturate therapy. Hyperventilation can acutely reduce the intracranial pressure but there are no proven or apparent advantages to a policy of sustained reduction in $Pa_{CO_2}$.

Fluid restriction and/or mannitol administration is a logical response to actual or suspected cerebral oedema but steroids are not known to be of benefit.

# Practical aspects of paediatric intensive care

### Assessment and prevention of critical illness

Diagnostic and procedural skills are only part of paediatric intensive care, although they may pose the greatest challenges for the inexperienced. Equally important is recognition that intensive care should be instituted early and escalated judiciously. Sudden death is unusual. Death is more commonly preceded by identifiable and measurable illness or injury, and deterioration can be alarmingly fast, such as with meningococcal septicaemia. Timely admission to the PICU allows pre-emptive action to be taken. Respiratory distress, cardiovascular instability, fluid imbalances, and neurological dysfunction can all be detected before preterminal events, such as acidosis and collapse, occur. The precise timing of PICU admission (and discharge) also depends upon the level of support offered by the paediatric ward or high dependency unit. Direct referral and involvement of senior clinical staff help avoid delayed or inappropriate admissions and discharges.

Common errors that delay PICU referral are a consequence of failure to take an adequate history and examination:

• Failure to appreciate the relevance of the child's age when interpreting physical signs, such as pulse and respiratory rate, blood pressure, or the degree of intercostal and subcostal recession in respiratory distress.
• Misinterpretation of, or failure to recognise, ominous physical signs, such as a silent chest on auscultation, or cyanosis or bradycardia, or an inappropriately passive child.
• Failure to anticipate or recognise the effects of fatigue.
• Failure to recognise early features of homeostatic compensation mechanisms, e.g. tachycardia, reduced peripheral perfusion, and elevation of diastolic blood pressure in hypovolaemia.

### Cardiopulmonary resuscitation

Cardiac arrest in childhood is usually precipitated by respiratory failure or fluid loss/maldistribution. Primary cardiac arrest is very unusual. Cardiopulmonary insufficiency should be suspected in any child who displays an abrupt deterioration in conscious level. There may be apnoea, hypoventilation, or respiratory distress. Specific causes, such as upper

Table 31.7 Ventilatory rates

| Age | Ventilatory rate (/min) |
| --- | --- |
| Neonate | 30 |
| 6 months | 25 |
| 1–5 years | 20 |
| > 5 years | 16 |

airway obstruction, may dictate specific action in addition to resuscitation. At this stage the commonest dysrhythmia is sinus tachycardia. Bradycardia is an ominous sign indicating severe hypoxaemia which must be immediately corrected.

Apnoea requires immediate artificial ventilation which, in smaller infants, without equipment, means mouth-to-mouth and mouth-to-nose resuscitation. As soon as possible more effective ventilation techniques (for example, bag and mask/endotracheal intubation) should be used to provide positive pressure ventilation with 100% oxygen. Ventilation should be of sufficient volume to cause appropriate chest movement and should be delivered at age-appropriate rates (Table 31.7). Circulation is assessed by palpation of the pulse in a major artery and external cardiac massage is required if the pulse is very weak or slow, as well as in asystole. Primary dysrhythmic events are very rare causes of cardiorespiratory arrest and the first treatment of all arrhythmias that are associated with circulatory compromise is artificial ventilation with oxygen and cardiopulmonary resuscitation. External cardiac massage is applied to the lower sternum and the best technique for babies is to grasp the thorax with both hands and apply pressure with adjacent thumbs while the finger tips support the vertebral column. Defibrillation should not be applied without ECG evidence of a shock-responsive rhythm. It is not used in asystole, which is the commonest ECG finding. Intravascular access should be attempted but, if unsuccessful, an early switch to the intraosseous route for fluids and the endotracheal route for drugs is indicated. Endotracheal doses are larger than intravenous doses and adrenaline is indicated in all paediatric pulseless arrhythmias. Intravenous bicarbonate may be required particularly if inadequate circulatory support has been applied, but doses should be metered. In general terms the correct treatment of acidosis is to treat the cause but, in situations where the measured base deficit is > 10, or the pH is <7·2, acidosis may compromise response to inotropes and slow "half correction" is recommended. Boluses of bicarbonate run the risk of exacerbating intracellular acidosis and are a hypertonic stress that small infants will not tolerate well. Formulae for calculating the amount of bicarbonate to give are given in Box 31.2.

> **Box 31.2** *Calculation of bicarbonate doses*
>
> Weight < 5 kg: deficit (mmol) = base excess × weight/2 (give half of this) slowly i.v.
>
> Weight > 5 kg: deficit (mmol) = base excess × weight/3 (give half of this) slowly i.v.

## Haemodynamic support

If rapid volume replacement is necessary, the intravenous cannula should be as big as possible: the 22 gauge cannula from the paediatric equipment trolley is often inappropriate. The placement and maintenance of central venous and peripheral arterial cannulae are core practical skills in PICU, but should not delay fluid resuscitation. An intraosseous needle for initial fluid and drug administration is simple to place in an emergency. It is easy to underestimate the intravascular volume deficit in children. For non-specific volume replacement, 4·5% human albumin solution or synthetic colloid solutions are preferred, in boluses of 10 ml/kg. Physiological saline (30 ml/kg) may be given initially while colloid is being obtained, the higher volume being required because saline diffuses into the interstitial space more rapidly than other plasma substitutes. It is very rare to require non-cross-matched blood. Beware concomitant hypoglycaemia.

Inotropic support should be used as part of a comprehensive approach to circulatory support which includes optimisation of preload and afterload. Invasive haemodynamic monitoring helps clinical decisions, with the proviso that measurements of cardiac output and haemodynamics are less reliable below two years of age. Inotropic agents do not work well in the face of intractable acidosis, which should be corrected more aggressively than described above if such a phenomenon is suspected. Low-dose dopamine administration confers no additional benefits to a comprehensive approach.

## Respiratory support

### Endotracheal intubation

All conscious children require an anaesthetic before attempts are made to instrument the airway, and many unconscious children benefit from the control and stability of general anaesthesia in that oxygenation is optimised and adverse autonomic responses to laryngoscopy and intubation are obtunded. The nasotracheal route is the most comfortable for the child and the easiest to fix securely. The few contraindications to this route include severe disorders of coagulation, and trauma to the nasopharynx or base of the skull.

Table 31.8 Endotracheal tube sizes and lengths

| Age | Weight (kg) | Endotracheal tube Size (mm) | At lip (cm) | At nose (cm) |
|---|---|---|---|---|
| Neonate | <1·0 | 2·0 | 5·0 | 6·0 |
| Neonate | 1·0 | 3·0 | 6·0 | 7·5 |
| Neonate | 2·0 | 3·0 | 7·0 | 9·0 |
| Neonate | 3·0 | 3·0 | 8·5 | 10·5 |
| Neonate | 3·5 | 3·5 | 9·0 | 11·0 |
| 3 months | 6·0 | 3·5 | 10·0 | 12·0 |
| 1 years | 10·0 | 4·0 | 11·0 | 14·0 |
| 2 years | 12·0 | 4·5 | 12·0 | 15·0 |
| 3 years | 14·0 | 4·5 | 13·0 | 16·0 |
| 4 years | 16·0 | 5·0 | 14·0 | 17·0 |
| 6 years | 20·0 | 5·5 | 15·0 | 19·0 |
| 8 years | 24·0 | 6·0 | 16·0 | 20·0 |
| 10 years | 30·0 | 6·5 | 17·0 | 21·0 |
| 12 years | 38·0 | 7·0 | 18·0 | 22·0 |
| 14 years | 50·0 | 7·5 | 19·0 | 23·0 |

Endotracheal tube (ETT) sizes and lengths for nasal and oral intubation are given in Table 31.8. The child's age is the best guide to tube size over two years, but one must have prepared a size above and below that predicted. The size may be several sizes below that predicted where there is significant airway oedema, but should nevertheless be of appropriate length for the child's age.

An uncuffed tube is used in young children because its cylindrical shape fits the funnel-shaped larynx snugly. Ideally there should be a small leak around this tube as too tight a fit causes ischaemia of the tracheal mucosa and may lead to subglottic stenosis. There will be an excessive leak of ventilatory gases around a tube that is too small. A cuffed tube is used for children older than 9 or 10 years of age, and this is managed in the same way as in adults. Children tolerate prolonged endotracheal intubation remarkably well and there are very few indications for elective tracheostomy.

Secure ETT fixation and meticulous endotracheal toilet are vital. As a general principle, the most secure fixation is to the most immobile part of the child's face, the maxilla. To avoid permanent soft tissue damage and disfiguration, care must be taken that the tube and its accessories do not press on the child's face. Figure 3.5 illustrates the method used in our PICU, which over the years has proved to be reliable.

## Ventilation

The type of mechanical ventilator used is less important than an understanding of what one is trying to achieve, and many modern ventilators are suitable for children provided the user is familiar with its basic design and function. Volume-controlled ventilation may be delivered by constant, decelerating or sinusoidal gas flow, depending on the ventilator and the pathophysiology. When lung compliance is poor, volume-controlled ventilation risks generating high airway pressures. Pressure-controlled ventilation avoids high pressure swing within the patient which would be hazardous if the patient is not in synchrony and if the volume of gas in the circuit is high compared to the tidal volume. The danger is, however, that tidal volume fluctuates when lung compliance changes. Pressure-controlled ventilation can be delivered by continuous or demand flow but for premature infants (and some term neonates) it has become standard practice to use continuous flow, pressure-regulated, time-cycled ventilators

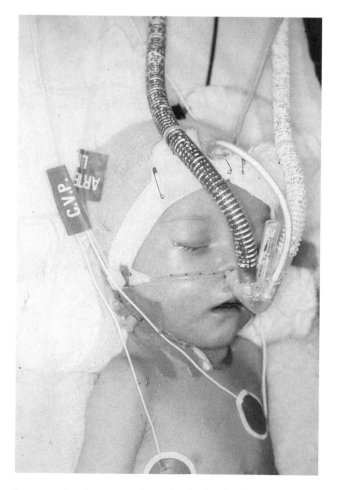

Fig 31.5    An example of secure endotracheal tube fixation.

Table 31.9 Management of continuous flow, pressure-regulated, time-cycled ventilation

| Ventilator adjustment | Expected effect upon $Pa_{O_2}$ | Expected effect upon $Pa_{CO_2}$ |
|---|---|---|
| Increase PIP | Increased | Decreased |
| Increase PEEP | Increased | Increased |
| Increase rate (I:E constant) | No change | Decreased |
| Increase insp. time (rate constant) | Increased | No change |
| Increase $F_{IO_2}$ | Increased | No change |
| Increase flow | Increased (marginal) | No change |
| Decrease PIP | Decreased | Increased |
| Decrease PEEP | Decreased | Decreased |
| Decrease rate (I:E constant) | No change | Increased |
| Increase exp. time (rate constant) | Decreased | No change |

Abbreviations: exp.: expiration; I:E inspiration to expiration ratio; insp.: inspiration; PEEP: positive end-expiratory pressure; PIP: peak inspiratory pressure.

(Table 31.9). These ventilators do not measure tidal volume and minute ventilation directly, and this necessitates simultaneous apnoea monitoring.

**Sedation and analgesia**

The indications for sedation and analgesia are similar to those in adult practice, and the most commonly prescribed drugs are morphine and midazolam, by infusion. Intermittent chloral hydrate (30 mg/kg) is a useful sedative in babies if the enteral route is available. As the intubated child in Figure 31.6 illustrates, a full stomach can also be a very effective sedative.

Many pharmacokinetic and pharmacodynamic processes are immature in the young child and it is the interplay between them that determines the dose of a given drug, its clinical effect, and the time taken for its elimination. Organ system failure complicates matters further. Considerable care should be taken with prescribing drugs for children, and it is never a sign of weakness to refer to a paediatric pharmacopoeia.

The neuromuscular junction is immature for the first two months after birth. Neonates are more sensitive to non-depolarising muscle relaxants, requiring significantly lower plasma concentrations to achieve equivalent depression of twitch height. The neonate's greater extracellular fluid volume, however, creates a greater volume of distribution for the drug, causing actual initial requirements to vary little with age. Subsequent doses of most non-depolarising muscle relaxants should be lower than the initial doses and are required at longer intervals in neonates because of slower elimination. An alternative in all children is to infuse relaxants of intermediate duration of action (atracurium or vecuronium) and monitor neuromuscular transmission when in doubt.

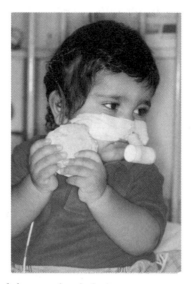

Fig 31.6   A full stomach is a good sedative!

**Transport of the critically ill child**

Whether by road or air, this is a job for specialist teams who have been shown to reduce adverse events and morbidity during transfer. Nevertheless, transfer must be preceded by comprehensive local resuscitation. The transport team can assist in this on their arrival or by giving telephone advice beforehand. Transport is a form of mobile intensive care with similar staffing, training, and equipment requirements. Personnel have to anticipate and be prepared for any deterioration during the move and have the skills to resuscitate, diagnose, and treat during transfer, rather than plead for a faster journey or police escort.

**Psychological support**

It requires considerable teamwork to provide an intensive care environment and clinical approach that takes account of the emotional and psychological needs of children of different ages. Those involved include not just medical and nursing staff, but also physiotherapists, play therapists, etc. Parents are usually constant bedside companions and observers. Whilst medical and nursing staff may become adept at working and communicating under such scrutiny, the clinical needs of the patient and the need for privacy and confidentiality for other patients and families must be considered. The death of a child in intensive care seems particularly tragic even if there had been a background of chronic illness. Staff are often skilled in counselling the bereaved or in supporting families during withdrawal and limitation of intensive care measures. Their own needs should not be forgotten.

### Outcome and assessment of paediatric intensive care

Children tend to have shorter stays in intensive care than adults or neonates and there are proportionately more survivors who have a qualitatively better outcome. In the development of severity of illness scores, paediatric intensive care has lagged behind. Nevertheless, the progression from "physiological stability index" (PSI) to "paediatric risk of mortality" (PRISM) mirrors the development of the APACHE from the "acute physiology score" in adult practice. PRISM has not been widely adopted because it has been criticised when applied outside the patient population to which it originally referred. Because of the brevity of most PICU admissions, our preference is for severity of illness scoring derived from criteria measured at time of admission rather than over the first 24 hours in the ICU. There is widespread agreement, however, that formal audit of paediatric intensive care is to be welcomed.

## Further reading

Crean PM. Neonatal physiology. In *Handbook of neonatal anaesthesia* (Hughes TDG, Mather TSJ, Wolf TAR, eds). London: Saunders, 1996.

Advanced Life Support Group. *Advanced paediatric life support*, 2nd edn. London: BMJ Publishing Group, 1997.

Kissoon N. Triage and transport of the critically ill child. *Crit Care Clin* 1992;**8**:37–57.

Shann F. *Drug doses*, 9th edn. Intensive Care Unit, Royal Children's Hospital, Melbourne, Australia, 1996.

# 32: Transport of the critically ill patient

P G M WALLACE

Moving critically ill patients may result in complications that adversely affect their outcome. These patients have deranged physiology, are closely monitored, and require organ support such as ventilation and inotrope infusions. Transfer may cause instability, and during transit monitoring and therapy are difficult. Physiological risks arise not only from the patient's condition but also from the effects of movement (tipping, vibration, acceleration/deceleration), barometric pressure, and temperature changes, which may further affect cardiorespiratory function and monitoring accuracy. There are also risks of injury from accidents to both patient and staff during the journey.

Risks are reduced when patients are supported by appropriate equipment and are accompanied by experienced personnel trained in transport medicine. In continental Europe, North America, and Australia dedicated transfer teams are common but in the UK, despite recommendations that retrieval teams be established, 90% of transferred patients are accompanied by staff from the referring hospital. Although over 10 000 adult ICU patients are transferred per year between hospitals in the UK, most hospitals transfer less than 20 patients per year.[1] Thus few hospitals or individual doctors have expertise or knowledge of transport medicine. Most transfers are organised in an infrequent *ad hoc* manner with attendants drawn from on-call anaesthetic trainees. Not only is the base hospital left with inadequate on-call staff, but the accompanying doctors have little experience.

Audits in the UK suggest that up to 15% of transferred patients are delivered to the receiving hospital with avoidable hypotension and/or hypoxaemia adversely affecting outcome;[2] 10% of patients will have "missed injuries". Critically ill patients transported within hospital may also suffer significant misadventures.[3] Other reports, however, indicate that, with experienced staff, suitable equipment, and careful preparation, these patients may be moved without deterioration.[4] This chapter will address the requirements for safe transfer of adult patients between hospitals[5] but the same principles will be required for transfer of these patients between departments within a hospital.

The *structure* of a safe transport system for intensive care patients requires:

- local and regional organisation
- liaison/coordination between hospitals and with ambulance services
- funding
- appropriate vehicles
- mobile equipment (trolley, monitors, ventilators, and other support)
- experienced accompanying personnel
- audit
- training.

The safe *process* of transfer requires:

- appropriate referral
- careful assessment
- comprehensive monitoring
- meticulous resuscitation
- stabilisation
- continuing care during transfer
- documentation
- handover.

## Structure

### Organisation

Each hospital should have clear guidelines and communication channels to initiate and undertake patient transport. A designated consultant must be available for advice. In addition a named individual should have responsibility for overall transport arrangements ensuring that equipment and staff are available, and that standards are audited.

Sufficient funding must be identified and made available. Provision for safe transfer of the critically ill should be a mandatory part of purchasing guidelines and policies for purchasing authorities.

Geographical areas may be defined where there are regular transfers of critically ill patients between hospitals. In each of these areas, ICU consultants should coordinate transport arrangements, guidelines/audit, and also negotiations with purchasers.

For emergency referrals to specialist hospitals, such as regional neurosurgical centres, facilities and staff must be available at each referring hospital to resuscitate, stabilise, and transfer patients, as the mobilisation time of retrieval or regional teams will often obviate their use for these urgent cases. Staffing levels must be sufficiently flexible within any hospital with an acute on-call function to allow 24-hour cover for emergency transfers.

Many interhospital transfers of critically ill patients, however, will be semi-elective in nature and, in these circumstances, transfer teams based at the receiving hospitals or regional transfer teams will generally provide the safest and most efficient service, and also maintain on-call staff levels in referring hospitals.

## Coordination/liaison

Clear guidelines and protocols for referral and transfer of patients should be available in all hospitals. Contact numbers should be on hand for referral, senior advice, and ambulance services. It is vitally important that close communication and cooperation are maintained with local ambulance services who will provide the vehicle, crew, and often other assistance. This is particularly important where helicopter or fixed-wing transfer is considered, and expert advice should be available on a 24-hour basis.

Close coordination between hospitals within local geographical areas will be required to integrate referral patterns, collect data, audit standards, and maintain a bed bureau if required. An area or regional approach may also be more fruitful in establishing a retrieval team and adequate funding.

At a national level, quality standards and guidelines have now been established by the Intensive Care Society (UK). These should form a basis for auditing local standards and applying corrective action where necessary.

## Vehicles

Vehicles should be designed with attention to trolley access and fixation, lighting, temperature control, space for medical attendants, adequate gases and electricity, storage space, and good communications. If there is sufficient workload, a dedicated, specially adapted vehicle may offer advantage in layout, augmented gas supplies, and storage of necessary equipment.

The mode of transport should take into account urgency, mobilisation time, geographical factors, weather, traffic conditions, and cost. Most ICU transfers will be in urban areas and within a distance of 20 miles and road transfer will be satisfactory for most, having the advantage over other vehicles of low cost, rapid mobilisation, less weather dependency, and easier patient monitoring.

Air transfer, however, should be considered for longer journeys or where access or road conditions are difficult and there is clinical urgency. Helicopters are recommended for journeys of 50–150 miles but they provide a less familiar and less comfortable environment than road ambulance or fixed-wing aircraft, are expensive, and have a poorer safety record.[6] Fixed-wing aircraft, preferably pressurised, should be selected for transfer distances over 150 miles.[7] Apparent speed must be tempered against organisational delays, mobilisation time, and also transfer between hospitals and airport/helicopter pad at beginning and end. Arrangements should be discussed with local ambulance control or specialised air medical providers.

## Equipment

Equipment must be robust, lightweight, and battery powered. There have been great advances in the design and provision of transport equipment, and most hospitals and ambulance services will now have the essentials.

Equipment for establishing and maintaining a safe airway must be available. A portable mechanical ventilator with disconnection and high pressure alarms is required, preferably with a means of providing positive end-expiratory pressure (PEEP), variable $F_{IO_2}$, I:E ratio, respiratory rate, and tidal volume. An oxygen supply sufficient to last the duration of the transfer plus a reserve of one to two hours is essential.

A portable monitor, battery powered with illuminated display, is required to record ECG, oximetry, non-invasive blood pressure (NIBP), invasive pressures, capnography, and temperature. Alarms should be visible as well as audible in view of extraneous noise levels.

Suction equipment and a defibrillator are needed as are appropriate drugs and a number of syringe pumps with long battery life. A mobile telephone for communication is advisable. A patient warming blanket is advantageous.

An individual should be responsible for ensuring that batteries are charged and supplies fully stocked. All those potentially involved in transfer should be aware of the location of equipment and should be familiar with equipment and drugs. Staff should be properly clothed for protection and identification.

With standard trolleys, designed for ordinary patient transfer, much of the above equipment must be carried by hand or laid on top of the patient. This is undesirable and dangerous. It is preferable that a special bed, trolley, or adaptor be designed which will allow these items to be secured to a metal pole or shelf system above or below the patient.

## Accompanying staff

The goal for these transfers, as far as possible, should be to move the ICU environment with the patient. To this end, in addition to the vehicle's crew, a critically ill patient should be accompanied by a minimum of two attendants.[8]

One should be an experienced doctor competent in resuscitation, airway care, ventilation, and other organ support. This doctor, often an anaesthetist, should have training in intensive care, have been involved in previous transfers, and preferably have at least two years' postgraduate experience. The fundamentals of safe transfer are basic but often ignored. The presence of experienced attendants will not only ensure that basics are undertaken but also help to resist the temptation to rush transfer without full preparation: this often requires a senior diplomatic voice.

The responsible doctor should be assisted by another doctor, nurse, paramedic, or technician familiar with intensive care procedures and equipment. This will usually be a nurse, and during the transfer he or she will carry independent professional responsibility towards the patient and should be qualified to ENB100 or equivalent level.

Provision must be made for adequate insurance cover, in the event of death or disability of accompanying staff, as a result of an accident during the course of their duties. Medical indemnity must be provided by the employing trust or health authority and personal Medical Defence cover is also recommended.

## Audit

Regular audit of transfers is necessary to maintain and improve standards. The consultant responsible should review all transfers in and out of the hospital, and a similar process should be established at regional and national levels.

## Training

All staff involved in transferring critically ill patients should be competent in intensive care medicine, familiar with the mobile equipment and, before taking responsibility for a transfer, should have received training and accompanied transfers as an observer. Currently there are few training opportunities, and resources are required to improve this; joint training courses should be set up locally and nationally.

# Process

The main components of the process of transferring critically ill patients safely are the essentials of resuscitation, stabilisation, communication, attention to detail, and commonsense. Too often these basics are ignored and patients suffer. Meticulous preparation of the patient before transfer is the key to avoiding complications during the journey.

## Referral

Transfer decisions should be made by consultant medical staff after full asssessment of the patient and discussion between staff at referring and receiving hospitals. Critically ill patients require transfer between hospitals:

- for an upgrade in their level of care, either to provide specialist therapy (for example, neurosurgery), or for complex organ support unavailable in the initial referring hospital;
- for a specialised investigation unavailable in the referring hospital;
- because there is a lack of staffed ICU beds in the referring hospital or repatriation of a patient taken ill at a distance from home.

A decision to transfer is based on assessment of the risk, benefit, and urgency associated with each individual patient. Benefit may be obvious where life-saving surgery will be performed by the receiving unit, but will be less clear where multiple medical problems coexist. The balance of risk and benefit requires liaison between senior referring, transferring, and receiving clinical staff.

The urgency of the transfer will be determined by the influence of delay on any definitive management in the receiving unit, for example, neurosurgical interventon. If delay may compromise the patient's outcome, then transfer must be performed quickly and efficiently without sacrificing preparation and exclusion of coexisting pathology. Inadequate resuscitation or missed or untreated injuries will result in instability during transfer and adversely affect outcome.[9]

Whether to retrieve or send the patient will depend on urgency of transfer, availability of experienced staff, equipment, and also possible delays in mobilising a retrieval team. Local policies should be prepared to reflect referral patterns, local expertise, and clinical circumstances.

The transfer process is the joint responsibility of the referring physician, receiving physician, and transfer personnel. Final authority to accept referral rests with the ICU consultant in the receiving unit. Relatives must be kept informed at all times.

### Assessment and monitoring

Full clinical details including medical, family, and social history must be obtained from medical staff, relatives, and the patient if possible. In addition to clinical examination, full assessment will require monitoring of ECG, $Sao_2$ (plus periodic blood gas analyses), blood pressure preferably by direct intra-arterial monitoring, central venous or pulmonary artery pressures (where circulating volume requires assessment), and urine output. Investigations should include chest radiograph, other appropriate radiographs or CT scanning, haematology, and biochemistry. If there is suspicion of intra-abdominal bleeding, peritoneal lavage should be undertaken.

### Preparation

The fundamental requirement before transfer is to ensure satisfactory and stable perfusion with adequate tissue oxygenation, by resuscitation and treatment of coexisting pathology.[10]

409

In transit, intubating conditions are difficult. The possibility of compromised airway or respiratory failure demands intubation of the trachea before departure. Intubated patients should be mechanically ventilated. Inspired oxygen should be guided by $Sao_2$ and blood gases to maintain a $Pao_2$ of > 13 kPa, and end-tidal $CO_2$ should be continuously monitored to achieve a $Paco_2$ of 4–4·5 kPa, although these may vary for individual patients. A disposable humidifying filter is recommended and a chest drain should be inserted if a penumothorax is present or a possibility, given the presence of fractured ribs. Appropriate drugs should be used for sedation and analgesia, and most patients will require muscle relaxation to achieve satisfactory ventilation.

Adequate venous access must be ensured preferably via two large-bore cannulae. To restore and maintain satisfactory blood pressure, perfusion, and urine output, intravenous volume loading will usually be required. Where necessary blood should be transfused to maintain a haematocrit of 30%. Inotropic infusions may be needed. In unstable patients central venous pressure or pulmonary artery catheterisation should be employed to optimise filling pressures and cardiac output. Hypovolaemic patients tolerate transfer poorly and circulating volumes should be normal or supranormal before transfer.

A patient persistently hypotensive despite resuscitation must not be moved until all possible sources of continued blood loss have been identified and controlled. It is important that these measures are not omitted in an attempt to speed transfer, as this may result in complications that are impossible to deal with once the journey has started.

Unstable long bone fractures should be splinted to provide neurovascular protection. A gastric drainage tube should be passed and all lines and tubes secured and fixed.

### Transfer

The travel arrangements should be discussed with relatives who normally should not expect to travel with the patient in the ambulance.

The transfer team should liaise with the local ambulance service to discuss a suitable mode of transfer, to arrange the availability of an appropriate vehicle with crew, and to confirm to the ambulance service anticipated time of departure and duration of transfer.

All equipment should be checked including battery charge status and oxygen availability against calculated requirements. Case notes, radiographs, and referral letter with investigation reports should be prepared, and blood or blood products collected. The receiving unit should be contacted to confirm that a bed remains available and be informed of the estimated time of arrival. Means of return to base hospital for attendants should be established. A mobile telephone and credit cards should be carried for emergencies.

When the patient is stable, adequately sedated, and fully investigated, monitoring and support functions should be transferred to the mobile equipment that will be used during transfer. The patient should be moved on to the transfer trolley, function of equipment rechecked, and only when further assessment has reconfirmed physiological stability should the journey commence.

## Care during transfer

Care should be maintained at as high a level as in the ICU. It must be remembered that many therapeutic interventions are difficult or impossible to perform in a moving ambulance. Monitoring of $Sao_2$, ECG, and arterial pressure should be continuous. As NIBP measurement is sensitive to motion artefact, intra-arterial monitoring is recommended. For patients receiving mechanical ventilation it is necessary to have a monitored oxygen supply, a means of detecting disconnection, and a monitor of airway pressure and end-tidal $CO_2$ concentration. Temperature should be monitored if the patient is suspected of having a temperature abnormality, during long journeys or in cold weather.

Transfer should be undertaken smoothly and not at high speed. All monitors and syringe drivers should be visible to accompanying staff. Patients should be well covered to ensure that they remain warm. Despite careful preparation, unforeseen clinical emergencies may occur; where possible the vehicle should be stopped at the first safe opportunity to facilitate patient management.

Transfers by air will bring further difficulties owing to altitude, noise, vibration, visibility, temperature control, and unfamiliar environment. Increasing altitude brings the potential for hypoxaemia and will also lead to an increase in the volume fo any gas-filled cavities in the patient. This is relevant in the presence of pneumothorax, pneumoperitoneum, and also of air in an endotracheal tube cuff, and care must be taken to prevent excessive expansion. Noise, vibration, and the unfamiliar environment are particularly prominent in helicopter transfers and, if attendants do not have specific training, they must be carefully supervised by the flight crew. The patient's monitors and visual alarms must be kept under continuous observation.

## Documentation

Clear notes should be maintained at all stages of transfer. Details of the clinical condition requiring transfer, reason for transfer, staff discussion, and details of transfer should be recorded on a standard form.

Physiological status and therapy prior to movement should be noted. A written record of clinical events, monitoring, and therapy during transfer should be made although vehicle motion makes this difficult.

## Handover

On arrival at the receiving hospital there must be direct communication between the transfer team and the receiving medical staff who will then assume responsibility for the patient's care. A record of the patient's history, therapy, and significant events during transfer should be added to the notes. Radiographs, scans and other investigations should be described and handed over.

A record of the transfer should be retained by the transfer team on a prepared pro forma for future audit. Refreshments should be provided for the transfer team and arrangements ensured for return to base.

# Conclusions

The purpose of secondary transfer of the critically ill is to reach a location where medical care and patient outcome will be improved. The aim of safe transport is to undertake the transfer while medical treatment is continued and without detrimental effect to the patient. Risks will be reduced by using apposite equipment, careful clinical preparation, and supervision by experienced staff familiar with the transfer environment.[11] This level of care will be required for critically ill patients whether they are transferred between departments within a hospital or between hospitals.

Any hospital with an acute receiving function must provide sufficient resources for the transfer of urgent cases. It would be beneficial in the UK, however, to establish dedicated transfer teams either at large receiving hospitals or within regions to deal with less urgent patients, who often have multi-organ failure and complex problems.

The number of transfers should be reduced, where possible, by sensible rationalisation of services and the provision of additional intensive care facilities in areas of shortage, to minimise transfers resulting from lack of staffed ICU beds.

1 Mackenzie PA, Smith EA, Wallace PGM. Transfer of adults between intensive care units in the UK. *BMJ* 1997;**314**:1455–6.
2 Gentleman D. Causes and effects of systemic complications among severely head injured patients transferred to a neurosurgical unit. *Int Surg* 1992;**77**:297–302.
3 Smith I, Fleming S, Cernaianu A. Mishaps during transport from the intensive care unit. *Crit Care Med* 1990;**18**:278–81.
4 Reeve WG, Runcie CJ, Reidy J, Wallace PGM. Current practice in transferring critically ill patients among hospitals in the west of Scotland. *BMJ* 1990;**300**:85–7.
5 Morton NF, Pollack MM, Wallace PGM (eds). *Stabilisation and transport of the critically ill.* London: Churchill Davidson, 1997.
6 Wilson A, Cross F. Helicopters. *J R Soc Med* 1992;**85**:1–2.
7 Bristow A, Toff NJ. A report – recommended standards for UK fixed wing medical air transport systems and for patient management during transfer by fixed wing aircraft. *J R Soc Med* 1992;**85**:767–71.
8 Intensive Care Society. *Guidelines for transfer of the critically ill adult in the UK.* London: Intensive Care Society, 1997.

9 The Neuroanaesthesia Society of Great Britain and Ireland. *Recommendations for the transfer of patients with acute head injuries to neurosurgical units.* London: Association of Anaesthetists of Great Britain and Ireland, 1996.

10 Runcie CJ, Reeve WR, Wallace PGM. Preparation of the critically ill patient for inter-hospital transfer. *Anaesthesia* 1992;47:327–31.

11 Guidelines Committee of the American College of Critical Care Medicine. Guidelines for the transfer of critically ill patients. *Crit Care Med* 1993;21:931–7.

# Index

Note: page numbers in **bold** type refer to figures; those in *italics* refer to tables or boxed material.